W0080148

CONTEMPORARY TOPICS IN IMMUNOBIOLOGY

VOLUME 7

CONTEMPORARY TOPICS IN IMMUNOBIOLOGY

General Editor

M. G. Hanna, Jr.
Frederick Cancer Research Center
Frederick, Maryland

Editorial Board:

Max D. Cooper
University of Alabama
Birmingham, Alabama

A. J. S. Davies
Chester Beatty Research Institute
London, England

John J. Marchalonis
Frederick Cancer Research Center
Frederick, Maryland

Victor Nussenzweig
New York University School of Medicine
New York, New York

George W. Santos
Johns Hopkins University
Baltimore, Maryland

Osias Stutman
Sloan-Kettering Institute for Cancer Research
New York, New York

Noel L. Warner
The Walter and Eliza Hall Institute
Victoria, Australia

William O. Weigle
Scripps Clinic and Research Foundation
La Jolla, California

A Continuation Order Plan is available for this series. A continuation order will bring delivery of each new volume immediately upon publication. Volumes are billed only upon actual shipment. For further information please contact the publisher.

CONTEMPORARY TOPICS IN IMMUNOBIOLOGY

VOLUME 7

T Cells

EDITED BY

OSIAS STUTMAN

Sloan-Kettering Institute for Cancer Research
New York, New York

PLENUM PRESS • NEW YORK AND LONDON

Library of Congress Cataloging in Publication Data

Main entry under title:

T cells.

(Contemporary topics in immunobiology; v. 7)
Includes bibliographies and index.
1. T cells. I. Stutman, Osias. II. Series. [DNLM: 1. T-Lymphocytes. W1 C077 v.
7/QW504 T114]
QR180.C632 vol. 7 [QR185.8.L9] 574.2'9'08s
                                    [616.07'9]   77-1933
ISBN 978-1-4684-3056-1   ISBN 978-1-4684-3054-7 (eBook)
DOI 10.1007/978-1-4684-3054-7

© 1977 Plenum Press, New York
Softcover reprint of the hardcover 1st edition 1977
A Division of Plenum Publishing Corporation
227 West 17th Street, New York, N.Y. 10011

All rights reserved

No part of this book may be reproduced, stored in a retrieval system, or transmitted,
in any form or by any means, electronic, mechanical, photocopying, microfilming,
recording, or otherwise, without written permission from the Publisher

Contributors

Edward Boyse   *Sloan-Kettering Institute for Cancer Research*
New York, New York

Hans Binz   *Department of Immunology, Uppsala University*
Biomedical Center, Uppsala, Sweden

Harvey Cantor   *Department of Medicine, Harvard Medical School*
Farber Cancer Center, Boston, Massachusetts

Leonard Chess   *Division of Tumor Immunology*
Sidney Farber Cancer Center
and Department of Medicine
Harvard Medical School, Boston, Massachusetts

Peter C. Doherty   *The Wistar Institute, Philadelphia, Pennsylvania*

Klaus Eichmann   *Institute for Immunology and Genetics*
Deutsches Krebsforschungszentrum, Heidelberg
West Germany

Pierre Golstein   *Department of Zoology, University College London*
London, England

Christopher S. Henney   *Departments of Medicine and Microbiology*
Johns Hopkins University School of Medicine, and
O'Neill Memorial Research Laboratories
Good Samaritan Hospital
Baltimore, Maryland

Eric Martz   *Department of Pathology, Harvard Medical School*
Boston, Massachusetts

Klaus Rajewsky   *Institute for Genetics, University of Cologne*
Cologne, West Germany

Terry G. Rehn   *Immunology Branch, National Cancer Institute*
Bethesda, Maryland

Stuart F. Schlossman   *Division of Tumor Immunology*
Sidney Farber Cancer Center, and
Department of Medicine, Harvard Medical School
Boston, Massachusetts

Gene M. Shearer   *Immunology Branch, National Cancer Institute*
Bethesda, Maryland

Anne-Marie Schmitt-Verhulst   *Immunology Branch, National Cancer Institute*
Bethesda, Maryland

Evan T. Smith   *Department of Zoology, University College London*
London, England

Osias Stutman   *Sloan-Kettering Institute for Cancer Research*
                     New York, New York
Hans Wigzell   *Department of Immunology*
                     Uppsala University Biomedical Center, Uppsala, Sweden
Rolf M. Zinkernagel *Department of Immunopathology*
                     Scripps Clinic and Research Foundation
                     La Jolla, California

Preface

> And even I can remember
> A day when historians left blanks in their writings,
> I mean for things they didn't know.
> —Ezra Pound, Canto XIII*

The prefaces to the previous volumes of this series have all expressed in various ways the actual motivation behind these collective efforts. There was agreement in most instances that we are facing some kind of publication explosion, and that the present type of compact and personalized reviews may be of help, from both a conceptual and a purely informational standpoint. The aims of the series were, and still are, to focus attention on the rapidly changing fields within the realm of immunology, and to present in each chapter the summation of results generated by an investigator or group of investigators, either as an analysis of their own work or as a correlation of such work with the general field in question. The present volume does not differ in its construction from its predecessors, although it does concentrate on a single target, the T lymphocyte and its biology.

The selection of subjects as well as contributors has been the sole responsibility of this editor; however, the actual format and length of the individual contributions was left to the discretion and inspiration of the different authors. Even the styles, ranging from the concise statement to the meticulously detailed review, attest to the freedom of format. Similarly, it was left to the discretion of the authors to include new information or to produce a thorough analysis of information already published during the past years. However, it is apparent from the well-thought-out discussion of the information in all the contributions that serious attempts at interpretation were made, albeit avoiding, in almost every case, any form of dogmatic stance. In some instances, this interpretative mood was coupled with an adequate dose of realistic critique, which made the editor's job awfully easy and which makes the quotation from Pound at the head of this preface highly appropriate.

*The Cantos of Ezra Pound, 1957, Faber and Faber, London, p. 64.

Prologues have been referred to by Jorge Luis Borges as a ". . . lateral kind of criticism"* in the sense that they offer the tempting opportunity to the author of producing some critical remarks without the formal responsibility of true criticism, and that the reader cannot help but accept such writings as an integral part of the book. In most cases, however, prologues serve as a brief introduction to the contents of a book. The contents of this volume are almost self-explanatory. The initial chapter on development of T cells describes mostly data on cell traffic and the experimental support for postthymic maturation as important factors in T-cell development and renewal. The newly developed characterization of different functional subsets of T cells is analyzed by Cantor and Boyse. Two contributions by Rajewsky and Eichmann and Binz and Wigzell discuss *in extenso* the present status of idiotypic recognition units as possible mechanisms for the specific reactivity and regulation of T-cell functions. The contributions by Zinkernagel and Doherty and Shearer *et alii* deal directly with some of the restrictions and requirements for effective interaction between cytotoxic T cells and their targets, while the contributions by Henney, Martz, and Golstein analyze the probable mechanisms of the lytic event. Finally, the chapter by Chess and Schlossman describes the approaches to defining T-cell functions in man.

In compiling this book, it was my aim to present a sampler of opinions and viewpoints on some aspects of T-cell biology, perhaps with excessive emphasis on the fully differentiated effector T cell (Volume 2 of this series, published in 1973, addressed the more general question of "thymus dependency"). Convincing the authors of the reality and urgency of deadlines seemed a frivolous occupation compared with the intellectual enjoyment that each arriving manuscript produced to this editor. Due to the rapidity of change within the field, and to prevent preprogrammed obsolescence, we tried to accelerate the usual process to its maximum, and all the chapters were written within a four-to-six-month period ending in August 1976. It is apparent that these contributions will stimulate and catalyze thought, among both newcomers and experts in the matter, especially in their capacity to focus attention on selected problems and questions, instead of serving merely as reference sources or general reviews. This new information, whether fashionable or not, as well as the reinterpretation of previously observed phenomena in the light of the new observations, does indeed represent a *continuum* that is constantly amplifying our understanding of the immune response and its regulation. However, we should also keep in mind to ". . . maintain a wise infidelity against the authority of (his) instructors . . . ,"† as recommended by Thomas Jefferson in his letter of 1807 to Dr. Caspar Wistar on the education of young doctors. This is the proper place to thank all the contributors for their efforts and Ms. Linda Stevenson for her invaluable help in preparing the book.

New York   Osias Stutman

*Jorge Luis Borges, *Prologos,* 1975, Torres Aquero Ed., Buenos Aires, p. 8.
†*Basic Writings of Thomas Jefferson,* 1944, John Wiley and Sons, New York, p. 672.

Contents

Chapter 3

Antigen Receptors of T Helper Cells

Klaus Rajewsky and Klaus Eichmann

Chapter 7
T-Cell-Mediated Cytolysis: An Overview of Some Current Issues
   Christopher S. Henney

Chapter 8
Mechanism of T-Cell-Mediated Cytolysis: The Lethal Hit Stage
   Pierre Golstein and Evan T. Smith

Chapter 9
**Mechanism of Specific Tumor-Cell Lysis by Alloimmune T Lymphocytes:
Resolution and Characterization of Discrete Steps in the Cellular Interaction**
  Eric Martz

Chapter 1

Two Main Features of T-Cell Development: Thymus Traffic and Postthymic Maturation

Osias Stutman

Sloan-Kettering Institute for Cancer Research
New York, New York

I. INTRODUCTION

One of the many reasons for the sustained interest in the ontogeny of T cells in mammals is the expectation that the process of adult differentiation and renewal of T cells should follow the same pathways as the development of the T-cell pool during early embryonation. In general, there is agreement between the major steps of ontogenic development and adult renewal of T cells. In this review, I will discuss two aspects of T-cell development, both of which appear critical for the generation of immunologically competent T cells: (1) the notion that there is further maturation of postthymic precursors in extrathymic lymphoid sites (i.e., the idea that what the thymus exports is not necessarily a fully competent T lymphocyte) and (2) the traffic of cells to and from the thymus (a necessary factor that requires a stream of stem cells derived from hemopoietic sites and an intact thymic stroma). Although there is general agreement that the generation of T cells is strongly thymus-dependent, there are still many unanswered questions concerning the graded steps of this differentiation, even within the intrathymic environment. The observation that the immunologically competent cells in thymectomized mice grafted with a thymus were almost entirely of host origin (Dalmasso *et al.*, 1963) was interpreted as indicating either that the thymus produced some humoral factor acting on host cells (Osoba and Miller, 1963) or that the host cells were modified into immunologic competence by migration through the thymus (Harris and Ford, 1963, 1964; C. E. Ford,

1966). Support for both views came after the description of several thymic extracts with apparent functional activity (four of the best-studied humoral thymic factors being those described by, in alphabetical order, Bach *et al.*, 1975a; A. L. Goldstein *et al.*, 1975; G. Goldstein, 1974, 1975; Trainin *et al.*, 1975) and the direct demonstration that hemopoietic precursors from marrow or from embryonic hemopoietic sites could become immunologically competent T lymphocytes after traffic through the thymus (Stutman, 1970, 1972a; Doenhoff *et al.*, 1970; Stutman and Good, 1971a,b).

II. POSTTHYMIC PRECURSOR CELLS

A. Effects of Late Treatment on Thymectomized Mice

During our studies on the restoration of immune functions in neonatally thymectomized mice, especially when using thymus enclosed in diffusion chambers (DC), we observed that the animals became refractory when such treatment was delayed for 40–60 days (depending on strains) after neonatal thymectomy (Stutman *et al.*, 1969a) or when the animals had overt postthymectomy wasting syndrome (Stutman *et al.*, 1967, 1969a). We proposed as interpretation for these results that a population of cells in the peripheral lymphoid tissues of these animals, which was sensitive to humoral thymic influence (i.e., thymus in DC), actually declined in the absence of a thymus through physiological attrition and strict thymus dependency for its renewal (Stutman *et al.*, 1969a). We termed this population *postthymic* on the basis of its requirements of a thymus for renewal, its sensitivity to humoral activity of the thymus, and the suggestive evidence that it may act as a precursor in the periphery for competent T cells (Stutman *et al.*, 1969a). We also assumed that these cells were generated during late embryonation, before thymectomy was performed at birth (Stutman *et al.*, 1967, 1969a,b). Using cell transfers in association with thymus in DC, we could demonstrate the presence of postthymic cells in the spleen of 5-day-old neonatally thymectomized mice (Stutman *et al.*, 1969a). In this context, "postthymic" meant that these cells had received some form of thymic influence, either through thymus traffic or directly in the periphery (in a way, they would represent the "committed" precursor of other hemopoietic systems; see Lajtha, 1975). It should be noted that the relative refractoriness observed with delay of treatment was found even when free thymus grafts were used, suggesting that the peripheral effects of the thymus on the postthymic compartment (as opposed to the intrathymic and import–export functions) was critical for the achievement of immunologic restoration (Stutman *et al.*, 1967, 1969a,b). Table I shows a summary of our studies on different restoration procedures in neonatally thymectomized animals treated at different times after thymectomy, as well as the cell types required for efficient restoration, types of restoration (donor or host), H2 requirements, tolerance induction, effect of age of thymus donors, dangers of graft-vs.-host disease, and other factors. Some of the problems observed in these studies using neonatally thymectomized hosts have been observed, and in some instances "rediscovered," in the studies on restoration of immune functions in athymic nude mice (Loor and Kindred, 1973; Kindred and Loor, 1974; Kindred, 1974, 1975, 1976; Seger *et al.*, 1974).

B. Restoration of Nude Mice

A comparison of our "late restoration" experiments with restoration of nude mice with thymus grafts may be illustrative. Based on our results with thymectomized animals, nude mice should be partially susceptible to restoration with thymus grafts (provided that truly inbred nude mice are used, thus preventing GVH by the allogeneic thymus graft) and should be resistant to treatment with humoral thymus such as thymus in DC. In general, both predictions have been observed. Nude mice can be restored by syngeneic thymus grafts in most instances, although quantitation and determination of actual incidence of restored animals per total animals treated are difficult (Pritchard and Micklem, 1972; Pritchard *et al.*, 1973; Wortis, 1974). Our own data indicate that the percentage of animals restored by thymus grafts in inbred BALB/C or in partially inbred CBA/H nudes averages 50% of the animals (Stutman, 1974, 1975a). It should also be noted, however, that we maintain our nudes in laminar flow units as partially pathogen-free animals, a procedure that was not used in our previous experiments with thymectomized animals, in which the animals were kept in conventional clean conditions. Treatment of nudes with thymus enclosed in cell-impermeable DC has been completely unsuccessful (Stutman 1974, 1975a; Pierpaoli and Besedovsky, 1975). Tables II–IV show some of our own results. Table II shows that nude mice with accepted allogeneic skin grafts could reject such grafts within 15–30 days after a thymus graft, but were unable to reject the grafts when treated with thymus in cell-impermeable DC. Table III shows that while nude mice grafted with thymus grafts of nu/+ or +/+ (CBA/HT6T6) origin could reject allogeneic skin normally, no such rejection capacity was observed when the mice were grafted with the nu/nu thymic rudiment or with thymus in DC. Table IV shows the effects of treatment on GVH capacity: thymus grafts restored such function when the test was performed at 20 days after grafting, but not when it was performed 5 days after a

Table I. Effect of Different Treatments on Restoration of Immune Functions in Mice Treated Early or Late after Neonatal Thymectomy

Treatment[a]	Donor–host combination[b]	Mice restored (%)[c]			Type of restoration[d]	Tolerance to donor[e]	Graft-vs.-host	References[f]
		Early (5–30)[a]	Late (+30)[a]	Wasting (+70)[a]				
Spleen cells[g]	Syn	95	85	80	Donor	–	–	1
Spleen cells[g]	$F_1 \to P$	95	85	80	Donor	Yes	No	1
Spleen cells	Allo (non-H2)	65	60	50	Donor	Yes	No[h]	1
Spleen cells	Allo (H2)	15	0	0	Donor	Yes	Yes	1
Lymph node or thoracic duct[i]	Syn	95	95	95	Donor	–	–	2
Thymus cells[j]	Syn	50	50	25	Donor	–	–	2
Marrow, newborn spleen, embryonic liver, etc.[k]	Syn	0	0	0	–	–	–	2
Thymus graft[l]	Syn	85	15	0	Host	–	–	3
Thymus graft	$F_1 \to P$	60	15	0	Host	Yes[m]	No	3
Thymus graft	$P \to F_1$	15	0	0	–	–	Yes[n]	4, 5
Thymus graft	Allo	15	0	0	–	Yes	Yes[n]	3, 6
Thymus grafts × 5	Syn	–	35	25	Host	Yes[m]	–	6
Thymus grafts × 5	$F_1 \to P$	–	25	15	Host	Yes[m]	No	6
Functional thymoma	Syn, Allo	65	15	0	Host	Yes[o]	No	7
Thymoma in DC	Syn, Allo	50	15	0	Host	No	No	8, 9
Thymus in DC	Syn, Allo	55	15	0	Host	No	No	9
Spleen, etc., in DC	Syn, Allo	0	0	0	–	–	–	9

[a] Time of treatment in days after thymectomy at birth indicated in parentheses in the "Mice restored" column (early, late, and after onset of wasting). Cells were usually injected intraperitoneally (i.p.). Thymus grafts as well as thymus in DC usually implanted i.p. Thymomas were implanted subcutaneously (for description of these functional thymomas, see reference 7). Most of these studies were done in C3H, CBA/H, or A strain mice.

b (Syn) syngeneic; (Allo) allogeneic; $(F_1 \to P)$ F_1 hybrid into parent strain.

c Restoration was measured in most of these experiments as capacity to reject allogeneic skin and respond in graft-vs.-host reactions (GVHR).

d Donor or host components were assayed either by chromosome markers in syngeneic combinations using CBA/H and CBA/HT6T6 or by discriminant GVHR assays in appropriate F_1 hybrids to test for host or donor components. When free thymus grafts are used, although most of the restoration is mediated by host cells (when tested 30 days or more after treatment), a donor component can usually be detected (especially in the late restorations or treatment of wasting using 5 thymuses).

e Tolerance is defined as acceptance of 60 days or more (usually permanent acceptance was the case) of skin from the same origin as the donor of "treatment" associated with the capacity to reject a third-party allogeneic skin graft.

f References: (1) Stutman et al., 1969c; (2) Stutman et al., 1970a; (3) Stutman et al., 1969d; (4) Stutman et al., 1968a; (5) Stutman et al., 1969e; (6) Stutman et al., 1967; (7) Stutman et al., 1968b; (8) Stutman et al., 1969a; (9) Stutman et al., 1969f.

g Optimal cell dose: 10^6–10^8. Unless otherwise stated, all studies used young adult donors (30–90 days).

h Presence of GVH depended on strain combination (no GVH observed in C3H treated with CE, CBA cells; mild GVH with AKR; severe with C58).

i Optimal dose: 10^6 cells.

j Adult or newborn cells; optimal dose: 10^8–10^9 cells.

k Highest dose tested: 5×10^8, 10^9 for adult marrow.

l Intraperitoneal and under-the-kidney capsule gave comparable results; subcutaneous grafts were less efficient. Most of the studies were done with newborn or young thymuses. Age of thymus donor is irrelevant in CBA or C3H strains (the ages tested–newborn to 3 years of age— usually give quite comparable results). However, strains such as A or NZB show an early decay (at 2–4 months of age) of capacity to restore immune functions in syngeneic neonatally thymectomized hosts (see Stutman and Good, 1974; Yunis et al., 1973).

m Tolerance to skin of same origin as thymus donor depends on strain combination, and in some combinations (i.e., C3H grafted with hybrids of C57BL/6), actual rejection of restored thymus graft is observed (see reference 3; Stutman and Good, 1974; Yunis et al., 1973). These findings correlate with recent observations in nude mice by Kindred (1975) and Seger et al. (1974), which described similar restrictions in restoration as well as tolerance induction.

n Thymus grafts of parental origin grafted into thymectomized F_1 hybrids can produce severe or lethal GVHR in some strain combinations (see references 4 and 5). Similarly, grafting of allogeneic thymuses in thymectomized hosts induced severe GVH (see references 3 and 6). However, grafting of embryonic thymus (from 14–16-day-old embryos) in some of these allogeneic or P to F_1 combinations prevents GVH development, and tolerance is usually observed (see Stutman et al., 1972).

o One functional thymoma of A origin could readily induce tolerance to A skin grafts when implanted into C3H or CBA animals, while restoring the capacity to reject third-party skin (see Biggar et al., 1972).

Table II. Rejection of Accepted Allogeneic Skin Grafts
by Nude Mice after Implantation of CBA/HT6T6 Thymus[a]

Experimental groups	Number of mice	Rejection of DBA/2 skin, days after thymus grafts					
		10	15	20	25	30	Total
Untreated	16	0	0	0	0	0	0/16
Thymus graft	29	0	22	3	2	2	29/29
Thymus in DC[b]	26	0	0	0	0	0	0/26

[a]All nude mice were grafted at 20 days of age with DBA/2 skin, and 30 days later were grafted intraperitoneally with a free thymus or a thymus enclosed in a diffusion chamber. The thymus grafts were from 15–17 day old CBA/HT6T6 embryos.
[b]Diffusion chambers with lucite rings and filters of 0.10 μm pore size.

thymus graft. Thymus in DC was completely ineffective. Similar effects were observed when the animals were tested for *in vitro* reactivity to phytohemagglutinin or Concanavalin A or in mixed leukocyte reactions (Stutman, 1974), or when tested for their ability to induce regression of Moloney-sarcoma-virus-induced tumors (Stutman, 1975a). The presence of "T-like" cells in nude mice as well as the effects of some thymic extracts will be discussed in Section II.E, to prevent this digression from running too long. In general, these results in nude mice support those observed in neonatally thymectomized mice treated late after thymectomy.

Table III. Effect of Thymus Replacement on
Allograft Skin Rejection in Nude Mice[a]

Treatment	Number of mice	Number of mice with DBA/2 skin grafts surviving for:		
		< 15 days	15–30 days	> 30 days
Nothing	17	0	0	17
Thymus graft (IP, nu/nu)	8	0	0	8
Thymus graft (IP, nu/+)	8	8	0	0
Thymus graft (IP, CBA/HT6T6)	8	8	0	0
Thymus in DC[b] (nu/+)	13	0	0	13
Thymus in DC[b] (CBA/HT6T6)	19	0	0	19

[a]The animals were implanted with thymus at 20 days of age and skin was grafted at 40 days of age. The thymi were derived from 15 to 17-day-old embryos.
[b]Diffusion chambers with lucite rings and filters of 0.10 μm pore size.

Table IV. Effect of Thymus Replacement
on GVH Capacity of Spleen Cells
from Nude Mice

Experimental groups	Cell dose tested $\times 10^6$	Number of mice giving a positive GVH/total[a]
Untreated	5	0/8
Untreated	10	0/8
Untreated	50	0/6
Thymus graft (day 5)	10	0/6
Thymus graft (day 5)	50	1/6
Thymus graft (day 20)	10	9/9
Thymus in DC (5)	10	0/8
Thymus in DC (20)	.10	0/10
Thymus in DC (20)	50	0/6

[a]The GVH was considered positive when the spleen index was higher than 1.30, or when there was one animal within an injected litter with an SI higher than 1.30. Tested in (CBA/H × C56BL/6) F_1 hybrids.

C. Characterization of a Postthymic Precursor Cell

When we studied the effects of various cell supplements in augmenting the capacity of thymus in DC to restore immune functions in 50-day-old neonatally thymectomized animals, we observed that (1) lymphoid and hemopoietic cells from adult or newborn animals (at cell dosages at which they were inefficient by themselves; see Table I) acted synergistically with thymus in DC in restoration of immune functions (Stutman *et al.*, 1969b, 1970a,b); (2) the actual content of immunologically competent lymphocytes in the different cell supplements was not a factor, since tissues with low or absent immunocompetent T lymphocytes (i.e., newborn liver or spleen, adult marrow) were as effective as adult spleen in such cooperative restoration (Stutman *et al.*, 1970a,b); and (3) embryonic hemopoietic cells (i.e., yolk sac, blood, liver), especially before day 14–16 of embryonation, cooperated in restoring immune functions *only* with free thymus grafts, and not with thymus in DC (Stutman *et al.*, 1969b, 1970b). It should be noted that all these embryonic cell types contain "prethymic" stem cells that can generate competent T cells via thymus traffic (see Section III).

The results of these ablation–replacement experiments, especially the restrictions for cooperation of different lymphohemopoietic tissues with either free thymus grafts or thymus in DC, were interpreted as being the consequence of the requirements of different subsets of T-cell precursors for either "humoral" (i.e., thymus in DC) or "cellular" (i.e., intrathymic environment differentiative influences (Stutman *et al.,* 1969a,b, 1970a,b). Thus, a subpopulation of T-cell precursors, termed *postthymic,* present in the lymphoid and hemopoietic tissues of adult and newborn mice was defined by its thymus dependency for renewal and for its sensitivity to the humoral influence of the thymus (Stutman *et al.,* 1969 a,b, 1970 a,b). On the other hand, the early embryonic hemopoietic tissues contained mainly a population of cells, termed *prethymic* (on a purely operational basis), that required contact with the thymic stroma through traffic for its further differentiation and was "insensitive" to the humoral activity of the thymus (Stutman *et al.,* 1970b). It is obvious that the intrathymic differentiation step may be, and probably is, mediated by humoral factors; thus, the quotation marks. These prethymic cells will be further discussed at the end of this section.

It is difficult at the present writing to define the actual magnitude and functional significance of these differentiation steps (i.e., intrathymic via traffic and the extrathymic via postthymic precursors), especially the possible quantitative or qualitative differences in ontogeny vs. adult life. It is obvious that such steps are not mutually exclusive, but most probably represent an integrated continuum that maintains homeostasis of T-cell production. Our own work shows that by temporary exposure to thymus, neonatally thymectomized animals can generate a pool of immunologically competent T cells within a relatively short period after exposure, but this pool of cells is depleted with time in absence of the thymus, i.e., is incapable of self-renewal (Stutman *et al.,* 1972). On the other hand, a "three-tier" system of pluripotent stem cells, committed precursors, and recognizable precursors (Lajtha, 1975) is the most probable mechanism of renewal of hemopoietic cells. We feel that most of the differentiation of the "recognizable precursor" for T cells occurs in the periphery and is not an intrathymic event.

Our hypothesis of a possible postthymic precursor in the periphery indicated that the actual postthymic pool was composed of both immunologically incompetent precursors (or early postthymic cells) and the pool of competent postthymic T lymphocytes (Stutman *et al.,* 1969a,b; 1970a,b). This idea was further developed and supported by the demonstration of a series of interactions among T cells, suggesting heterogeneity of the competent T compartment as well as the possible existence of peripheral T precursors (or T regulators), the most popular proposal being that of Raff and Cantor (1971). There have even been some actual attempts to compare the properties of some of these T-cell subsets (Bach *et al.,* 1975b), which will be discussed in more detail in Section II.D (also see Chapter 2). These ideas also prompted our work to attempt to define and characterize the postthymic precursor (Stutman, 1975b–d). Table V presents a summary of the properties of the postthymic precursor cell and compares such properties with those of both the prethymic stem cell and the postthymic immunologically competent T cell (Stutman, 1975b–d).

Table V. Some Characteristics of a Postthymic Precursor Cell in the Mouse (Compared with Prethymic Precursor and Competent Postthymic T Cell)

Biological characteristics	Prethymic precursor	Postthymic precursor	Postthymic T cell
Tissue distribution			
adult	Marrow	Spleen, marrow	Lymphoid tissues
newborn	Liver, marrow	Spleen, liver	—
embryo	Yolk sac, liver, blood	Liver	—
Time of appearance, ontogeny (days)	9 (embryo)	15 (embryo)	Birth?
Traffic patterns	Spleen-seeking	Spleen-seeking	Lymph-node-seeking
Migration to thymus?	Yes	No	No
Recirculation (presence in TD)?	No	No	Yes
Immunologic competence?[a]	No	No	Yes
Restoration of Tx animals:			
alone?	No	No	Yes
with thymus graft?	Yes	Yes	Yes
with humoral thymus?	No	Yes	Yes
Effect of neonatal thymectomy	None?	Depletion	Depletion
Effect of adult thymectomy	None	Depletion (30–40 days)	None (within 60 days)
Present in nu/nu?	Yes	No	No
Effect of short-term ALS	None	None	Depletion
Sensitivity to high-dose steroids	None?	Depletion	Mostly none
Proliferative rate ($3H$ thymidine suicide?)	No?	Yes	No
Life span (probable)	?	30–60 days	Long, usually
Density (in BSA gradients)[b]	Low	Low	High
Sedimentation rates (unit gravity)[c]			
adult spleen	5.0 mm/hr	5.9 mm/hr	3.7 mm/hr
adult marrow	4.6 mm/hr	5.4 mm/hr	3.6 mm/hr
newborn spleen	4.8 mm/hr	5.8 mm/hr	3.5 mm/hr[d]
liver (15-day embryo)	8.0 and 10.5 mm/hr	5.9 mm/hr	—
Adherence to nylon wool (45 min)?	No	Yes	No
Surface markers			
Thy.1	No	Yes	Yes
TL	No	No?	No
Ly 1, 2, 3[e]	None	1, 2, 3+	1+; 2, 3+; 1, 2, 3+
Ig	No	No	No
Fc	No	No	No, usually

[a]Measured as mitogen responses (PHA, Con A), graft-host reactivity, capacity to react in mixed leukocyte cultures (against major histocompatibility differences), and helper activity (primary antibody response to sheep red cells).

[b]BSA discontinuous gradients, low density (A-B layers, 10–26% BSA), high density (C-D layers, 26–35% BSA).

[c]Velocity sedimentation in fetal calf serum gradients (lower values when separated in ficoll gradients). Data for "prethymic" actually apply to hemopoietic stem cells and are in accordance with values obtained by Haskill and Moore (1970).

[d]Con A reactivity only, negative to PHA or MLR. Low reactivity in GVH.

[e]Similar results for postthymic precursor cells whether tested in CBA/H, C3H, or DBA/2 (Ly.1.1; Ly.2.1; Ly.3.2) and BALB/C or C57BL/6 strains (Ly.1.2; Ly.2.2; Ly.3.2).

Before discussing in detail the characteristics of the cells described in Table V, I will make a brief presentation of the basic experimental model. The work was done using 50–60 day old neonatally thymectomized C3Hf, CBA/H, or A/J mice (see Stutman *et al.*, 1967, for details on strains and animal care), which were injected intraperitoneally with cells derived from syngeneic mice of different ages or types (newborn spleen or adult marrow was used in most of the experiments). In some instances, the cells were derived from animals that had received some form of treatment *in vivo* (adult thymectomy, treatment with antilymphocyte serum or high doses of steroids) or were manipulated *in vitro* (treatment with different alloantisera and complement, different cell separation procedures, etc.). Some of these animals were subsequently grafted intraperitoneally with an empty DC or a DC containing a thymic lobe or a spleen fragment (for details on preparation of DC and controls, see Stutman *et al.*, 1969f). At different times after treatment, starting at 7 days (although most of the animals were tested at 30 days after treatment), the immune responses were measured in spleen, nodes, or thoracic duct as capacity to generate graft-vs.-host reactions *in vivo*, as well as responses *in vitro* to phytohemagglutinin or in mixed lymphocyte reactions (for details on procedures, see Stutman, 1975b–d).

1. Tissue Distribution of Postthymic Precursors (Table V)

In the adult, marrow and spleen are the main sources of postthymic precursors, while spleen, marrow, and liver contain a high proportion of postthymic precursors in the newborn mouse. Postthymic precursors are present in liver even for a few days after birth (Stutman *et al.*, 1970b). In the embryo, postthymic precursors are detected with ease by day 17, although experiments using 15–16 day old embryonic liver gave some positive results (Stutman *et al.*, 1970b; Stutman, 1975b).

2. Time of Appearance in Ontogeny (Tables V and VI)

Table VI presents a summary of most of the critical events in the development of lymphoid and hemopoietic tissues in mice. This timing would serve to put in perspective some of the discussion in later sections. We have indicated day 15 as a tentative date for the appearance of postthymic precursor cells in embryonic liver (i.e., 5 days after development of the thymus anlage, and about 3 days after the appearance of lymphoid cells in the thymus). Table VI also shows that the only source of stem cells that can be considered to be truly prethymic would be yolk sac (if we assume that the effects of humoral factors from the mother's thymus do not play any role, even though placental passage of at least one of the thymic factors that can be demonstrated in serum has been reported by Bach *et al.*, 1975a).

Table VI. Ontogeny of Hemopoiesis and Lymphopoiesis
in the Mouse[a,b]

Event	Age (days)[c]														
	7	8	9	10	11	12	13	14	15	16	17	18	19	Br	+1
Yolk sac hemopoiesis[d]	+	+	+	+	+	+	+	+	+	+	+	±	±	−	−
Liver hemopoiesis[d]					+	+	+	+	+	+	+	+	+	±	±
B cells in liver								+	+	+	+	+	+	±	±
Postthymic cells in liver									+	+	+	+	+	+	−
Epithelial thymus			+	+	+	+	+	+	+	+	+	+	+	+	+
Lymphoid cells in thymus					±	+	+	+	+	+	+	+	+	+	+
Spleen hemopoiesis						+	+	+	+	+	+	+	+	+	+
Lymphoid cells in spleen[e]										±	+	+	+	+	+
Marrow hemopoiesis										±	+	+	+	+	+
Lymphoid cells in nodes											±	+	+	+	+
Lymphocytes in blood[f]										±	+	+	+	+	+
Lymphocytes in gut														±	+

[a]Based on Metcalf and Moore, 1971; Owen, 1972, 1974; Stutman and Calkins, 1976 (which are review articles containing the actual references).

[b]A general note concerning detection of some of the surface antigens characteristic for T cells: When tested for Thy.1 positivity, 14-day-old embryonic thymus was consistently negative (Owen and Raff, 1970), although a high proportion of cells became positive after 4 days in culture. Similarly, detectable levels of Thy.1-positive cells can be found in the periphery at about birth, and lymph nodes precede spleen (Raff and Owen, 1971). It is obvious that these results are dependent on the sensitivity of the serological methods used (cytotoxicity with antibody and complement).

[c]Based on a 19–21 day gestation period. Most of the data were obtained with CBA/H mice.

[d]Both yolk sac and liver contain precursors for both T and B lineage (see Section III).

[e]The first lymphoid cells that appear in spleen are B cells.

[f]Blood contains totipotential stem cells, as well as T and B precursors, at the earliest possible time tested (day 14 or 15 of embryonation).

3. Traffic Patterns (Table V)

When unfractioned newborn spleen or purified fractions containing mainly postthymic precursors are labeled with ^{51}Cr and injected intravenously into syngeneic mice, the main component is detected in the spleen, either 4 or 24 hr after injection. Thus, the precursor cells are mainly *spleen-seeking*, while the competent postthymic T cells are *lymph-node-seeking*, using an accepted terminology proposed by Zatz and Lance (1970). Postthymic precursor cells do not migrate back to the thymus (as will be discussed further in Section III), while a population within the prethymic pool has thymus migration capacity (i.e., dividing progeny of cells derived in thymus grafts by the use of chromosome markers; see Stutman, 1970, 1972a, and Section III). The postthymic precursor is not a recirculating cell (i.e., is absent from lymph), but can be detected in blood, especially in late embryos and newborn mice (Stutman, 1975b). The capacity of the precursor to become a recirculating cell (i.e., as detected in the thoracic duct lymph) was used in some of our experiments as one of the markers for differentiation under thymic influence (Stutman, 1975b–d).

4. Immunologic Competence (Table V)

The postthymic precursor is immunologically incompetent (Stutman, 1975b). Purified preparations from newborn spleen were unable to generate GVH *in vivo* or help B cells to respond *in vivo* to sheep red cells (even at doses 100-fold larger than those required for competent T cells; Stutman, unpublished data), and do not respond *in vitro* to phytohemagglutinin (PHA), Concanavalin A (Con A), or allogeneic cells.

A brief comparison with the known immune capabilities of newborn spleen cells is pertinent. Specific antigen-binding cells are detected by day 15–17 of embryonation and reach adult levels by day 7 after birth (Dwyer and MacKay, 1972; Spear *et al.*, 1973). Response to PHA appears by day 7 after birth and reaches adult levels by day 30–60, depending on mouse strains (Stobo and Paul, 1972). Con A reactivity usually appears at birth and reaches adult levels by day 30 (Stobo and Paul, 1972). Table V also shows that by velocity sedimentation at unit gravity, it is possible to separate the postthymic immunologically incompetent precursor from the Con-A-responsive T cell detected in newborn spleen. The response to allogeneic cells in mixed lymphocyte reactions (MLR) has been detected in some cases at birth (Wu *et al.*, 1975), and in most cases at 7 days after birth, and reaches adult levels by 1 month of age (Adler *et al.*, 1970a; Howe and Manziello, 1972). The capacity to stimulate MLR also appears by day 7 and reaches adult levels by 30 (Adler *et al.*, 1970b). Similarly, the capacity to generate cytotoxic cells in an MLR reaction also appears by day 7 and reaches adult levels by 30–60 days of age (Wu *et al.*, 1975). The capacity to produce GVH reactions is detectable at birth, but is at least 10 times lower than the adult level (Sosin *et al.*, 1966), and reaches adult levels at approximately 1 week after birth (Chiscon and Golub, 1972). Again, Table V shows that by velocity sedimentation at unit gravity, these GVH-active cells can be separated from the postthymic precursor. Helper activity appears by day 4 after birth and reaches adult levels by day 8–10 (Claman *et al.*, 1966; Chiscon and Golub, 1972; Arrenbrecht, 1973). Mosier and Johnson (1975) showed that newborn spleen contains suppressor cells that can regulate the response of T helper cells. We have been unable to detect suppressive effects on fractions enriched for postthymic precursors (most of the activity detectable in the slower migrating, smaller cells), but this aspect needs further study. Postthymic precursor cells had no suppressive effect on the parent F_1 model of GVH described by Gershon *et al.* (1972), in which thymocytes proved effective. If anything, the only observed effect was some increase of GVH reactivity of the normal spleen cells (Stutman, unpublished data). The capacity to restore immune functions in neonatally themectomized mice was discussed in previous sections, and, especially in the adoptive restoration (i.e., restoration by donor cells alone; see Table I), it correlates with the presence of competent T cells, and, as expected, postthymic precursors are inefficient by themselves.

5. Effects of Neonatal Thymectomy (Table V)

These effects have been discussed in the previous sections. Both precursor and competent postthymic T compartments are depressed by neonatal thymectomy. Concerning the prethymic stem cell, a question mark has been inserted in Table V. When measured as totipotential stem cells using colony-forming assays in spleens of irradiated recipients (the spleen-colony-forming unity, CFU-S, being a direct measure of stem-cell numbers; see Metcalf and Moore, 1971, for details), the CFU-S content of marrow or spleen from neonatally thymectomized animals of different ages and their controls showed no significant differences (Stutman et al., 1968c). The only positive finding in this study was the decrease of CFU-S in marrow in animals with overt wasting disease. Wasting is a complex syndrome observed in neonatally thymectomized mice kept in conventional conditions that has an infectious etiology and can be prevented by the germ-free state (McIntire et al., 1964). We also found a correlation between presence of viral hepatitis and marrow depression in neonatally thymectomized animals (Yunis et al., 1972). Other laboratories have observed a depression of CFU in hemopoietic tissues of neonatally thymectomized mice, and have proposed some form of thymus-dependent feedback control of marrow activity (Resnitzky et al., 1971; Trainin, 1974; Trainin et al., 1975). However, the possible role of infections, such as mouse hepatitis, secondary to the immune deficiency induced by thymectomy cannot be excluded. Similarly, some studies on CFU-S in nude mice have shown either normal values (Pritchard and Micklem, 1973) or depressed functions (Zipori and Trainin, 1973), perhaps as a consequence of the differing infectious backgrounds in the nude colonies.

6. Effects of Adult Thymectomy (Table V)

When the cell donors were thymectomized as adults (usually at 30 days of age or more) and their spleens or marrow cells were used in the restoration models, it was apparent that the postthymic precursor was depleted within 20–30 days after thymectomy (Stutman, 1975b). Adult thymectomy has no effect on prethymic precursors (see Section III) and little or no effect on postthymic competent T cells (measured within 60 days after thymectomy). This statement needs some qualification, however, since some early effects of adult thymectomy on immune functions have been described (see Section II.D for additional discussion of this point).

7. Presence in Nude Mice (Table V)

As discussed before, nude mice lack postthymic precursor cells, based on restoration experiments (see also Tables III–V). Using cooperation with thymus in DC, we observed that while newborn spleen from nu/+ or +/+ animals can produce good restoration of immune functions in 60-day-old neonatally thymectomized CBA/H or BALB/C mice, nude spleen cells, syngeneic to the host, showed no cooperative effect (Stutman, unpublished data) comparable to the lack of effect obtained with spleens from 50-day-old neonatally thymectomized animals (Stutman et al., 1969a). On the other hand, nude mice have detectable prethymic precursors (Pritchard and Micklem, 1973).

8. Effects of ALS and Steroids (Tables V and VII)

Short-term treatment with ALS (0.5 ml i.p. and cells obtained 24 or 48 hr later; Stutman, 1975b) had no detectable effect on the postthymic precursors in adult spleen or marrow. These results support the tissue distribution and the "fixed" (i.e., nonrecirculating) nature of the postthymic precursor. Conversely, high doses of steroids (250 mg hydrocortisone kg injected i.p. and cell collection 48 hr later) produced a marked decrease in the capacity of adult marrow to restore immune functions in 60-day-old neonatally thymectomized hosts in association with a thymus in DC. Table VII shows the actual results on the effects of pretreatment of the cell donor with high doses of hydrocortisone (HC). It is apparent that marrow cells from HC-treated donors had no ability to restore immune functions in the thymectomized hosts (Table 7, lines 3 and 4). Since a redistribution of mature T cells toward marrow has been reported as a consequence of high-dose steroid treatment (Cohen, 1972), we tested higher dosages of HC-treated marrow cells by themselves or associated with thymus in DC (Table 7, lines 6 and 7). The results show that while HC-treated marrow at higher dosages could induce adoptive restoration in 30% of the animals, no differences were detected when the cells were associated with thymus in DC. These results support the idea of a redistribution of competent postthymic T cells to marrow after HC treatment, but also indicate that the incompetent postthymic precursor is sensitive to the HC treatment.

9. Life Span (Table V)

Due to the complexities of the in vivo models used, it is difficult to determine actual half-lives of the postthymic precursor; however, the disap-

Table VII. Effect of Hydrocortisone on the Capacity of Bone Marrow Cells to Restore Immune Functions in 60-day-old Neonatally Thymectomized CBA/H Mice When Associated with Thymus in Diffusion Chambers

Treatment of cell donor[a]	Cell dosage	Thymus in DC[b]	Restoration[c]
None	20×10^6	Yes	7/10 (70%)
None	20×10^6	No	0/10
HC	20×10^6	Yes	1/10 (10%)
HC	20×10^6	No	1/10 (10%)
None	100×10^6	No	0/10
HC	100×10^6	No	3/10 (30%)
HC	100×10^6	Yes	3/12 (25%)
None	None	Yes	0/12

[a]Donors 50–70 days old were injected i.p. with 250 mg hydrocortisone/kg body weight, and marrow cells were collected 48 hr later.
[b]One thymus lobe from a 10-day-old CBA/HT6Tt donor was enclosed in chambers prepared as described in Stutman *et al.* (1969f), using filters with 0.10 μm pores. The chambers were implanted i.p. Marrow cells were also injected i.p.
[c]Restoration was measured 30 days after treatment, as the capacity to produce GVH *in vivo.* when spleen cells were injected into (CBA $\times$ C57BL/6) F_1 hybrids, and by the capacity to react *in vitro* to PHA. The number of animals restored per total treated is indicated. In every instance, both immune tests were restored. There was no instance of only one test being positive.

pearance rate after adult thymectomy would indicate a rapid turnover (Stutman, 1975b). Supporting this view is the fact that the precursor is contained within a rapidly dividing population that can commit "thymidine suicide" when exposed to a relatively short pulse of $[^3H]$thymidine of high specific activity (Stutman, 1975b).

10. Physical Characteristics (Table V)

Using bovine serum albumin (BSA) gradients, the precursor cells are detected mainly in the A–B layers (10–26% BSA), while the competent T cells are denser and mostly concentrated in the C–D layer (26–35% BSA). These results were comparable (i.e., the precursor appeared in the A–B layer) when adult spleen or marrow or newborn spleen or newborn liver was studied (Stutman, 1975 b,c). It should be noted that the less dense bands (i.e., the A–B layers) also contain the cells that can be induced to express T-cell-surface antigens by thymic extracts, using the same fractionation techniques (Scheid et al., 1973, 1975a; see also Section II.E).

By velocity sedimentation at unit gravity (R. G. Miller and Phillips, 1969) using either fetal calf serum or ficoll gradients, a good characterization of the three different cell types is obtained: the postthymic precursor cell is a cell of intermediate volume with a migration velocity of 5.4–5.9 mm/hr, while the immunologically competent postthymic T cell is a smaller cell with a velocity of 3.5–3.7 mm/hr. These values are quite constant regardless of the type of tissue studied (i.e., adult spleen or marrow, newborn spleen, or even embryonic liver). On the other hand, the prethymic stem cell (studied mostly as CFU-S) is quite a heterogeneous group of cells of intermediate size that are either smaller or larger than the postthymic precursor (these values are in accordance with those obtained for CFU by Worton et al., 1969 and Haskill and Moore, 1970, using comparable techniques).

11. Adherence to Nylon Wool (Table V)

The method described by Julius et al. (1973) for the rapid enrichment of competent T cells from spleen or other sources showed another difference between the postthymic precursor and the competent T cell: while the former is retained within the column (together with B and other cell types), the later passes through (Stutman, 1975b).*

12. Surface Markers (Table V)

Some cell-surface antigens such as Thy.1, TL, and the Ly series are characteristic for murine T cells at different stages of maturation (Boyse and Bennett, 1974; Boyse and Abbott, 1975; Chapter 2). Our studies indicate that the surface phenotype of the immunologically incompetent postthymic precursor is: Thy.1+;TL−;Ly 1+;Ly 2+;Ly 3+ (for details on Thy.1 and TL data, see Stutman, 1975b–d). The results for the Ly antigens are being prepared for publication.† The Thy.1 results, especially those using newborn spleen or adult marrow,

---

*In an in vitro system in which normal T cells in spleen are capable of suppressing the response of primed cells after reexposure to antigen (Calkins et al.,1976), we observed that nylon filtration did not remove suppression when either 1-week-old or newborn spleens were used as a source of suppressor cells, suggesting that the suppressor cell in this system is different from the postthymic precursor (Calkins and Stutman, unpublished data).

†The sera were provided by Drs. F. W. Shen and E. A. Boyse, Sloan-Kettering Institute, New York, New York, who collaborated in some of the experiments.

indicate that the postthymic precursor is present in low quantities, and that it is actually effective in cooperating with thymus in DC at low dosages. For example, in experiments using newborn spleen cells separated in BSA gradients, 10^7 cells were effective in restoring immune functions in association with thymus in DC (Stutman, 1975c), and such activity was abolished by pretreatment *in vitro* with the appropriate anti Thy.1 antiserum and C; however, the actual percentage of cells destroyed by such treatment was never above 15% of the total nucleated cells (indicating that approximately 1.5×10^6 cells were sufficient for generating competent T cells, a cell dosage that is rarely effective by itself, even using competent postthymic T cells; see Table I). That the postthymic precursor population is a minority makes it difficult to enrich on a quantitative basis, and does not permit determination of the actual amounts of Thy.1 present on their surfaces (see Section II.D for further discussion of the amounts of Thy.1 on T cells). Concerning the TL data discussed in Stutman (1975d), our present results suggest that it may be due to a contaminant in our TL serum (which was not prepared in congenic strains), since absortion of such serum with C57BL/6 thymocytes (which do not express TL surface antigens) absorbed out the ability of the antibody to decrease the restoration of immune functions in 50-day-old neonatally thymectomized A/J mice (Stutman, unpublished data); hence the question mark in Table I. The results in the *Ly* antisera are of interest for two main reasons: (1) Ly1,2,3+ cells were the first and only cells detected early in ontogeny (tested at 1 week of age by Cantor and Boyse, 1975a), and (2) Ly 1,2,3+ cells decline rather rapidly after adult thymectomy, as opposed to either Ly 1+,2,3− or Ly 1−,2,3+ cells (Cantor and Boyse 1975a,b; Chapter 2). Both observations fit well with the characteristics of the postthymic precursor described in Table V. Thus, it seems that the Ly 1,2,3 compartment contains, among other possible functional subsets, the immunologically incompetent postthymic precursor. It should be noted that in the adult spleen, Ly 1,2,3+ cells represent approximately 50% of the T cells (Cantor and Boyse, 1975a,b; Chapter 2).

The postthymic precursor has no detectable surface immunoglobulin or receptors for the Fc portion of the Ig molecule (Yoshida and Andersson, 1972; Stout and Herzenberg, 1975).

None of these antigens and surface markers is present in the prethymic cell or on the "prothymocytes" that can be activated to display these surface markers *in vitro* (Komuro and Boyse, 1973a,b; Komuro *et al.,* 1975; Boyse and Abbott, 1975). On the other hand, competent postthymic T cells, although they are a heterogeneous population with respect to function, have the phenotype Thy.1+, TL−, Ly+ (which can be Ly 1,2,3+; Ly 1+2,3−; Ly 1−, Ly 2,3+, depending on functional subclass; see Chapter 2), and some T cells show Fc receptors (Yoshida and Andersson, 1972; Stout and Herzenberg, 1975).

13. Direct Demonstration That the Postthymic Precursor Can Become a Competent T Cell

When purified postthymic precursor cells obtained from the spleens of newborn CBA/HT6T6 mice were injected into 60-day-old neonatally thymectomized CBA/H mice that also had a thymus in DC, we could show that the precursor cells indeed differentiated into competent T cells in the peripheral tissues of the hosts (Stutman, 1975b,c). When tested 30 days after treatment, a high proportion of cells in the lymph nodes and thoracic duct that were responding *in vitro* to PHA or to allogeneic cells had the T6T6 chromosomes of the postthymic precursor (Stutman, 1975b,c). These experiments indicate that as a consequence of a "maturation" event that is most probably regulated by thymic humoral factors (i.e., by thymus in DC and not by spleen in DC) and that is time-dependent (the earliest detectable responding population was observed 6–8 days after treatment), cells with the chromosome marker of the injected postthymic precursor (1) showed recirculating capacities (i.e., detected in thoracic duct, while no such cells could be detected in the controls receiving cells alone or cells plus either an empty DC or spleen in DC) and (2) could respond to PHA and to allogeneic cells in MLR, indicating immunologic competence.

14. Antigen Reactivity

Although we have stressed in the preceding pages that the postthymic precursor is immunologically incompetent, we have been able to show that either the postthymic precursor itself or a subpopulation within those cells could be driven into specific differentiation by repeated exposure to antigen (Stutman, 1975c,d). However, the design of the experiments and the limitations of the cell-separation techniques may permit the actual cloning of small numbers of immunologically competent T cells, which may be mediating the response. The experiments consisted in the injection of purified (by velocity sedimentation) postthymic precursors from newborn spleen into syngeneic 50-day-old neonatally thymectomized mice, which were subsequently immunized with tissues from allogeneic or xenogeneic (rat) origin. After one or three immunizations, the spleen cells from the recipients were tested for cytotoxic activity against the appropriate target. Cytotoxicity, which was mediated by Thy.1+ cells, could be detected only after three or more immunizations, suggesting the need for expansion of the primed population. These results should be taken with caution, as indicated above.

15. Summary

It appears from the results presented in Table V and discussed in the preceding pages that a precursor population of immunologically competent T cells can be characterized and defined by multiple biological criteria as being probably of postthymic origin and substantially different from either the immunologically competent T lymphocyte or the prethymic stem cells. On the basis of recent data on functional characteristics of different subsets of T cells, which suggest parallel lines of differentiation (see Chapter 2), it is possible that the postthymic precursor compartment may also show heterogeneity; however, this cannot be presently asserted from our results.

D. T-Cell Subsets

It is accepted that the population of small recirculating T lymphocytes, once considered the prime example of a homogeneous lymphoid population (Gowans and McGregor, 1965), is heterogeneous and represents, together with the nonrecirculating fixed lymphoid cells, a complex system with different functional classes of T cells that interact with each other as precursor, regulator, amplifier, suppressor, and effector cell subsets. In addition, the precursor cell described in the preceding pages, which is capable of differentiating into some of the functional subsets (probably into all of them, but this point needs clarification), may either behave as a strict precursor (i.e., generating new competent cells of a determined type) or may also act as regulator of the differentiated T-cell sets (this last aspect still needs intensive study). Our results with chromosome markers showing that the postthymic precursor can generate cells capable of producing a mitogenic response to phytohemagglutinin or allogeneic cells (Stutman, 1975b,c) would indicate, although they do not prove, that the Ly 1,2,3+ precursor can generate competent T cells of different Ly phenotype. The issue is far from clear, however, since in both such mitogenic responses, there is participation of both Ly 1+ and Ly 2,3+ cells (see Chapter 2), and our model is absolutely dependent on mitogenic responses to determine the chromosome type of the responding cell. However, since Ly 1+ cells respond in MLR mainly to I-region determinants, while Ly 2,3+ cells respond to $K–D$ regions of the $H2$ complex (see Chapter 2), this point can be tested experimentally using the appropriate mixtures of responding and stimulator cells, thus allowing definition of the actual precursor of the subsets of effector T cells that express different Ly phenotypes. The issue of one single lineage giving rise to different effector subsets vs. separate, albeit interacting, lineages (perhaps with a common precursor) is still unresolved. Concerning lineages, it should be noted that in some of the experiments using Ly sera (Cantor and Boyse, 1975a,b), the lymphoid cells were separated before treatment with the *Ly* antisera in nylon wool columns, possibly removing the Ly 1,2,3+ postthymic precursors (see Table V and Section II.C.).

The field of T-cell heterogeneity has developed rapidly in the past five years, and two basic "systems" have emerged: (1) the rather simple differentiation system of peripheral precursor giving rise to competent postthymic T cells (Stutman *et al.,* 1969a,b; 1970 a,b; Bach and Dardenne, 1972, 1973); and (2) the T–T interactions of the amplifier–effector or regulator–effector type (Cantor and Asofsky, 1970, 1972; Asofsky *et al.,* 1971; Raff and Cantor, 1971; Cantor, 1972a,b; Fathman *et al.,* 1975; Cantor *et al.,* 1975), which suggested "two stages in development of lymphocytes" (Cantor, 1972b), or at least a clear "functional heterogeneity" of lymphoid populations in the periphery (Stobo *et al.,* 1972, 1973; Stobo and Paul, 1972, 1973; Dutton, 1972, 1973). Most of these systems have been associated with either a $T_0-T_1-T_2$ (Bach and Dardenne, 1972, 1973) or a T_1-T_2 (Raff and Cantor, 1971; Cantor 1972a,b) terminology.

Comparisons between the biological and functional characteristics of some of these T-cell subsets have shown some similarities and some discrepancies (see Cantor 1972a,b; Kappler *et al.,* 1974; and especially Bach *et al.,* 1975b, the only collective effort by different investigators to compare these subsets). In general, both the postthymic precursor (Stutman, 1970, 1975b–d) and the T_0(and T_1) of Bach and Dardenne (1972, 1973) and the T_1 amplifier or regulator cells of most of the other systems (Cantor and Asofsky, 1970, 1972; Asofsky *et al.,* 1971; Raff and Cantor, 1971; Cantor 1972a,b; Dutton, 1972, 1973; Kappler *et al.,* 1974) decline relatively quickly after adult thymectomy, are mostly spleen-seeking, and are resistant to short-term treatment with ALS. The exception is the cells studied by Stobo *et al.* (1972, 1973) and Stobo and Paul (1972, 1973), which were relatively refractory to adult thymectomy and capable of responding to mitogens.

All these different cell types are Thy.1 positive. Concerning the amounts of Thy.1 antigen, it appears that the T_1 subsets have higher surface concentrations of the antigen than the T_2 cells (Cantor, 1972a,b; Stobo and Paul, 1972; Bach and Dardenne, 1972, 1973; Fathman *et al.,* 1975; Cantor *et al.,* 1975), and probably some of the T_1 regulatory cells also have some degree of reactivity to Concanavalin A, with low reactivity to phytohemagglutinin (Stobo and Paul, 1972, 1973). It also appears that most of the regulatory T_1 cells are Ly 1,2,3+ or Ly 1+, 2,3– (see Chapter 2). Thus, there is a large degree of overlapping between the postthymic "precursor" and the postthymic "regulatory" compartment in the periphery. To complicate matters even more, many of the studies cited above do not differentiate between those cell types within the thymus proper and outside the thymus, and in some instances (Cantor and Asofsky,

1970, 1972), the T_1 subset is termed *precursor*, while it probably is an amplifier for the effector-cell population.

A paraphrase of the discussion of one of the Cantor and Asofsky papers (1972) actually summarizes the two main hypotheses proposed for the different T–T interactions. The first hypothesis states that both the interacting T lymphocytes belong to a single line of differentiation, but differ in their degree of maturation. Thus, the T_1 cells differentiate from thymocytes within the thymus and then mature further to T_2 cells "within the thymus or more commonly in the periphery" (Cantor and Asofsky, 1972). The second hypothesis (termed an "alternative" hypothesis by Cantor and Asofsky, 1972) states that there are at least two separate differentiated lines of T lymphocytes in peripheral tissues and thymus, and the observed properties of the T_1 and T_2 subsets would be properties belonging to each of such lines. It appears that both hypotheses are probably correct, in the sense that the first may be pertinent to the postthymic precursor-differentiated T-cell model discussed in the previous section, while the "independent subline" theory (supported strongly by the *Ly* data; see Chapter 2) would apply mainly to some of the T–T functional interaction resulting in a defined immune response. The first hypothesis would predict that if the supply of new T cells in the adult is removed by thymectomy, amplifiers (T_2) will arise at the expense of the T_1 compartment (a hypothesis that is supported by some of the experimental data; see Cantor 1972a,b). The second hypothesis would predict that after adult thymectomy, both T_1 and T_2 (or *amplifier* and *precursor* as used in Cantor and Asofsky, 1972) would decline, although perhaps at "somewhat different rates" (Cantor and Asofsky, 1972). Such predictions cannot be strongly enunciated, however, due to the marked differences in life span (or of thymus-dependent renewal rate) of these different populations, plus the fact that the actual postthymic precursor compartment has a relatively short life after adult thymectomy (see Table V and Section II.C). A brief summary of the effects of adult thymectomy in some of the systems discussed in previous paragraphs would support our view (the numbers represent theoretical half-lives, based on the adult thymectomy data): T_1 and T_2 in GVH, 30–40 and more than 300 days, respectively (Cantor and Asofsky, 1972; Asofsky *et al.,* 1971); T cell required for priming activity for secondary responses, 30–40 days (Cantor, 1972a,b); Thy.1-positive rosette-forming cells in spleen (or background RFC), 5–7 days (Bach and Dardenne, 1972, 1973); mild depression of cell-mediated lympholysis, 15 days (Andersson *et al.,* 1974); increased antibody response to thymus-independent antigens (loss of suppressor T cells; see Gershon, 1974, for a review), 30 days; depression of cells required to prime for delayed hypersensitivity and helper activity, 30 days (Kappler *et al.,* 1974); helper activity in primary IgM or IgG responses, more than 200–300 days (Kappler *et al.,* 1974); Concanavalin-A-activated suppressors or stimulators of humoral responses, 200 days (Dutton, 1972, 1973); delays in skin graft rejection, depression of graft-vs.-host reactivity, more than 300 days (Stutman *et al.,* 1972; Stutman and Good, 1974). Indeed a complex picture.

Concerning the intrathymic T cells, different subpopulations have been described, based especially on size–volume–density, corticosteroid sensitivity, division rate, density of surface antigens and functional properties (Mosier and Cantor, 1971; Dyminsky *et al.,* 1974; Weissman *et al.,* 1975a). It appears that a class of large cells with bright Thy.1 fluorescence (i.e., high amounts of surface Thy.1) may serve as progenitors for all other classes of cells within the thymus (Weissman *et al.,* 1975a). Two other classes have been described: small cells with intermediate Thy.1 fluorescence and mid size cells with low but above-background Thy.1 fluorescence (Weissman *et al.,* 1975a; Fathman *et al.,* 1975). The corticosteroid-resistant population is a minority present mostly in the low-Thy.1 fraction (Fathman *et al.,* 1975). These authors indicate, however, that there is no clear evidence that sequential maturation from high-Thy.1 progenitor cells must proceed through any subclass to any other subclass (Weissman *et al.,* 1975a). Although the immunologic competence of the small pool of steroid-resistant cells in the thymus is well accepted (see Dyminsky *et al.,* 1974, for additional references), it appears from *in vivo* transfer experiments that these cells require some additional factors when outside the thymus to express immune competence (Mosier and Cantor, 1971). These results suggest that the thymus may contain two corticosteroid-resistant subpopulations, one a "non-reactive precursor" that matures in the periphery in the transfer experiments and one a reactive T cell that has already matured in the thymus (Mosier and Cantor, 1971). The main problem (which will be discussed in Section III) is that most probably, neither of these two corticosteroid-resistant populations actually leaves the thymus. However, *in vitro* culture of embryonic thymus can generate Thy.1-positive cells (Owen and Raff, 1970), as well as T cells capable of immunologic activity (Owen, 1974; Robinson and Owen, 1976), and in some cases show enrichment of such T cells (suggesting actual "accumulation" in the absence of true export).

Finally, a relatively new cell has been added to the list. This cell has some characteristics that are similar to those of the postthymic precursor (see Bach *et al.,* 1975b, for a direct comparison); however, it has been termed *prethymic* due to its presence in nude mice (Roelants *et al.,* 1975, 1976; Sato *et al.,* 1976). This cell is characterized by being Thy.1+ weak (as opposed to the conventional T lymphocyte, which is Thy.1+ strong; see Roelants *et al.,* 1975, 1976). The unique features of this cell are that it actually increases (or accumulates) after thymectomy and decreases after thymus grafting; it also expresses TL antigen, has a very short life span (of 1–2 days), and does not recirculate (Roelants *et al.,* 1975, 1976). A similar cell obtained from nude mice (characterized by low amounts of Thy.1) can be differentiated further into Concanavalin-A-responding cells by incubation on thymus epithelium, and was termed a *pre-T cell* (Sato *et al.*, 1976). It should be noted that an increase of TL+ Thy.1+ as well as TL− Thy.1+ cells in nodes and spleen has been described in nude mice after infection with mouse hepatitis virus as well as after treatment with some thymic extracts (Scheid *et al.*, 1975b). These *prethymocytes* (Roelants *et al.*, 1975) or *prothymocytes* (Scheid *et al.*, 1975b), which appear to be cells that are already committed to the T pathway of differentiation independently of thymic influence, but needing the thymus for further differentiation, will be discussed in Section II.E.

Some final remarks concerning T cells in nude mice are appropriate here. It appears that some lymphocytes with detectable amounts of Thy.1 surface antigen can indeed be found in nude mice (see *Nature*, 1973); however, it is also clear that no detectable T cells with T-cell functions can be found in such mice (see Wortis, 1974, for a review, and Section II.B). It is apparent that these findings could be interpreted in more than one way, and that they raise such questions as: Is there any transitory thymic function during fetal life in nude mice? What is the role of thymic humoral factors in the heterozygote breeding of nude mice (i.e., the nu/nu being exposed to its mother as well as its siblings' thymuses)? Is there a blockade of differentiation of the pre-T cell in nude mice? How good a marker for T cells is Thy.1? It is also apparent that some of these questions were presented in a 1973 editorial (*Nature*, 1973) that was signed H. S. M. (i.e., H. S. Micklem?), but are still unanswered. The significance of the induction of surface markers is discussed further in Section II.E.

E. *In Vitro* Induction

An important recent development was the demonstration that hemopoietic cells of adult or embryonic origin (as well as from nude mice) could express an array of cell-surface antigens characteristic of T cells (i.e., TL, Thy.1, and *Ly* series) after incubation *in vitro* for short periods of time with various thymus extracts (Komuro and Boyse, 1973a,b). It also became apparent, however, that a wide variety of substances that had in common the ability to increase the intracellular levels of cyclic AMP were also capable of inducing the same changes (Scheid *et al.*, 1973, 1975a,b; Goldstein *et al.*, 1975). This last set of results suggested that elevation of cyclic AMP may be the physiological mechanism of action of the thymic hormones (this fact was also observed in other *in vitro* systems and using other thymic preparations and assays by Bach *et al.*, 1975a; Trainin *et al.*, 1975; and Singh and Owen, 1975), and also pointed toward the strict controls that are required for determining that a tissue extract (whether derived from thymus or not) has some physiological properties and echoes some of our own early criticisms of the field of "thymic hormones" (Stutman and Good, 1973).

The actual target cell for this *in vitro* induction has been considered to be a predetermined T-cell precursor, probably prethymic, that is termed a *prothymocyte* in most of the publications (Komuro and Boyse, 1973a,b; Scheid *et al.,* 1973, 1975a,b; Goldstein *et al.,* 1975). It should be stressed, however, that the *in vitro* induction assays mimic to a large degree the intrathymic step of differentiation (including the appearance of TL antigen) and usually produce cells with T-cell-surface characteristics, but devoid of immunologic competence (Scheid *et al.,* 1973, 1975a,b) or with a modest response to Concanavalin A (Basch and Goldstein, 1975), which also resembles the situation of the nude mouse (see Scheid *et al.,* 1975b, and Sections II.B and II.D). The short-term event (assays are usually 2-hr incubations) as well as the need for transcription and translation for expression of surface phenotype (Storrie *et al.,* 1976) indicate that the induction *in vitro* is triggered by the inducing substance and that it is an inherent property of the responding cell. However, none of the experiments so far performed formally rules out that the commitment of the stem cell to T differentiation (i.e., to become a prothymocyte) is a thymus-independent or a prethymic event. As a matter of fact, yolk sac cells apparently are not inducible (i.e., are not induced to express T-cell markers after *in vitro* incubation with purified thymic extracts such as thymopoietin; reported in a personal communication to this author by Drs. Komuro and Boyse from Sloan-Kettering Institute and by Dr. Ross Basch from New York University). It is apparent that additional work is required to clarify these issues. It is also clear that thymic humoral factors may mediate both the intrathymic and the extra-thymic events, perhaps by mediation of different products or by differences in concentration of the same factor.

F. A Matter of Terminology

In this section, I will try to present a brief vocabulary that may help to situate and define the meaning of most of the terms used to designate T cells and their precursors, and attempt to correlate such terms with the different nomenclatures. All these terms are purely operational and mostly descriptive. And although they are less appealing than some of the prevalent "symbols" (i.e., T_1-T_2, etc.), they may be more accurate.

Prethymic: In our original presentations, this term designated a cell that had not received thymic influence, i.e., a stem cell that had the capacity either to migrate to the thymus or to be influenced by the thymus (Stutman *et al.,* 1969a; 1970a,b; Stutman, 1972a). Obviously, such a prethymic compartment may include everything from the totipotential stem cell to the "prothymocyte" (i.e., probably equivalent to a committed stem cell, committed to the T-cell lineage; see Komuro and Boyse, 1973a,b; Komuro *et al.*, 1975; Scheid *et al.*, 1973, 1975a). In a strict sense, the only true prethymic hemopoietic cell would be that found in the yolk sac, before the epithelial anlage of the thymus develops (see Table VI). However, even such early hemopoietic stem cells in yolk sac may be influenced by the mother's thymic humoral factors. Two important features of the prethymic compartment as a whole are its ability to traffic to the thymus (Stutman, 1972a,b; Komuro *et al.*, 1975; see also Section III) and the absence of detectable T-cell surface markers (see Table V).

Postthymic: This term is also a purely operational one to designate all the different cell subsets that have received some form of thymic influence (most probably through traffic) and that are presently in an extrathymic location. The two main characteristics of this group of cells are their incapacity to traffic back to thymus (see Section III) and the presence on their surfaces of easily detected antigenic markers characteristic of the T-cell series. This group of cells includes: (1) the postthymic *precursor*, extensively discussed in the previous sections, which may be termed a "recognizable" precursor using Lajtha's terminology (Lajtha, 1975); (2) postthymic *regulatory* cells probably representing most of the Ly 1,2,3+ subset and exerting regulatory functions on either the generation or the activity of effector cells, of the type described by Beverly *et al.*, (1976); (3) postthymic *amplifier* cells, perhaps an artificial category that may be fused to the regulatory group; however, it seems to have some bearing as functional amplifiers of GVH and probably also in cytotoxic responses (see Cantor 1972a,b; Cantor and Asofsky, 1972; Cantor *et al.*, 1975; (4) postthymic *suppressor* cells (Gershon, 1974), considered here as a separate entity on a functional basis and due to some of the *Ly* data discussed in Chapter 2; and (5) postthymic *effector* cells, which are the classic categories of cytotoxic, helper T cells (see also Chapter 2), representing most of the T_2 compartments discussed in previous paragraphs. Since there is sufficient evidence to support the idea of a true postthymic precursor in the periphery (see Section II.C) that behaves like a committed or "recognizable" precursor such as those defined in the differentiation of other hemopoietic cells (see Lajtha, 1975), it would be helpful to restrict this term to such a cell type and clearly separate it from other cell types that may be regulating or modifying in some way the reactivity of the differentiated effector cells.

III. TRAFFIC

The term *traffic* is used here to indicate the traffic of cells to and from the thymus, probably as part of a maturational pathway (C. E. Ford, 1966; Stutman, 1972a). By the use of cells with chromosome markers in irradiated mice, it has been demonstrated that there is a migration of cells from hemopoietic origin (marrow) via the thymus to lymph nodes (C. E. Ford and Micklem, 1963; Micklem *et al.*, 1966; C. E. Ford, 1966). This journey has a probable duration of weeks, and the thymus seems to play a role in instructing the migrating cells (Harris and Ford, 1963, 1964; C. E. Ford, 1966; Stutman, 1970, 1972a; Doenhoff *et al.*, 1970). Most of the original observations on thymus traffic dealt exclusively with the finding of the cells (with the chromosome marker) dividing in different anatomic locations such as lymph nodes and other sites (C. E. Ford and Micklem, 1963; Harris and Ford, 1963, 1964; Micklem *et al.*, 1966; C. E. Ford, 1966), or as dividing cells derived from thymus grafts in the periphery showing some quantitative changes in response to immunologic stimuli (Davies *et al.*, 1966, 1971; Davies, 1969). Later studies actually showed that cells capable of responding to phytohemagglutinin in the peripheral tissues of reconstituted mice were derived from the thymus (Davies *et al.*, 1968; 1971; Davies, 1969; Doenhoff *et al.*, 1970). The subsequent step in clarification of this peculiar biological traffic was the direct demonstration that hemopoietic precursors could become immunologically reactive T cells (capable of responding to phytohemagglutinin and allogeneic cells) after traffic through thymus and subsequent export to the periphery (Stutman, 1970, 1972a, 1976; Stutman and Good, 1969, 1971a,b). This last set of findings will be briefly discussed in this section.

The term "traffic" has also been used to describe the rapid recirculation of small mature lymphocytes (mostly T) from blood into lymphoid tissues and back to blood, which takes place in hours (W. L. Ford and Gowans, 1969). As will be seen in the following sections, this second type of "traffic" is a property of the mature T lymphocyte and is a consequence of the first type of traffic (i.e., traffic of hemopoietic cells through the thymus).

A. A Brief Description of Methods

The use of CBA/H and CBA/HT6T6 mice (and their F_1 hybrids) allows the detection of three different cell types, characterized by their chromosome types: no markers (CBA/H), two small chromosomes (CBA/HT6T6), and one single small chromosome (the F_1 hybrid, CBA/HT6). For details on these strains, see most of the previously quoted references; for details on the CBA sublines used in the present study, see Stutman (1970). Our sublines are syngeneic to each other (the proper term would be congenic for the T6 marker), and skin grafts are accepted permanently when exchanged between CBA/H and CBA/HT6T6 of CBA/HT6 animals. It must be stressed that this model permits only the study of cells in division, either spontaneous or induced after exposure to mitogens. Our own work is interpreted exclusively on a qualitative basis, with no attempts at actual quantitation of cell populations. Some authors have attempted to make quantitative estimates of T-cell compartments (and renewal rates) using chromosome-marked populations (Davies *et al.,* 1971).

The basic models used (Stutman 1970, 1972a,b; Stutman and Good, 1969, 1971a,b) are:

Model 1: 50—60 day old neonatally thymectomized CBA/H grafted intraperitoneally (or under the kidney capsule) with a thymus lobe from newborn CBA/HT6 (or CBA/H donors) and subsequently injected intraperitoneally with hemopoietic cells of CBA/HT6T6 origin. The T6T6 cells are derived from adult marrow, newborn liver, or spleen, embryonic 14—17 day old liver, 14—17 day old embryonic blood, or 10—13 day old yolk sac cells, and the cell dosages ranged from 5×10^5 to 5×10^6.

At 20—90 days after treatment, chromosome preparations were made of the thymus grafts and other lymphohemopoietic tissues of the host. This model was used mainly to study traffic of hemopoietic cells to the thymus proper.

Model 2: This model consisted of 50—60 day old neonatally thymectomized CBA/H secondary hosts grafted intraperitoneally with the thymus from the Model 1 animals. Such as thymus graft, 20—30 days after cell injection in the primary host, contains migrating CBA/HT6T6 cells in transit (Stutman 1970, 1972a; Stutman and Good 1971a,b). At 20—90 days after thymus grafting, chromosome preparations are made of lymph nodes or thoracic duct lymphocytes (and other lymphoid tissues) of the secondary hosts. These cells are studied either unstimulated or after stimulation with phytohemagglutinin or allogeneic cells. In this model, the only source of T6T6 cells is the thymus graft itself, and the design permits the study of the export of cells from the thymus to the periphery.

Other additions to or changes in the basic models will be discussed in the appropriate paragraphs.

Since there was no detectable difference in the proportion of T6T6 cells migrating to the thymus graft, regardless of the source of hemopoietic cells (whether embryonic, newborn, or adult), or in the export of such cells from the thymus graft, the results will be discussed for "hemopoietic precursors" as a group, unless otherwise stated. Although there is evidence that hemopoietic cells migrate to tissues of irradiated hosts (Micklem *et al.,* 1966), the proportion of migrating cells is much lower when hemopoietic cells are injected into normal hosts, usually only 1—2% of the dividing cells (Micklem *et al.,* 1968). On the other hand, the rate of entry of hemopoietic cells into thymus grafts is quite comparable for normal or thymectomized hosts (Leuchars *et al.,* 1967). The advantage of our model is that by using 50—60 day old neonatally thymectomized hosts, which are also deprived of postthymic precursors, both the traffic of cells to the graft and the export of such cells to the periphery appear to be increased, or at least to reach levels at which useful numbers of mitoses can be scored. Perhaps the observation that the traffic of cells to and from the thymus is determined "more by the thymus itself than by peripheral shortage of cells of thymic origin" (Leuchars *et al.*, 1967) may be explained by the fact that the thymectomized animals used in those experiments at the time of thymus grafting had an intact compartment of postthymic precursors (the hosts were thymectomized at 8–10 weeks of age and grafted 1 week later; see Leuchars *et al.*, 1967; Davies, 1969; and Davies *et al.*, 1971).

B. Migration of Hemopoietic Precursors to Thymus

With Model 1, the results showed that 20 days after cell injection, 10–25% of the dividing cells within the thymus grafts were of CBA/HT6T6 type, i.e., derived from the injected probe of hemopoietic precursors of embryonic or adult origin (Stutman 1970, 1972a, 1976; Stutman and Good, 1969, 1971a,b). Donor type T6T6 cells could be detected as early as 10 days after injection (Stutman, 1976), although the exception to this case will be discussed in Section III.C. The T6T6 dividing cells were also found in the marrow (usually 3–6% of the dividing cells), but were absent from lymph nodes or thoracic duct (Stutman, 1972a; Stutman and Good, 1971a,b). T6T6 metaphases were detected in nodes or thoracic duct only when tested after 30 days of treatment (Stutman, 1972a), which fits rather well with the timing observed in radiation chimeras (Micklem *et al.*, 1966). The ability of hemopoietic precursors to migrate to nodes or appear in thoracic duct (i.e., to recirculate) was not observed in thymectomized animals that were injected with cells but had not received a thymus graft, or that were grafted with a thymus in a cell-impermeable diffusion chamber (Stutman and Good, 1971a,b). In these animals, the T6T6 cells were detected almost exclusively in marrow and spleen (3–7% of the dividing cells). These results indicate that a viable and accessible thymus stroma is a requirement for the production of lymph-node-migrating or recirculating T cells or both. In a way, these cells behave like prethymic precursor cells (see Table V and Section II). This thymus requirement was also observed in radiation chimeras, and based on transfer of thymus cells, Micklem *et al.*, (1966) discussed the possibility of "apprentice" thymocytes (not yet able to colonize lymph nodes) and "trained" thymocytes (able to colonize nodes).

Another interesting observation was that the migration of hemopoietic precursors to thymus grafts in Model 1 animals was highly sensitive to histocompatibility differences between cells and thymus graft, even weak non-*H2* differences (Stutman and Good, 1969). When cells and thymus were incompatible, the percentage of dividing cells of donor origin in the grafts dropped to 0–3% (Stutman and Good, 1969). In these experiments, the model was reversed and CBA/HT6T6 hosts and thymus grafts were used, while the injected cells had normal chromosome types. These experiments indicate that in the presence of competing syngeneic hemopoietic precursors (from the marrow of the host), allogeneic cells are at a clear disadvantage in repopulating the thymus graft.

Our preliminary studies, still unpublished, concerning the effects of some of the procedures listed in Table V (which were useful for the study of the postthymic precursor) on the ability of hemopoietic precursors to migrate to thymus indicate that: (1) Adult thymectomy does not change the capacity of marrow cells to migrate to thymus (studied at 30–160 days after thymectomy). (2) Treatment with antilymphocyte serum of the marrow donor also had no significant effect. (A note of caution: Some ALS preparations contain contaminants that are cytotoxic for hemopoietic stem cells; such contaminants can be absorbed with hemopoietic fetal liver cells.) (3) Treatment with steroids (see also Table VII) at dosages and timings that affected postthymic precursors in marrow had no effect on the capacity of those cells to migrate to thymus grafts. (4) Preliminary separation procedures indicate that the hemopoietic precursor capable of thymus traffic (and colonization) has density and volume characteristics similar to those of the totipotential colony-forming unit (described in Table V in the "Prethymic precursor" column). These studies are presently under way, and should be considered as preliminary.

C. Need of Yolk Sac Cells for an Additional "Step" before Thymus Migration

Our initial observations, testing the animals at 20–30 days after cell injection, did not show any differences in thymus migration among the different cell types tested, including yolk sac. When the grafts were studied early after cell injection, however, a marked difference was apparent (Stutman, 1976). For example, while 7–14% of adult marrow or embryonic liver were detected by day 10 within the grafts, no detectable yolk sac cells were observed at that period. Table VIII shows some of these results. This gap suggested that yolk sac cells required an additional step before being able to migrate to thymus (i.e., possibly a sojourn in a secondary hemopoietic site such as liver in the physiological situation and marrow in the present experimental conditions).

To test this hypothesis, we used the effects of strontium-89, a bone-seeking isotope that produces a functional obliteration of the marrow cavity (Fried *et al.*, 1966) with retention of spleen hemopoiesis. Table IX shows that while the marrow or 14–15-day-old embryonic liver cells could migrate to thymus in the ^{89}Sr-treated animals, yolk sac cells were incapable of such migration in the absence of a functional marrow cavity, and apparently the spleen could not replace such a deficit (the main site in these animals where yolk sac cells could be found was indeed the spleen; see Stutman, 1976, for more details). We also

Table VIII. Chromosome Analysis
of Dividing Cells Within CBA/H Thymus Grafts
in Thymectomized Hosts Injected with
CBA/HT6T6 Hemopoietic Cells

Days after cell injection[a]	T6T6 metaphases in thymus grafts (%)[b]		
	Marrow	Liver	Yolk sac
5	4	4	0
10	14	13	0
15	17	16	5
20	16	17	12
25	22	20	16
30	18	20	18
35	13	10	14
40	5	3	3
50	2	1	1
75	2	2	1

[a]CBA/HT6T6 cells from adult marrow (40–60 days of age), liver (14–15 days of embryonation), and yolk sac (10–13 days of embryonation) were injected intravenously (10^6) into 60-day-old neonatally thymectomized CBA/H mice, grafted with a CBA/H thymus under the kidney capsule, 30 days prior to cell injection.
[b]Three mice per point for the different cell types and days; 100–400 metaphases per mouse scored.

showed that in the ^{89}Sr-treated animals, competent T cells capable of responding to phytohemagglutinin (and recirculating, i.e., detected in thoracic duct) could be found in the animals injected with marrow or liver, but not with yolk sac (Stutman, 1976). On the other hand, we showed that yolk sac cells can indeed become competent T cells after thymus traffic, provided there is an intact marrow in the host (Stutman, 1976), or when transferred as intrathymic in transit cells (Stutman and Good, 1971a,b).

These results could be interpreted as indicating that the capacity of the hemopoietic precursor to migrate to thymus may in itself be mediated via thymus products, since truly prethymic hemopoietic precursors such as yolk sac seem unable to migrate directly to the thymus, without a previous step in the peripheral secondary hemopoietic sites. This interpretation fits rather snugly with the observation that the "prothymocyte," which can be induced in vitro to express T-cell surface antigens, also has the ability to migrate to the thymus

Table IX. Chromosome Analysis
of Dividing Cells Within CBA/H Thymus Grafts
in Thymectomized Hosts Treated with [89]Sr
Injected with CBA/HT6T6 Hemopoietic Cells

Days after cell injection[a]	T6T6 metaphases in thymus graft (%)[b]		
	Marrow	Liver	Yolk sac
5	5	2	0
10	12	12	0
15	15	14	0
20	17	14	0
25	17	17	1
30	20	19	1
35	14	15	0
40	4	10	0
45	2	3	2
50	2	2	0
55	3	2	0
60	2	2	0
70	1	1	0
75	1	1	0

[a]CBA/HT6T6 cells from adult marrow, embryonic liver, and yolk sac were injected intravenously (10^6) into 60-day-old neonatally thymectomized CBA/H mice grafted at 30 days of age with a CBA/H thymus under the kidney capsule and injected at 50 days of age with 100 μCi [89]Sr.
[b]Three mice per point, 100–400 metaphases per mouse scored.

(Komuro *et al.,* 1975). Thus, the prothymocyte could in reality be a postthymic cell (i.e., a cell that received some sort of thymic influence) present in liver and marrow, but absent from yolk sac. The only evidence supporting this interpretation is (1) the timing of events in ontogeny (see Table VI) and (2) the unpublished evidence that yolk sac cells are noninducible *in vitro* (see Section II.E). It is also apparent that the marrow precursors described by El-Arini and Osoba (1973) fit within the category of prethymic cells that probably restore the T-cell compartment in irradiated (nonthymectomized) animals via thymus traffic (in these experiments, the source of "precursors" was T-depleted adult marrow, treated *in vitro* with anti-Thy.1 and C; see El-Arini and Osoba, 1973). It seems that additional study is necessary for clarification of these problems.

Table X. Chromosome Analysis of CBA/HT6
Thymus Grafts in 50-Day-Old Neonatally
Thymectomized CBA/H Hosts Injected with
CBA/HT6T6 Fetal Liver Cells

Days after treatment[a]	Metaphases in thymus graft (%)[b]		
	CBA/HT6T6 (liver)	CBA/HT6 (thymus)	CBA/H (host)
7	4	92	3
15	14	32	54
30	19	0.5	80
45	1	1	98
60	1	1	98
75	1	1	98

[a]Thymus graft under the kidney capsule and subequent injection of 5×10^6 liver cells from 15–16-day-old embryos.
[b]Five to eight thymi were analyzed per point. The number of
metaphases scored per graft ranged from 125 to 301.

D. Time of Intrathymic Residence

Table X shows the actual timing of dilution of the migrant T6T6 cells by
the host hemopoietic cells that migrate to the thymus. It is apparent that most
of the injected cells that had migrated to thymus had disappeared by 45 days
after cell injection and were replaced by migrants of host origin. However, a
small population of dividing cells of donor origin remained. This population can
be associated with the corticosteroid-resistant population in the medulla of the
thymus (see Section III.H and Table XIII for further details). On the other hand,
donor cells in the lymph nodes or thoracic duct of the Model 2 recipients, i.e.,
exported cells, have been detected for as long as we tested (most of our
unpublished studies tested animals at 30–180 days after thymus transfer however, we studied some animals at 600–700 days posttransfer and detected T6T6
donor cells in 8 of 12 animals studied, and the percentages ranges ranged from 4
to 9%; see also Section III.G).

E. Emigration from the Thymus

When thymus grafts containing migrating hemopoietic cells of CBA/HT6T6
origin (including yolk sac cells) were transplanted to secondary thymectomized
CBA/H hosts (Model 2), dividing cells of T6T6 type could be detected in lymph
nodes or thoracic duct within 20 days after intraperitoneal grafting (Stutman,

1972a; Stutman and Good, 1971a,b). By day 20–30 after grafting, the proportion of T6T6 cells was 5–20% in nodes, 9–15% in blood, and 10–26% in thoracic duct. T6T6 cells were also found in spleen (12–14%), in Peyer's patches (15–10%), and in some animals also in bone marrow, supporting our previous data on a postthymic compartment in marrow (see Section II). For more details on thes results, see Stutman (1970, 1972a) and Stutman and Good (1971a,b).

Using different radio labeling procedures (including *in situ* intrathymic), most of the evidence indicates that there is export of thymus-derived cells to the periphery, and that such export is higher during early perinatal stages and that can also be increased by external stimuli (Joel *et al.*, 1972; Bryant, 1972; Bryant *et al.*, 1975; Laissue *et al.*, 1976); however, most of the labeled thymocytes die within the thymus or have a very short life in the periphery. Our data, although not quantitative, suggest that a good proportion of the dividing cells, and especially of the competent T cells in the periphery (see Section III.I), are derived from postthymic cells exported by the thymus. These seemingly discrepant results could be explained by the expansion in the periphery of a relatively small pool of postthymic precursors (see Section II) and/or by the constant daily output of relatively small numbers of short-lived lymphocytes that accumulate in the periphery. (A third possibility would be that the endogenous labeling alters the normal behavior of the cells.)

F. Unidirectional Emigration of Postthymic Cells

A set of experiments was designed to test whether the cells exported by the thymus grafts in Model 2 animals would return to the thymus. To study this possibility, Model 2 animals were modified and either had a CBA/H thymus graft implanted before the thymus from Model 1 animals was grafted (Model 2.A) or were grafted simultaneously with a CBA/H thymus and a thymus from Model 1 donors (Model 2.B). Some of these results were presented in Stutman (1972a). In both instances, no T6T6 cells could be detected in the second CBA/H thymus, while T6T6 could be detected in lymph nodes or thoracic duct, i.e., were exported to the periphery, but did not return to the thymus. Table XI shows some of these results. Again, we should stress that in these experiments, the only source of T6T6 cells is the thymus graft from the Model 1 animals. In summary, the export of postthymic cells to the periphery is unidirectional.

G. Short- and Long-Lived Emigrant Lymphocytes

Using Model 2 animals and subsequent injections of [^{3}H] thymidine in schedules that will preferentially label short- and long-lived cells (Everett *et al.*,

Table XI. Cells Exported by Thymus Do Not Return to Thymus: CBA/HT6T6 Metaphases in Lymph Nodes and Thymus Grafts in Model 2.A and 2.B CBA/H Hosts

Tissues studied[a]	T6T6 metaphases per total metaphases[b]	
	Model 2.A	Model 2.B
CBA/H thymus graft	0/976	0/1233
CBA/H thymus graft (PHA)	0/699	0/873
Lymph nodes	98/899 (11%)	76/801 (9%)
Lymph nodes (PHA)	168/902 (19%)	159/863 (18%)

[a]Results from 4 experiments (8–10 animals) 20–30 days after transplantation of a thymus from a Model 1 animal (injected with hemopoietic T6T6 cells). PHA indicates the results after incubation of the cells with phytohemagglutinin (see Stutman, 1970, for details). "Thymus graft" indicates the second thymus, derived from a normal CBA/H implanted under the kidney capsule, either 20 days before intraperitoneal implantation of the Model 1 thymus (Model 2.A) or simultaneously with the Model 1 thymus (Model 2.B).
[b]Pooled results. Numbers in parentheses indicate percentages of T6T6 metaphases.

Table XII. Short- and Long-Lived Lymphocytes in Lymph Nodes of Model 2 Animals Grafted with a CBA/H Thymus Containing CBA/HT6T6 Hemopoietic Immigrants

Labeling procedure[a]	Number of T6T6 metaphases per total metaphases	Number labeled T6T6 metaphases
Short	47/390 (12%)	26/47 (55%)
Long	57/299 (19%)	3/57 (2%)

[a][³H]Thymidine (0.75 μCi/g body weight) was administered every 6 hr for 6 days (Short) or daily for 17 days (Long), and the animals were sacrificed 4–6 hr after the last injection in the former case (Short) and 20–30 days after the last injection in the latter case (Long). Metaphases, after autoradiography, were scored for combined presence of radioactive grains and T6T6 chromosome markers.

1964; Rieke and Schwartz, 1967; see Table XII for details), we tried to determine whether both types of lymphocytes were generated from hematopoietic precursors after thymus traffic and subsequent export (Stutman, 1972b). The association of radioactive grains with the T6T6 chromosome markers in lymph node lymphocytes would determine, depending on the labeling schedules, whether short- or long-lived cells or both were generated after traffic. Table XII shows some of the results. It is apparent that both cell types are generated, although most of the cells bearing both markers seem to be short-lived. When the same experiments were performed using phytohemagglutinin for further stimulation of mitoses (Stutman, unpublished data), comparable results were obtained; i.e., most of the responding cells were short-lived (however, it has been shown in rats that the cell that responds to phytohemagglutinin is a short-lived lymphocyte; see Rieke and Schwartz, 1967). These results can also be interpreted as suggesting that the short-lived population may give rise, in the periphery, to the long-lived recirculating population. It is obvious that these results need further study.

As was indicated in Section II.D, however, thymus emigrants can be detected in the lymph nodes and thoracic duct of Model 2 recipients for long periods of time, even at 600–700 days after thymus transfer (Stutman, unpublished data). These results support the view that long-lived recirculating lymphocytes are also generated through thymus traffic of hemopoietic precursors.

H. Steroid Resistance and Sensitivity

In Section II, we showed that the postthymic precursor was sensitive to high doses of corticosteroids. The sensitivity or resistance to steroids was also tested in the traffic model, and our unpublished results indicate that (1) the population of corticosteroid-resistant thymocytes within thymus grafts is in part derived from hemopoietic immigrants and (2) when thymus grafts from Model 1 animals pretreated with high doses of hydrocortisone (25 μg/kg body weight) were transferred to secondary thymectomized hosts, there was no evidence of export of the corticosteroid-resistant intrathymic population. Table XIII shows some of our results on the inability of corticosteroid-resistant thymus cells (derived from T6T6 hemopoietic precursors in transit) to migrate outside the thymus graft. Table XIII also shows that the corticosteroid-resistant population within the thymus has the ability to respond mitotically to phytohemagglutinin, and that it is a long-lasting population in residence (still detectable at 180 days after grafting and when the donor T6T6 cells are mostly diluted by host-derived cells; see also Table X).

Data from *in situ* labeling of the thymic cortex indicate that the medullary thymocytes that are corticosteroid resistant appear to be derived from the

Table XIII. Hemopoietic Origin of Intrathymic Corticoresistant Cells—A Resident
Population Incapable of Traffic Outside the Thymus (Model 2 Animals Grafted
with Thymus with T6T6 Hemopoietic Cells in Transit Derived from Untreated
or from Model 1 Animals Injected with Hydrocortisone)

Days after thymus grafting[a]	Hydrocortisone treatment of thymus donor[b]	T6T6 metaphases per total metaphases scored[c]			
		Thymus graft		Lymph nodes	
		No PHA	PHA	No PHA	PHA
30	No	82/736 (11%)	ND	ND	132/869 (15%)
30	Yes	22/246 (9%)	198/769 (26%)	0/532	2/998 (0.2%)
60	No	12/439 (3%)	56/390 (14%)	69/733 (9%)	298/799 (37%)
60	Yes	9/298 (3%)	69/435 (16%)	0/499	0/763
180	No	2/442 (0.4%)	29/456 (6%)	58/792 (7%)	155/1875 (8%)
180	Yes	3/520 (0.5%)	39/483 (8%)	0/532	0/777

[a]50–60 day old neonatally thymectomized CBA/H grafted under the kidney capsule with a thymus
derived from a Model 1 animal (20–30 days after injection of 5×10^5 15-day-old CBA/HT6T6 fetal
liver cells).
[b]Thymus donors were either untreated or pretreated, 48 hr before thymus transfer, with 250 μg of
hydrocortisone/kg body weight.
[c]Pooled results for 6 animals. (PHA) Phytohemagglutinin; (ND) not done.

cortical thymocytes (Weissman, 1973; Weissman et al., 1975a,b). On the other
hand, mature T cells in the periphery show both sensitivity and resistance to
high dosages of steriods (Claman and Moorhead, 1972). The present results
indicate that the intrathymic steroid-resistant population of thymocytes is also
derived from hemopoietic precursors. They also indicate (together with our
previous data, discussed in Section II) that the bulk of the postthymic cells
derived from the thymus graft are corticosteroid-sensitive cells (which apparently become steroid-resistant in the periphery), and that there is no detectable
evidence of export of the intrathymic corticosteroid-resistant population to the
periphery (supporting the observation by Elliott et al., 1971, and Elliott, 1973).

The presence of the mature T-like lymphocytes within the thymus has
usually been interpreted as indicative of the compartment that represents the
immediate precursors of the thymus cell migrants, and as the source of peripheral T lymphocytes (see, for example, Raff, 1971; Leckband and Boyse, 1971;
Dyminsky et al., 1974; Shortman et al., 1975). The experiments of Elliott et al.
(1971) indicate that the cortisone-resistant PHA-responsive subpopulation in
thymus grafts is of donor origin for at least 28 days after transplantation (this
finding was interpreted as indicating that such cells were generated within the
graft). These results, as well as those of Elliott (1973) and our present results,

indicate that the "mature" subpopulation is not undergoing rapid replacement (or any detectable export to the periphery) for a relatively long period of time. Thus, it appears that only a small proportion of the "immature" thymus lymphocytes may differentiate to become the "mature" subpopulation in the medulla. It is most probable that the majority of the "immature" corticosensitive rapidly dividing cells must either die within the thymus or migrate from it.

I. Generation of Competent T Cells Through Thymus Traffic

To test whether this peculiar traffic implies a true differentiative process toward immunologic competence, the lymph nodes, blood, or thoracic duct cells from the Model 2 animals were tested for their ability to respond *in vitro* to phytohemagglutinin or Concanavalin A, or to allogeneic cells in mixed lymphocyte cultures (usually using C57BL/6 cells as stimulators). The results obtained (and mostly published) indicated that a substantial fraction (at least a readily detectable one) of the responding cells (ranging from 10 to 38% of the dividing cells; see Stutman, 1970, 1972a, 1976; Stutman and Good, 1971a,b) were of the T6T6 type, i.e., derived from embryonic or adult hemopoietic precursors after thymus traffic and subsequent export. The property of recirculation (i.e., detection in thoracic duct lymph) is characteristic of T lymphocytes (J. F. A. P. Miller and Sprent, 1971), and by itself also indicates a specific change after thymus traffic (since none of the hemopoietic precursors has such an ability by itself). Thus, the traffic represents a true maturation process that is operative in the generation of the peripheral T-cell population, including immunologically competent T cells. No differences in the generation of competent T cells were observed with the different sources of hemopoietic precursors (i.e., embryonic, newborn, or adult).

It should be indicated that the same hemopoietic compartments, including yolk sac, also contain precursors of B cells that differentiate via a thymus-independent pathway (Tyan and Herzenberg, 1968; Stutman, 1973).

IV. EPILOGUE

At the risk of being repetitious, I will discuss our present opinions on T-cell development. At least from the mouse experiments (and also suggested by the human immunodeficiency data), the thymus is an obligatory step for the generation of competent T cells. Some of the exceptions, such as sheep, have been discussed by Bryant (1974) as possible suggestive evidence of alternative differentiation pathways. It is apparent from most of the work discussed in

Section II that neonatal thymectomy leaves behind, even in the mouse, a population of postthymic cells, probably generated through thymus traffic. It is also apparent, from the data in both Sections II and III, that the thymus most probably exports a postthymic precursor that differentiates further in the periphery, and that through actual thymus traffic, the final competent T cell is generated. I also discussed in Section III the evidence indicating that the immunologically competent set of intrathymic T cells seems to be a resident population and is *not* the final product of thymus export. This interpretation, which was favored by us in our initial studies on postthymic precursors (Stutman *et al.*, 1969a,b, 1970a,b), was not the prevalent view, although it appears to be progressively rediscovered and incorporated into the corpus of present experimental data. As Weissman *et al.* (1975b) indicated: "At face value, it would seem that the thymus generated two "mature" subpopulations: one immunocompetent, which is retained in the thymus, and one immunoincompetent, which migrates to the periphery. . . ." Weissman *et al.* (1975b) also added that such evidence was "exactly the opposite of what would be predicted by 'conventional wisdom.' " We could not have described the evidence in better terms in 1969–1970! What Weissman *et al.* (1975b) consider "conventional wisdom" is the prevalent view of a single lineage of differentiation from cortical thymocyte to medullary thymocyte and then to the periphery.

It is apparent that the increasing evidence on peripheral T-cell heterogeneity brought forth the idea, albeit slowly, of a more complex thymus-dependent differentiation scheme. Three possible schemas can be proposed: (1) several differentiation steps in a single developmental pathway (the "conventional wisdom" approach); (2) branched pathways leading to different specialized end points (this probably is the most convincing model, since it is probable that there is indeed a single stem cell precursor for the different lineages; however, it is not apparent where the branching takes place, i.e., intrathymically or in the periphery, as either a prethymic or a postthymic event); and (3) the possibility of entirely specialized lymphocyte lineages (without any common precursors).

The advantages of Model 2, especially the availability in the periphery of a postthymic precursor compartment that can be driven into further differentiation by thymic influence (and perhaps by other influences), is that it seems the most economical way of maintaining homeostasis of the T-cell compartment (for additional remarks on this possibility, see Section II; for other thoughts on the role of the thymus in lymphoid homeostasis, see Bryant, 1974).

It is apparent that significant progress toward an understanding of T-cell differentiation has been generated in the past years, especially compared with the simple ablation–replacement experiments that laid the groundwork for this present knowledge. Concerning "unified theories," it is clear that at our present stage of incomplete understanding of the process, it is probably healthier to retain the heterogeneity, even on a purely theoretical basis.

ACKNOWLEDGMENTS

The experimental work described in this paper has been supported by U.S. Public Health Service grants CA-08748, CA-15988, and CA-16889. I would like to thank Ms. Linda Stevenson for her invaluable help in preparing this manuscript and Dr. Catherine Calkins for her collaboration on some parts of the work as well as for her criticism of the manuscript. Finally, I would like to thank all the able technical help that has been involved in the present and past work, both from the University of Minnesota and from the Sloan-Kettering Institute.

V. REFERENCES

Adler, W.H., Takiguchi, T., Marsh, B., and Smith, R.T., 1970a. Cellular recognition by mouse lymphocytes *in vitro*. I. Definition of a new technique and results of stimulation by phytohemagglutinin and specific antigens. *J. Exp. Med.* **131**:1049.

Adler, W.H., Takiguchi, T., Marsh, B., and Smith, R.T., 1970b, Cellular recognition by mouse lymphocytes *in vitro*. II. Specific stimulation by histocompatibility antigens in mixed cell culture, *J. Immunol.* **105**:984.

Andersson, L. C., Hayry, P., Bach, M.A., and Bach, J.C., 1974, Differences in the effects of adult thymectomy on T-cell mediated responses *in vitro, Nature* **252**:252.

Arrenbrecht, S., 1973, Normal development of the thymus-dependent limb of humoral immune responses in mice, *Eur. J. Immunol.* **3**:506.

Asofsky, R., Cantor, H., and Tigelaar, R.E., 1971, Cell interactions in the graft-versus-host response, in: *Progress in Immunology,* pp. 369–381 (D.B. Amos, ed.), Academic Press, New York.

Bach, J.F., and Dardenne, M., 1972, Antigen recognition by T lymphocytes. II. Similar effects of azathioprine, antilymphocyte serum and anti-theta serum on rosette-forming lymphocytes in normal and neonatally thymectomized mice, *Cell. Immunol.* **3**:11.

Bach, J.F., and Dardenne, M., 1973, Antigen recognition by T lymphocytes. III. Evidence for two populations of thymus-dependent rosette-forming cells in spleen and lymph nodes, *Cell. Immunol.* **6**:394.

Bach, J.F., Bach, M.A., Charriere, J., Dardenne, M., Fournier, C., Papiernik, M., and Pleau, J.M., 1975a, The circulating thymic factor (TF). Biochemistry, physiology, biological activities and clinical applications. A summary, in: *The Biological Activity of Thymic Hormones,* pp. 145–158 (D.W. Van Bekkum, ed.), Kooyker Science Publications, Rotterdam.

Bach, J.F., Cantor, H., Roelants, G., and Stutman, O., 1975b, T cell subsets: Terminology problems, in: *The Biological Activity of Thymic Hormones,* pp. 159–168 (D.W. Van Bekkum, ed.), Kooyker Science Publications, Rotterdam.

Basch, R.S., and Goldstein, G., 1975, Thymopoietin-induced acquisition of responsiveness to T cell mitogens, *Cell. Immunol.* **20**:218.

Beverly, P.C.L., Woody, J., Dunkley, M., Feldmann, M., and McKenzie, I., 1976, Separation of suppressor and killer T cells by surface phenotype, *Nature* **262**:495.

Biggar, W.D., Stutman, O., and Good, R.A., 1972, Morphological and functional studies on fetal thymus transplants in mice, *J. Exp. Med.* **135**:793.

Boyse, E.A., and Abbott, J., 1975, Surface reorganization as an initial inductive event in the differentiation of prothymocytes to thymocytes, *Fed. Proc. Fed. Amer. Soc. Exp. Biol.* **34**:24.

Boyse, E.A., and Bennett, D., 1974, Differentiation and the cell surface: Illustrations from work with T cells and sperm, in: *Cellular Selection and Regulation in the Immune Response*, pp. 155–176 (G.M. Edelman, ed.,), Raven Press, New York.

Bryant, B.J., 1972, Renewal and fate in the mammalian thymus: Mechanisms and inferences of thymocytokinetics, *Eur. J. Immunol.* **2**:38.

Bryant, B.J., 1974, Thymic and bursal microenvironments in the context of alternative pathways of immunogenesis, in: *Progress in Immunology* II, Vol. 3, pp. 5–14 (L. Brent and J. Holborow, eds.), North-Holland, Amsterdam.

Bryant, B.J., Hess, M.W., and Cottier, H., 1975, Thymus lymphocytes: Efflux and restoration phases after peripheral exposure of mice to phytohemagglutinin, *Immunology* **29**:115.

Calkins, C.E., Orbach-Arbouys, S., Stutman, O., and Gershon, R.K., 1976, Cell interactions in the suppression of *in vitro* antibody responses, *J. Exp. Med.* **143**:1421.

Cantor, H., 1972a, T cells and the immune response, *Prog. Biophys. Mol. Biol.* **25**:71.

Cantor, H., 1972b, Two stages in development of lymphocytes, in: *Cell Interactions,* 3rd Lepetit Colloquium, pp. 172–182 (L.G. Silverstri, ed.), North-Holland, Amsterdam.

Cantor, H., and Asofsky, R., 1970, Synergy among lymphoid cells mediating the graft-versus-host response. II. Synergy in graft-versus-host reactions produced by BALB/C lymphoid cells of differing anatomic origin, *J. Exp. Med.* **131**:235.

Cantor, H., and Asofsky, R., 1972, Synergy among lymphoid cells mediating the graft-versus-host response. III. Evidence for interaction between two types of thymus derived cells, *J. Exp. Med.* **135**:764.

Cantor, H., and Boyse, E.A., 1975a, Functional subclasses of lymphocytes bearing different Ly antigens. I. The generation of functionally distant T cell subclasses is a differentiative process independent of antigen, *J. Exp. Med.* **141**:1376.

Cantor, H., and Boyse, E.A., 1975b, Functional subclasses of T lymphocytes bearing different Ly antigens. II. Cooperation between subclasses of Ly+ cells in the generation of killer activity, *J. Exp. Med.* **141**:1390.

Cantor, H., Simpson, E., Sato, V.L., Fathman, C.G., and Herzenberg, L.A., 1975, Characterization of subpopulations of T lymphocytes. I. Separation and functional studies of peripheral T cells binding different amounts of fluorescent anti-Thy.1.2 (Theta) antibody using a fluorescence-activated cell sorter (FACS), *Cell. Immunol.* **15**:180.

Chiscon, M.O., and Golub, E.S., 1972, Functional development of the interacting cells in the immune response. I. Development of T cell and B cell function, *J. Immunol.* **108**:1379.

Claman, H.N., and Moorhead, J.W., 1972, Heterogeneity of thymus-dependent lymphoid cell functions in the mouse, in: *Cell Interactions,* 3rd Lepitit Colloquium, pp. 132–142 (L.G. Silvestri, ed.), North-Holland, Amsterdam.

Claman, H.N., Chaperon, E.A., and Triplett, R.F., 1966, Immunocompetence of transferred thymus marrow cell combinations, *J. Immunol.* **97**:828.

Cohen, J.J., 1972, Thymus-derived lymphocytes sequestered on the bone marrow of hydrocortisone-treated mice, *J. Immunol.* **108**:841.

Dalmasso, A.P., Martinez, C., Sjodin, K., and Good, R.A., 1963, Studies on the role of the thymus in immunobiology. Reconstitution of immunologic capacity in mice thymectomized at birth, *J. Exp. Med.* **118**:1089.

Davies, A.J.S., 1969, The thymus and the cellular basis of immunity, *Transplant. Rev.* **1**:43.

Davies, A.J.S., Leuchars, E., Wallis, V., and Koller, P.C., 1966, The mitotic response of thymus-derived cells to antigenic stimulus, *Transplantation* 4:438.

Davies, A.J.S., Festenstein, H., Leuchars, E., Wallis, V.J., and Doenhoff, M.J., 1968, A thymic origin for some peripheral blood lymphocytes, *Lancet* 1:183.

Davies, A.J.S., Leuchars, E., Wallis, V., and Doenhoff, M.J., 1971, A system for lymphocytes in the mouse, *Proc. R. Soc. London Ser. B* 176:369.

Doenhoff, M.J., Davies, A.J.S., Leuchars, E., and Wallis, V., 1970, The thymus and circulating lymphocytes of mice, *Proc. R. Soc. London Ser. B* 176:69.

Dutton, R.W., 1972, Inhibitory and stimulatory effects of Concanavalin A on the response of mouse spleen cell suspensions to antigen. I. Characterization of the inhibitory cell activity, *J. Exp. Med.* 136:1445.

Dutton, R.W., 1973, Inhibitory and stimulatory effects of Concanavalin A on the response of mouse spleen cell suspensions to antigen. II. Evidence for separate stimulatory and inhibitory cells, *J. Exp. Med.* 138:1496.

Dwyer, J.M., and Mackay, I.R., 1972, The development of antigen binding lymphocytes in fetal tissues, *Immunology* 25:871.

Dyminsky, J.W., Forbes, J., Gebhardt, B., Nakao, Y., Konda, S., and Smith, R.T., 1974, Relationship between structure and function of human and mouse thymus cell subpopulations, in: *Progress in Immunology II,* pp. 35–47, North-Holland, Amsterdam.

El-Arini, M.O., and Osoba, D., 1973, Differentiation of thymus-derived cells from precursors in mouse bone marrow, *J. Exp. Med.* 137:821.

Elliott, E.V., 1973, A persistent lymphoid cell population in the thymus, *Nature (London) New Biol.* 242:150.

Elliott, E.V., Wallis, V., and Davies, A.J.S., 1971, Origin of PHA-responsive cells in the mouse thymus after treatment of the animal with hydrocortisone, *Nature (London) New Biol.* 234:77.

Everett, N.B., Caffrey, R.W., and Rieke, W.O., 1964, Recirculation of lymphocytes, *Ann. N. Y. Acad. Sci.* 113:887.

Fathman, C.G., Small, M., Herzenberg, L.A., and Weissman, I.L., 1975, Thymus cell maturation. II. Differentiation of three "mature" subclasses *in vivo, Cell. Immunol.* 15:109.

Ford, C.E., 1966, Traffic of lymphoid cells in the body, in: *The Thymus: Experimental and Clinical Studies,* pp. 131–152 (G.E.W. Wolstenholme and R. Porter, eds.), Little, Brown & Co., Boston.

Ford, C.E., and Micklem, H.S., 1963, The thymus and lymph nodes in radiation chimaeras, *Lancet* 1:359.

Ford, W.L., and Gowans, J.L., 1969, The traffic of lymphocytes, *Semin. Hematol.* 6:67.

Fried, W., Gurney, C.W., and Swatek, M., 1966, The effect of strontium-89 on the stem cell compartment of the spleen, *Radiat. Res.* 29:50.

Gershon, R.K., 1974, T cell control of antibody production, in: *Contemporary Topics in Immunobiology,* Vol. 3, pp. 1–40 (M.D. Cooper and N.L. Warner, eds.), Plenum Press, New York.

Gershon, R.K., Cohen, P., Hencin, R., and Liebhaber, S., 1972, Suppressor T cells, *J. Immunol.* 108:586.

Goldstein, A.L., Thurman, G.B., Cohen, G.H., and Hooper, J.A., 1975, Thymosin: Chemistry, biology and clinical applications, in: *The Biological Activity of Thymic Hormones,* pp. 173–197 (D.W. Van Bekkum, ed.), Kooyker Science Publications, Rotterdam.

Goldstein, G., 1974, Isolation of bovine thymin: A polypeptide hormone of the thymus, *Nature (London)* 247:11.

Goldstein, G., 1975, The isolation of thymopoietin (thymin), *Ann. N.Y. Acad. Sci.* **249**:177.

Goldstein, G., Scheid, M., Hammerling, U., Boyse, E.A., Schlesinger, D.H., and Niall, H.D., 1975, Isolation of a polypeptide that has lymphocyte differentiating properties and is probably represented universally in living cells, *Proc. Natl. Acad. Sci. U.S.A.* **72**:11.

Gowans, J.L., and McGregor, D.D., 1965, The immunological activities of lymphocytes, *Prog. Allergy* **9**:1.

Harris, J.E., and Ford, C.E., 1963, Role of the thymus: Migration of cells from thymic grafts to lymph-nodes in mice, *Lancet* **1**:389.

Harris, J.E., and Ford, C.E., 1964, Cellular traffic of the thymus: Experiments with chromosome markers. Evidence that the thymus plays an instructional part, *Nature (London)* **201**:884.

Haskill, J.S., and Moore, M.A.S., 1970, Two dimensional cell separation: Comparison of embryonic and adult hemopoietic stem cells, *Nature (London)* **226**:853.

Howe, M.L., and Manziello, B., 1972, Ontogenesis of the *in vitro* response of murine lymphoid cells to cellular antigens and phytomitogens, *J. Immunol.* **109**:534.

Joel, D.D., Hess, M.W., and Cottier, H., 1972, Magnitude and pattern of thymic lymphocyte migration in neonatal mice, *J. Exp. Med.* **135**:907.

Julius, M., Simpson, E., and Herzenberg, L.A., 1973, A rapid method for the isolation of functional thymus-derived lymphocytes, *Eur. J. Immunol.* **112**:420.

Kappler, J.W., Hunter, P.C., Jacobs, D., and Lord, E., 1974, Functional heterogeneity among the T-derived lymphocytes of the mouse. I. Analysis by adult thymectomy, *J. Immunol.* **113**:27.

Kindred, B., 1974, Rejection of skin grafts from different inbred strains by nude mice reconstituted with allogeneic or congenic thymus cell suspensions, *Eur. J. Immunol.* **4**:388.

Kindred, B., 1975, The failure of allogeneic cells to maintain an immune response in nude mice, *Scand. J. Immunol.* **4**:653.

Kindred, B., 1976, Lymphocytes which differentiate in an allogeneic thymus. I. Response to MLC determinants and skin grafts from the thymus donor, *Cell. Immunol.* **25**:189.

Kindred, B., and Loor, F., 1974, Activity of host-directed T cells which differentiate in nude mice grafted with co-isogenic or allogeneic thymuses, *J. Exp. Med.* **139**:1215.

Komuro, K., and Boyse, E.A., 1973a, *In vitro* demonstration of thymic hormone in the mouse by conversion of precursor cells into lymphocytes, *Lancet* **1**:740.

Komuro, K., and Boyse, E.A., 1973b, Induction of T lymphocytes from precursor cells *in vitro* by a product of the thymus, *J. Exp. Med.* **138**:479.

Komuro, K., Goldstein, G., and Boyse, E.A., 1975, Thymus-repopulating capacity of cells that can be induced to differentiate to T cells *in vitro*, *J. Immunol.* **115**:195.

Laissue, J.A., Chanana, A.D., Cottier, H., Cronkitte, E.P., and Joel, D.D., 1976, The fate of thymic radioactivity after local labeling with 125-iododeoxyuridine, *Blood* **47**:21.

Lajtha, L.G., 1975, Annotation: Haemopoietic stem cells, *Br. J. Haematol.* **28**:529.

Leckband, E., and Boyse, E.A., 1971, Immunocompetent cells among mouse thymocytes: A minor subpopulation, *Science* **172**:1258.

Leuchars, E., Morgan, A., Davies, A.J.S., and Wallis, V.J., 1967, Thymus grafts in thymecto-mized and normal mice, *Nature (London)* **214**:801.

Loor, F., and Kindred, B., 1973, Differentiation of T cell precursors in nude mice demonstrated by immunofluorescence of T cell membrane antigens, *J. Exp. Med.* **138**:1044.

McIntire, K.R., Sell, S., and Miller, J.F.A.P., 1964, Pathogenesis of the post-neonatal thymectomy wasting syndrome, *Nature (London)* **204**:151.

Metcalf, D., and Moore, M.A.S., 1971, *Haemopoietic Cells,* North-Holland Publishing Co., Amsterdam.

Micklem, H.S., Ford, C.E., Evans, E.P., and Gray, J., 1966, Interrelationships of myeloid and lymphoid cells: Studies with chromosome-marked cells transfused into lethally irradiated mice, *Proc. R. Soc. London Ser. B* **165**:78.

Micklem, H.S., Clarke, C.M., Evans, E.P., and Ford, C.E., 1968, Fate of chromosome-marked mouse bone marrow cells transfused into normal syngeneic recipients, *Transplantation* **6**:299.

Miller, J.F.A.P., and Sprent, J., 1971, Thymus-derived cells in mouse thoracic duct lymph, *Nature (London) New Biol.* **230**:267.

Miller, R.G., and Phillips, R.A., 1969, Separation of cells by velocity sedimentation, *J. Cell. Physiol.* **73**:191.

Mosier, D., and Cantor, H., 1971, Functional maturation of mouse thymic lymphocytes, *Eur. J. Immunol.* **1**:459.

Mosier, D.E., and Johnson, B.M., 1975, Ontogeny of mouse lymphocyte function. II. Development of the ability to produce antibody is modulated by T lymphocytes, *J. Exp. Med.* **141**:216.

Nature (London), 1973, T. lymphocytes in nude mice? (editorial), **246**:328.

Osoba, D., and Miller, J.F.A.P., 1963, Evidence of a humoral thymus factor responsible for the maturation of immunological faculty, *Nature (London)* **199**:653.

Owen, J.J.T., 1972, The origins and development of lymphocyte populations, in: *Ontogeny of Acquired Immunity, A Ciba Foundation Symposium,* pp. 35–54, Elsevier, Amsterdam.

Owen, J.J.T., 1974, Ontogeny of the immune response, in: *Progress in Immunology II,* pp. 163–173 (L. Brent and J. Holborow, eds.), North-Holland, Amsterdam.

Owen, J.J.T., and Raff, M.C., 1970, Studies on the differentiation of thymus-derived lymphocytes, *J. Exp. Med.* **132**:1216.

Pierpaoli, W., and Besedovsky, H.O., 1975, Failure of "thymus factor" to restore transplantation immunity in athymic mice, *Br. J. Exp. Pathol.* **56**:180.

Pritchard, H., and Micklem, H.S., 1972, Immune response in congenitally thymus-less mice. I. Absence of response to oxazolone, *Clin. Exp. Immunol.* **10**:151.

Pritchard, H., and Micklem, H.S., 1973, Haemopoietic stem cells and progenitors of functional T lymphocytes in the bone marrow of nude mice, *Clin. Exp. Immunol.* **14**:597.

Pritchard, H., Riddaway, J., and Micklem, H.S., 1973, Immune responses in congenitally thymus-less mice. II. Quantitative studies of serum immunoglobulins, the antibody response to sheep erythrocytes and the effect of thymus allografting, *Clin. Exp. Immunol.* **13**:125.

Raff, M.C., 1971, Evidence for a subpopulation of mature lymphocytes within mouse thymus, *Nature (London) New Biol.* **229**:182.

Raff, M.C., and Cantor, H., 1971, Subpopulations of thymus cells and thymus-derived lymphocytes in: *Progress in Immunology,* pp. 83–93 (D.B. Amos, ed.), Academic Press, New York.

Raff, M.C., and Owen, J.J.T., 1971, Thymus-derived lymphocytes: Their distribution and role in the development of peripheral lymphoid tissues of the mouse, *Eur. J. Immunol.* **1**:27.

Resnitzky, P., Zipori, D., and Trainin, N., 1971, Effect of neonatal thymectomy on hemopoietic tissue in mice, *Blood* **37**:634.

Rieke, W.O., and Schwartz, M.R., 1967, The types of rat thoracic duct lymphocytes which respond to phytohemagglutinin *in vitro, Acta Haematol.* **38**:121.

Robinson, J.H., and Owen, J.J.T., 1976, Generation of T cell function in organ culture of foetal mouse thymus. I. Mitogen responsiveness, *Clin. Exp. Immunol.* **23**:347.

Roelants, G.E., Loor, F., von Boehner, H., Sprent, J., Haag, L.B., Mayor, K.S., and Ryden, A., 1975, Five types of lymphocytes characterized by double immunofluorescence and electrophoretic mobility: Organ distribution in normal and nude mice, *Eur. J. Immunol.* **5**:127.

Roelants, G.E., Mayor, K.S., Haag, L.B., and Loor, F., 1976, Immature T lineage lymphocytes in athymic mice. Presence of TL, lifespan and homeostatic regulation, *Eur. J. Immunol.* **6**:75.

Sato, V.L., Waksal, S.D., and Herzenberg, L.A., 1976, Identification and separation of pre T cells from nu/nu mice: Differentiation by preculture with thymic reticuloepithelial cells, *Cell. Immunol.* **24**:173.

Scheid, M.P., Hoffman, M.K., Komuro, K., Hammerling, U., Abbott, J., Boyse, E.A., Cohen, G.H., Hooper, J.A., Schulof, R.S., and Goldstein, A.L., 1973, Differentiation of T cells induced by preparations from and by non-thymic agents. The determined state of the precursor cell, *J. Exp. Med.* **138**:1027.

Scheid, M.P., Goldstein, G., Hammerling, U., and Boyse, E.A., 1975a, Lymphocyte differentiation from precursor cells *in vitro, Ann. N. Y. Acad, Sci.* **249**:531.

Scheid, M.P., Goldstein, G., and Boyse, E.A., 1975b, Differentiation of T cells in nude mice, *Science* **190**:1211.

Seger, R., Rogers, K., and Catty, D., 1974, Differentiation of T cell percursors in nude mice. Rejection of heart grafts of thymus donor strain, *Eur. J. Immunol.* **4**:524.

Shortman, K., von Boehmer, H., Lipp, J., and Hopper, K., 1975, Subpopulations of T lymphocytes. Physical separation, functional specialization and differentiation pathways of sub-sets of thymocytes and thymus-dependent peripheral lymphocytes, *Transplant. Rev.* **25**:163.

Singh, U., and Owen, J.J.T., 1975, Studies on the effect of various agents on the maturation of thymus stem cells. *Eur. J. Immunol.* **5**:286.

Sosin, H., Hilgard, H., and Martinez, C., 1966, The immunologic competence of mouse thymus cells measured by the graft-versus-host spleen assay, *J. Immunol.* **96**:189.

Spear, P.G., Wong, A.L., Rutishauser, U., and Edelman, G.M., 1973, Characteristics of splenic lymphoid cells in fetal and newborn mice, *J. Exp. Med.* **138**:557.

Stobo, J.D., and Paul, W.E., 1972, Functional heterogeneity of murine lymphoid cells. II. Acquisition of mitogen responsiveness and of theta antigen during ontogeny of thymocytes and T lymphocytes, *Cell. Immunol.* **4**:367.

Stobo, J.D., and Paul, W.E., 1973, Functional heterogeneity of murine lymphoid cells. III. Differential responsiveness of T cells to phytohemagglutinin and Concanavalin A as a probe for T cell subsets, *J. Immunol.* **110**:362.

Stobo, J.D., Rosenthal, A.S., and Paul, W.E., 1972, Functional heterogeneity of murine lymphoid cells. I. Responsiveness to and surface binding of Concanavalin A and phytohemagglutinin, *J. Immunol.* **108**:1.

Stobo, J.D., Paul, W.E., and Henney, C.S., 1973, Functional heterogeneity of murine lymphoid cells. IV. Allogeneic mixed lymphocyte reactivity and cytolytic activity as functions of distinct T cell subsets, *J. Immunol.* **110**:652.

Storrie, B., Goldstein, G., Boyse, E.A., and Hammerling, U., 1976, Differentiation of thymocytes: Evidence that induction of the surface phenotype requires transcription and translation, *J. Immunol.* **116**:1358.

Stout, R.D., and Herzenberg, L.A., 1975, The Fc receptor on thymus-derived lymphocytes. I. Detection of a subpopulation of murine T lymphocytes bearing the Fc receptor, *J. Exp. Med.* **142**:611.

Stutman, O., 1970, Hemopoietic origin of cells responding to phytohemagglutinin in mouse lymph nodes, in: *Fifth Leukocyte Culture Conference*, pp. 671–681 (J. Harris, ed.), Academic Press, New York.

Stutman, O., 1972a, Traffic of cells and development of immunity, in: *Membranes and Viruses in Immunopathology*, pp. 437–450 (S.B. Day and R.A. Good, eds.), Academic Press, New York.

Stutman, O. 1972b, Hemopoietic origin of short and long-lived lymphocytes in mouse lymph nodes after thymus traffic, *Fed. Proc. Fed. Amer. Soc. Exp. Biol.* **31**:776 (abstract).

Stutman, O., 1973, Hemopoietic origin of B cells in the mouse, in: *Microenvironmental Factors of Immunity*, pp. 19–26 (B.D. Jankovic and K. Isakovic, eds.), Plenum Press, New York.

Stutman, O., 1974, Inability to restore immune functions in nude mice with humoral thymic function, *Fed. Proc. Fed. Amer. Soc. Exp. Biol.* **33**:736 (abst.).

Stutman, O., 1975a, Delayed tumor appearance and absence of regression in nude mice infected with murine sarcoma virus, *Nature (London)* **253**:142.

Stutman, O., 1975b, Humoral thymic factors influencing postthymic cells, *Ann. N. Y. Acad. Sci.* **249**:89.

Stutman, O., 1975c, Characterization of a T cell precursor in mouse spleen, *Transplant. Proc.* **7**:291.

Stutman, O., 1975d, The postthymic precursor cell, in: *The Biological Activity of Thymic Hormones*, pp. 87–94 (D.W. van Bekkum, ed.), Kooyker Science Publications, Rotterdam.

Stutman, O., 1976, Migration of yolk sac cells to thymus grafts: Requirement of prior sojourn in bone marrow (or liver?), *Ann. D'Immunol. (Inst. Pasteur)* **127C**:943.

Stutman, O., and Calkins, C.E., 1976, Ontogenetic aspects, in: *Transplantation, Handbuch der Allgemeinen Pathologie*, VI/8, pp. 169–193, Springer-Verlag, Heidelberg,

Stutman, O., and Good, R.A., 1969, Traffic of hemopoietic cells to the thymus: Influence of histocompatibility differences, *Exp. Hematol.* **19**:12.

Stutman, O., and Good, R.A., 1971a, Immunocompetence of embryonic hemopoietic cells after traffic to thymus, *Transplant. Proc.* **3**:923.

Stutman, O., and Good, R.A., 1971b, Immunocompetence of cells derived from hemopoietic liver after traffic to thymus, in: *Morphological and Functional Aspects of Immunity*, pp. 129–133 (K. Lindahl-Kiessling, G. Alm, and M.G. Hanna, eds.), Plenum Press, New York.

Stutman, O., and Good, R.A., 1973, Thymus hormones, in: *Thymus Dependency, Contemporary Topics in Immunobiology*, pp. 299–319 (A.J.S. Davies and R.L. Carter, eds.), Plenum Press, New York.

Stutman, O., and Good, R.A., 1974, Duration of thymic function, *Ser. Haematol.* **7**:505.

Stutman, O., Yunis, E.J., Martinez, C., and Good, R.A., 1967, Reversal of post-thymectomy wasting disease in mice by multiple thymus grafts, *J. Immunol.* **98**:79.

Stutman, O., Yunis, E.J., Teague, P.O., and Good, R.A., 1968a, Graft-versus-host reactions induced by transplantation of parental strain thymus in neonatally thymectomized F_1 hybrid mice, *Transplantation*, **6**:514.

Stutman, O., Yunis, E.J., and Good, R.A., 1968b, Carcinogen induced tumors of the thymus. I. Restoration of neonatally thymectomized mice with a functional thymoma, *J. Natl. Cancer Inst.* **41**:1431.

Stutman, O., Yunis, E.J., and Good, R.A., 1968c, Colony-forming capacity of hemopoietic cells from thymectomized mice, *Exp. Hematol.* **16**:18.

Stutman, O., Yunis, E.J., and Good, R.A., 1969a, Carcinogen-induced tumors of the thymus. IV. Humoral influences of normal thymus and functional thymomas and influence of post thymectomy period on restoration, *J. Exp. Med.* **130**:809.

Stutman, O., Yunis, E.J., and Good, R.A., 1969b, Thymus: An essential factor in lymphoid repopulation, *Transplant. Proc.* **1**:614.

Stutman, O., Yunis, E.J., and Good, R.A., 1969c, Reversal of postthymectomy wasting in mice with immunocompetent cells: Influence of histocompatibility differences, *J. Immunol.* **102**:87.

Stutman, O., Yunis, E.J., and Good, R.A., 1969d, Tolerance induction with thymus grafts in neonatally thymectomized mice, *J. Immunol.* **103**:92.

Stutman, O., Yunis, E.J., and Good, R.A., 1969e, Effect of parental strain thymus grafts on neonatally thymectomized F_1 hybrids, *Transplantation,* **7**:420.

Stutman, O., Yunis, E.J., and Good, R.A., 1969f, Carcinogen-induced tumors of the thymus. III. Restoration of neonatally thymectomized mice with thymomas in cell impermeable chambers, *J. Natl. Cancer Inst.* **43**:499.

Stutman, O., Yunis, E.J., and Good, R.A., 1970a, Studies on thymus function. I. Cooperative effect of thymic function and lymphohemopoietic cells in restoration of neonatally thymectomized mice, *J. Exp. Med.* **132**:583.

Stutman, O., Yunis, E.J., and Good, R.A., 1970b, Studies on thymus function. II. Cooperative effect of newborn and embryonic hemopoietic liver cells with thymus function, *J. Exp. Med.* **132**:601.

Stutman, O., Yunis, E.J., and Good, R.A., 1972, Studies on thymus function. III. Duration of thymic function, *J. Exp. Med.* **135**: 339.

Trainin, M., 1974, Thymic hormones and the immune response, *Physiol. Rev.* **54**:272.

Trainin, N., Small, M., Zipori, D., Uniel, T., Kook, A.I., and Rother, V., 1975, Characteristics of THF, a thymic hormone, in: *The Biological Activity of Thymic Hormones,* pp. 117–144 (D.W. van Bekkum, ed.), Kooyker Science Publications, Rotterdam.

Tyan, M.L., and Herzenberg, L.A., 1968, Immunoglobulin production by embryonic tissues thymus independent, *Proc. Soc. Exp. Biol. Med.* **128**:952.

Weissman, I.L., 1973, Thymus cell maturation: Studies on the origin of cortisone-resistant thymic lymphocytes, *J. Exp. Med.* **137**:504.

Weissman, I.L., Small, M., Fathman, C.G., and Herzenberg, L.A., 1975a, Differentiation of thymus cells, *Fed. Proc. Fed. Amer. Soc. Exp. Biol.* **34**:141.

Weissman, I.L., Masuda, T., Olive, C., and Friedberg, S.H., 1975b, Differentiation and migration of T lymphocytes, *Isr. J. Med. Sci.* **11**:1267.

Wortis, H.H., 1974, Immunological studies of nude mice, in: *Contemporary Topics in Immunobiology,* Vol. 3, pp. 243–263 (M.D. Cooper and N.L. Warner, eds.), Plenum Press, New York.

Worton, R.G., McCulloch, E.A., and Till, J.E., 1969, Physical separation of hemopoietic stem cells differing in their capacity for self-renewal, *J. Exp. Med.* **130**:91.

Wu, S., Bach, F.H., and Auerbach, R., 1975, Cell-mediated immunity: Differential maturation of mixed leukocyte reaction and cell-mediated lympholysis, *J. Exp. Med.* **142**:1301.

Yoshida, T.O., and Andersson, B., 1972, Evidence for a receptor recognizing antigen complexed immunoglobulin on the surface of activated mouse thymus lymphocytes, *Scand. J. Immunol.* **1**:401.

Yunis, E.J., Fernandes, G., Teague, P.O., Stutman, O., and Good, R.A., 1972, The thymus, autoimmunity and the involution of the lymphoid system, in: *Tolerance, Autoimmunity and Aging,* pp. 62–119 (M.M. Sigel and R.A. Good, eds.), Charles C Thomas, Springfield, Illinois.

Zatz, M.M., and Lance, E.M., 1970, The distribution of chromium 51-labeled lymphoid cells in the mouse. A survey of anatomical compartments, *Cell Immunol.* **1**:3.

Zipori, D., and Trainin, N., 1973, Defective capacity of bone marrow from nude mice to restore lethally irradiated recipients, *Blood* **42**:671.

Chapter 2

Regulation of the Immune Response
by T-Cell Subclasses

Harvey Cantor*

Department of Medicine, Harvard Medical School, Farber Cancer Center
Boston, Massachusetts

and

Edward Boyse

Sloan-Kettering Institute for Cancer Research
New York, New York

I. INTRODUCTION

Purified T lymphocytes mediate a wide variety of immunologic functions. These cells can generate cytotoxic responses to alloantigens (Cerottini and Brunner, 1974; Cantor *et al.*, 1975a), exert helper (Transplantation Reviews, 1969) and suppressive (Gershon, 1974) effects on the production of antibody, and initiate graft-vs.-host (Cantor, 1972) and delayed-type inflammatory responses (David and David, 1972). One may ask whether this diversity of function reflects a functional heterogeneity of T cells existing prior to antigen stimulation. According to this model, each T-cell function might be mediated by a subclass of T cells that has been programmed during differentiation to express a single or limited type of immune response. Alternatively, a single mature pluripotent T cell may be induced by antigen to give rise to cells capable of mediating the complete range of T-dependent responses.

We have approached this problem by asking whether or not it is possible to separate subclasses of T cells from nonimmune animals that are already deter-

*Scholar of the Leukemia Society of America. Supported by NIH Grants AI 13184 and AI 13600.

mined to express a limited range of immune activities on contact with antigen. Until recently, separation techniques such as velocity gradient sedimentation, limiting dilutions of anti-Thy-1.2 + complement (C), antilymphocyte serum, mitogen reactivity, and adult thymectomy have been used in an attempt to purify functionally different T-cell subclasses (reviewed in Cantor and Weissman, 1976). Although these approaches have suggested that T cells represent a functionally heterogeneous population, they have not allowed definitive conclusions since the techniques used do not permit direct identification and complete separation of relevant T-cell subclasses.

We therefore attempted a more direct approach, based on the development by Boyse and colleagues of alloantisera that define a panel of cell-surface differentiation antigens, called *Ly antigens,* found on mouse thymocytes and a fraction of peripheral lymphocytes (Boyse *et al.,* 1968; Boyse *et al.,* 1971). Since these alloantigens have not yet been detected on the surfaces of non-lymphoid cells (Boyse *et al.,* 1968, 1971), we hoped that they might represent components expressed exclusively on the surfaces of cells undergoing thymus-dependent differentiation, and potentially might be expressed selectively on the surfaces of sublines of T cells. Each of the *Ly* loci is expressed as one of two alternative alleles. *Ly-1* has been located on chromosome 19, and *Ly-2* and *Ly-3* are closely linked on chromosome 6 (Itakura *et al.,* 1972).

Examination of the expression of *Ly* antigens on lymphocytes from C57BL/6 (B6) mice (*Ly* phenotype 1.2, 2.2, 3.2), using different *Ly* antisera + rabbit complement, revealed the presence of three major T-cell subclasses that express different *Ly* phenotypes and display a unique set of biological properties and immune functions. The preparation and use of *Ly* antisera to distinguish T-cell subclasses has recently been reported (Shen *et al.,* 1975). The following account summarizes current information concerning the functional and biological characteristics of the three T-cell subclasses that have been defined so far using these techniques. In addition, the contribution of each T-cell subclass to the immune response to both foreign material and "altered-self" will be discussed.

II. PROPERTIES OF THREE MAJOR T-CELL SUBCLASSES

A. T_H (*Ly1*) Subclass

1. Functional Properties

These cells account for approximately one-third of the peripheral T-cell population. Evidence to date suggests that cells of this subclass are especially programmed to help or amplify the functional activity of other cells after stimulation by antigen associated with *I*-region determinants (Cantor and Boyse, 1975a,b; Shevach, 1976; Katz *et al.*, 1973). The amplifying effects of cells of this subclass have been demonstrated in relation to the three target cells described below.

(a) B Cells. Generation of T_H activity by *Ly1* cells has been noted for the antibody response to a variety of antigens such as SRBC (Cantor and Boyse, 1975a; Cantor *et al.*, 1975b), BSA, HGG (Cantor, unpublished data), and KLH (Herzenberg *et al.*, 1976). These studies also show that *Ly1* cells are already programmed to generate helper function, prior to overt immunization (Cantor and Boyse, 1975a; Jandinski *et al.*, 1976; Cantor *et al.*, 1975b). Similarly, after immunization with either SRBC or KLH, helper memory activity resides almost entirely in the *Ly1* population (Herzenberg *et al.*, 1976; Cantor *et al.*, 1975b). Evidence that *Ly1* T_H cells are programmed to help B cells, *independently* of their ability to interact with antigens, comes from experiments with Concanavalin A (Con A) (Jandinski *et al.*, 1976). Polyclonal activation of resting *Ly-1* cells by Con A results in the generation of nonspecific T-helper activity, as indicated by the ability of graded numbers of Con-A-activated *Ly1* cells to help B lymphocytes produce antibody to sheep erythrocytes. The development of helper activity and not suppressor activity after polyclonal activation of *Ly1* cells is in contrast to the suppressive effects generated after stimulation of *Ly23* T cells by Con A in an identical fashion. These findings have effectively eliminated the possibility that suppressor T-cell activity is due to a "hyperactivated" population of helper T cells.

(b) $T_{C/S}$ (Ly-23) Killer Cells. Under appropriate circumstances, *Ly-1* T_H cells can enhance the generation of $T_{C/S}$ (*Ly23*) killer–effector cells from *Ly23* prekillers during the mixed lymphocyte response (Cantor and Boyse, 1975b). *Ly1* cells also account for the major portion of the proliferative reaction in mixed lymphocyte culture, but do not themselves directly contribute to the cytotoxic effector cell pool (Cantor and Boyse, 1975a,b).

(c) Macrophages and Monocytes. The provision of T_H *Ly1* cells to thymus-deprived mice restores the ability of these cells to mount a delayed-type hypersensitivity response to sheep erythrocytes, while the provision of other subclasses of T cells does not (Huber *et al.*, 1976a).

2. H-2 Reactivity of T_H Cells

In mixed lymphocyte culture, the *Ly1* population is primarily concerned with responding to *I*-region differences, at least as judged by thymidine incorporation. This is shown most clearly in one-way cultures in which the responding cell differs from the stimulator cell by a defined *I*-region difference (Cantor and Boyse, 1975a). In the several examples investigated so far [B10.T6R cells vs.

AQR, B10.4R vs. B10.A(4R), and ATH vs. ATL), this *I*-region-incompatible proliferative response is mediated solely by *Ly1* cells. Preliminary experiments by M. Nabholz and B. Elliot also indicate that following mixed lymphocyte stimulation, *Ly1* responder cells can be shown to specifically bind allogeneic Ia molecules from the stimulator-cell population. It is therefore likely from these and other data (Rosenthal *et al.*, 1975; Katz *et al.*, 1973) that T_H *Ly1* cells are stimulated by Ia differences in the form of either alloantigen or self-Ia associated with foreign determinants.

3. Production of Helper Factors

T cells stimulated in mixed lymphocyte culture produce factors that can amplify the response of other T cells to antigen (Dutton *et al.*, 1971; Armerding and Katz, 1974). This factor, called *allogeneic effector factor* (AEF), is thought to contain Ia components (Armerding and Katz, 1974). Recent studies have indicated that *Ly1* cells are required for AEF production (Cantor, unpublished data), but further work is necessary to determine whether these materials are in fact produced by *Ly1* cells.

B. $T_{C/S}$ (*Ly23*) Cells

These cells account for approximately 5–10% of the total peripheral T-cell pool. They have been shown to develop both alloreactive cytotoxic activity and the capacity to suppress both humoral and cell-mediated immune responses.

1. Killer Function

Ly23 cells in lymph node (LN) account for virtually all the prekiller and killer activity seen after stimulation of LN cells with allogeneic lymphocytes (Cantor and Boyse, 1975 a,b). In addition, these cells account for one-half to three-fourths of splenic prekiller activity; the remaining activity may reflect the contribution of *Ly123* cells (Cantor and Boyse, 1975b, and unpublished data). Killer effector cell activity, generated from either LN or spleen, is mediated almost solely by *Ly23* cells.

2. Immunosuppressive Activity

Ly23 cells play a major suppressive role after stimulation by polyclonal activators such as Con A (Jandinski *et al.*, 1976). In addition, cells of this subclass exert substantial antigen-specific suppressive effects after immunization with high doses of antigen, such as sheep erythrocytes (Cantor *et al.*, 1975b).

Other studies have shown that F_1 hybrid mice that have been exposed during perinatal life to the Ig1b allotype of one parent develop $Ly23$ T cells that suppress the production of this Ig1b immunoglobulin subclass (allotype suppression) (Herzenberg *et al.*, 1976). Recent studies of this phenomenon also indicate that the target of $Ly23$ T suppression is an $Ly1$ T_H cell that is programmed to interact selectively with Ig1b$^+$ B lymphocytes ($T_S \rightarrow T_H$ suppression) (Herzenberg *et al.*, 1976). In general, $Ly23$ $T_{C/S}$ cells have been shown to possess suppressive activity *after* stimulation by antigen. It is likely that the generation of $Ly23$ $T_{C/S}$ activity is in part the result of signals from $Ly1$ T_H cells and T_E cells (see below). This T–T interaction is *not* essential for $T_{C/S}$ generation after strong polyclonal stimulus; thus, exposure of isolated $Ly23$ cells to Con A is sufficient to generate strong suppressive activity (Jandinski *et al.*, 1976). These findings also indicate that $Ly23$ $T_{C/S}$ cells, prior to activation, are programmed to develop suppressive activity independent of their ability to recognize antigen (Jandinski *et al.*, 1976).

3. H-2 Reactivity of $T_{C/S}$ Cells

This subclass of T cells does not contribute to the proliferative response to *I*-region differences in mixed lymphocyte culture, although these cells are activated in the presence of K/D differences in mixed cultures (Cantor and Boyse, 1975a; also see below). Experiments by Nabholz and Elliott have recently shown that following mixed lymphocyte stimulation, $Ly23$ cells *specifically* bind K/D molecules from the stimulator-cell population. We do not know whether $Ly23$ surface components contribute directly to such binding.

4. Production of Suppressive Factors

Following Con A stimulation, T cells can produce a suppressive factor called *soluble immune response suppressive factor* that can inhibit the generation of PFC activity to sheep erythrocytes (Jandinski *et al.*, 1976). This substance, which has not been shown to contain *H-2* molecules, is produced by $Ly23$ cells after Con A activation (Jandinski *et al.*, 1976). The role of this factor in the regulation of *in vivo* responses has not been established.

C. Development of and Functional Relationship between T_H (*Ly1*) and $T_{C/S}$ (*Ly23*) Cells

Possibly, cells of these two subclasses represent different stages of cell maturation within the same line of thymus-dependent differentiation. Alterna-

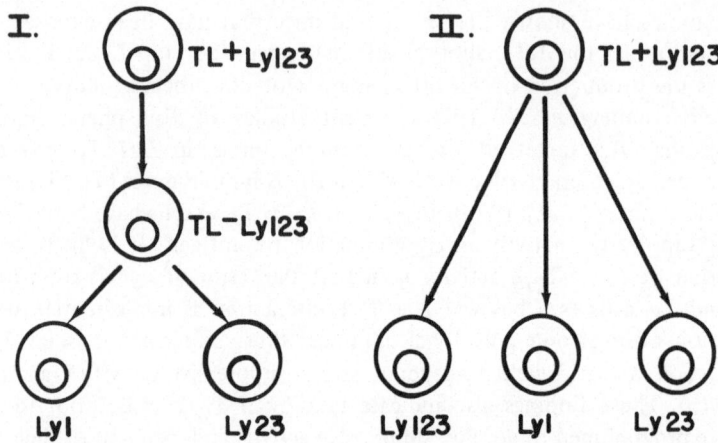

Fig. 1. Alternative developmental models for *Ly* subclasses. The two models are based on recent findings indicating that *Ly1* T_H cells and *Ly23* $T_{C/S}$ cells are stable and apparently do not give rise to one another (Huber *et al.*, 1976b). We currently favor Model I in view of evidence that at least after stimulation by chemically modified autologous cells, TL-Ly123$^+$ cells may give rise to *Ly23* cells.

tively, these cells may represent the products of distinct lines of differentiation. Recent studies by B. Huber in our laboratory have indicated that separated cells of either the T_H or the $T_{C/S}$ subclass that have been "parked" in syngeneic B recipients remain functionally stable for as long as 6 months after parking (Huber *et al.*, 1976b). These findings therefore indicate that cells of these two subclasses do not give rise to one another and suggest that they represent products of separate sublines of thymus-dependent maturation (see Fig. 1).

Recent studies have also indicate that the net helper response after immunization with SRBC is determined by the relative proportions of SRBC-specific *Ly1* T_H activity and *Ly23* T_S activity present in the primed cell population (Cantor *et al.*, 1975b). This finding implies that (1) the level of response to a given antigenic determinant may reflect the relative proportions of T_S and T_H cells with specificity for that determinant and (2) unresponsiveness to a given antigenic determinant may reflect a preponderance of antigen-specific T_S cells, rather than a lack of specifically reactive T_H cells. In view of recent indications that genetic unresponsiveness to antigen may in some cases be caused by preferential activation of antigen-specific T_S cells (Kapp *et al.*, 1974; Debre *et al.*, 1975), it is possible that at least some immune response (*Ir*) genes may act by channeling the differentiation of antigen-reactive T-cell clones toward the T_H of the T_S pathways, high-responder *Ir* alleles favoring the former, and low-responder alleles the latter. Indeed, preliminary experiments done in collaboration with J. Kapp, C. Pierce, and B. Benacerraf have indicated that DBA/1 mice, which do not normally respond to the GAT terpolymer, develop substantial levels of $Ly-2^+ Ly-1^-$ GAT-specific suppressor cells following immunization with that antigen.

D. T_E ($Ly123$) Cells

Cells of this subclass account for approximately half of all peripheral T cells. They have several characteristics that suggest they may be less mature than $Ly-1$ and $Ly23$ cells; $Ly123$ cells appear first during ontogeny and can be demonstrated within the first week of life, while $Ly1$ and $Ly23$ cells are not apparent until the second and third weeks of life in both B6 and BALB/c mice. In addition, a portion of $Ly123$ cells is sensitive to the short-term effects of adult thymectomy: at 4 weeks after adult thymectomy, the proportions of $Ly123$ cells in the spleen have diminished by approximately 50% (Cantor and Boyse, 1975a). These findings suggest either that a portion of this subclass is lost after adult thymectomy or that the thymus is required for maintenance of the cell-surface phenotype of at least a portion of cells of this T-cell subclass. Moreover, it is not clear whether this reduction 4 weeks after thymectomy reflects the half-life of the whole population of $Ly123$ cells or whether cells of this subclass are themselves heterogeneous, at least with respect to life span. Nonetheless, the most likely possibility at this time is that at least a portion of T_E ($Ly123$) cells corresponds to the subpopulation previously designated "T_1" (Raff and Cantor, 1971; Bach et al., 1976), i.e., it is a short-lived precursor population that may give rise to either T_H or $T_{C/S}$ activity.

The functional activities of T_E cells are currently being studied. Recent evidence obtained by B. Huber suggests that they play an essential role in the induction of graft-vs.-host responses, probably in collaboration with one of the mature subclasses mentioned above (Kapp et al., 1974). Preliminary evidence also indicates that these cells may be important both in the induction of helper memory cells and in the generation of T suppressor activity. To date, however, the best-studied function of T_E cells involves the generation of both cellular and humoral immunity to "modified-self."

E. Role of T-Cell Subclasses in the Response to "Modified-Self"

There is increasing evidence that cytotoxic T lymphocytes are generated after exposure to syngeneic cells expressing either viral antigens or antigens that have been chemically added to the surface lymphocytes (Shearer et al., 1975; Zinkernagel and Doherty, 1975). Studies of the specificity of these killer cells have indicated that efficient lysis was obtained only when the target expressed $H-2K$

or *H-2D* phenotypes identical to those of the sensitizing cells, in addition to the added (viral or hapten) determinant. It has been suggested that immunity to "modified-self" may play an important role in the control of tumor development, viral infections, and autoimmune disease. However, we know less about the cellular basis of this reaction than about the comparatively less biologically useful response to allogeneic cells.

We have therefore investigated the types of T cells that participate in both the induction phase and the effector phase of the response to modified-self. Our studies show that in contrast to the generation of killers after allogeneic stimulation, the generation of killers to TNP-conjugated syngeneic spleen cells requires the presence of *Ly123* (T_E) cells in both spleen and lymph node for induction of significant cytotoxic activity (Table I). Once generated, however, killer cells to TNP-modified targets express the *Ly23* phenotype, similar to killer cells generated after stimulation by allogeneic lymphocytes (Table II). These findings indicate that $Ly123^+$ T_E cells play an essential role in the generation of *Ly23* killer cells having specificity for altered *K/D* cell-surface components. Preliminary experiments also indicate that the *Ly123* cells serve as precursors of *Ly23* killer-effector cells, rather than performing an essential "helper" function for the maturation of *Ly23* cells. The essential role of T_E cells in the generation of this response stands in marked contrast to their modest or insignificant contribution to the generation of *allo*reactive killers. In the latter instance, virtually all alloreactive prekiller activity in lymph node is found in the *Ly23* $T_{C/S}$ population, and most (60–80%) of prekiller activity in spleen also resides mainly in the *Ly23* subclass (the rest being accounted for by *Ly123* cells).

The role of different T-cell subclasses in the generation of antibody of TNP-conjugated syngeneic spleen cells was also investigated. To this end, different populations of spleen cells were incubated 5 days with irradiated TNP-conjugated spleen cells, and then tested for TNP–PFC activity. B cells incubated alone with irradiated TNP-conjugated autologous cells produced few PFC. More-

Table I. T-Cell Subclasses Responsible for Generation of Killer Cells to TNP-Modified Self and Alloantigen

B6 T cells in culture	Number of cells ($\times 10^6$)	Sensitized vs. irradiated B6-TNP % Lytic activity vs. TNP-EL-4 (10:1 attacker/target ratio)	Sensitized vs. irradiated BALB/c % Lytic activity vs. P815 ($H\text{-}2^d$) (10:1)
Unselected	6	41	55
Ly-1	6	3	4
Ly23	6	7	61
Ly1 + Ly23	3 + 3	4	59

Table II. T-Cell Subclasses Responsible
for Lysis of TNP-Modified Autologous Targets
and Allogeneic Targets

Attacker population (10:1 A/T ratio)	% Lysis (10:1 A/T ratio)	
	Target EL-4-TNP	Target P815 (H-2^d)
Unselected T	36	54
$Ly1$	1	8
$Ly23$	41	51

over, B cells incubated with unselected T cells also produced very few anti-TNP PFC. In contrast, B cells incubated with Ly-1 cells alone (after removal of Ly-2^+ cells) produced substantial numbers of anti-TNP PFC. Since only a partial reduction of the activity was seen in groups containing both $Ly1$ and $Ly23$ cells, these findings indicate that *both* $Ly23$ and $Ly123$ cells may normally suppress the generation of anti-TNP PFC.

These experiments taken together indicate that $Ly123$ T_E cells play a central role in the generation of both cellular and humoral immunity to hapten-modified "self," insofar as these cells (1) are essential (probably as cytotoxic precursors) for the generation of cell-mediated cytotoxicity to hapten-modified autologous targets and (2) can suppress the generation of antibody to TNP-modified autologous cells.

F. Regulatory Effects of *H-2* Activated T-Cell Subclasses on Antibody Responses

In view of the reactivity of Ly-2^+ cells to allogeneic K/D structures, as judged both by proliferative activity in mixed lymphocyte culture (Cantor and Boyse, 1975a) and by specificity, studies of $Ly23$ killer cells (Alter et al., 1971), it is likely that the Ly-2^+ suppression of the PFC response to hapten-modified self described above reflects stimulation of the Ly-2^+ T-cell system by antigen associated with autologous K/D molecules. According to this idea, trinitrophenylated K/D cell-surface structures activate T_E and $T_{C/S}$ cells to develop both killer and suppressor activity (see above). Haptenated Ia surface structures, on the other hand, may selectively stimulate $Ly1$ T_H activity (Cantor and Boyse, 1975a; Shevach, 1976; Katz et al., 1973; Cantor et al., 1975b). One prediction of this hypothesis is that T cells might cooperate in an optimal fashion with allogeneic B cells (incompatible at both I and K/D regions) *provided* that Ly-2^+ cells were removed. We tested this prediction in collabora-

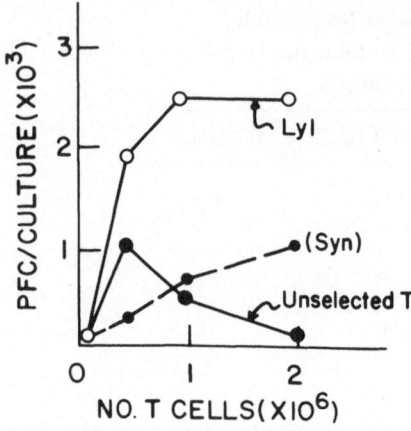

Fig. 2. Primary PFC response of SRBC-stimulated cultures containing graded doses of B6 unselected T cells (●———●) or *Ly-1* cells (○———○) and 5×10⁶ BALB/c "B" cells (obtained after treatment with anti-Thy-1 + C), compared with the response of syngeneic (B6 T cells + B6 B cells) mixtures (●———●).

tion with R. K. Gershon by determining the ability of graded numbers of B6 T cells to help 5×10^6 BALB/c B cells produce a primary PFC response to sheep erythrocytes in Mishell–Dutton cultures (Chao *et al.,* 1976). These experiments show that small numbers of allogeneic T cells provide effective primary helper function that is greater than that of syngeneic T cells at low concentrations ("positive" allogeneic effect); the addition of larger numbers of allogeneic T cells results in a "shut-off" of the response ("negative" allogenic effect). (Fig. 2).

In contrast, the addition of graded numbers of purified *Ly1* T cells to allogeneic B cells resulted in progressively increasing numbers of PFC; these PFC responses were far greater than those produced by mixtures of syngeneic T and B lymphocytes. These findings indicate that the "positive" and "negative" aspects of the allogeneic effect reflect the separate amplifying and suppressive influence of the *Ly1* and *Ly-2⁺* systems, respectively.

To determine whether *Ly1* helper activity and *Ly-2⁺* suppressive activity was selectively activated by *I*-region and *K/D*-region incompatibilities, respectively, the SRBC response of mixtures of T and B cells differing at either *I, D,* or *I + K/D* were then determined. Cultures containing *I + K/D* incompatible T and B cells again produced a slightly enhanced response when small numbers of unselected T cells were added to the cultures, followed by a shutoff effect with increasing numbers of T cells. Again, removal of *Ly-2⁺* cells permitted a vigorous PFC response, even when large numbers of T cells were present in culture. Cultures containing mixtures of T and B cells differing only at *H-2D* produced a modest response; this response was again shut off when larger numbers of T cells were added to cultures. Removal of the Ly-2^+ population completely removed the shutoff effect, permitting increasing PFC responses in direct proportion to increasing numbers of T cells in culture, similar to responses of cultures containing mixtures of syngeneic T and B cells. Finally, the response of T and B mixtures differing only at the I region was tested. In this case, *unselected* T cells provided substantial helper activity ("positive" allogeneic effect), which was considerably in excess of that noted in syngeneic T/B combinations. Thus, substantial enhancement of the PFC response was noted even in the presence of Ly-2^+ cells, simply by removing the K/D incompatibility from the system.

These findings indicate that (1) Ly-1 T_H cells can be activated by I-region incompatibilities to generate nonspecific helper activity and (2) the Ly-2^+ suppressor system is activated by K/D differences. The results of experiments in which $Ly23$ ($T_{C/S}$) cells were "added-back" to $Ly1$ cells indicate that the major source of Ly-2^+ K/D reactive suppression in this system is the $Ly23$ $T_{C/S}$ subclass.

Finally, it should also be noted that there was some decrease in the PFC response in I-different T–B cultures when large doses of unselected T cells are used. This falloff may reflect either (1) saturation of the system or (2) stimulation of $T_{C/S}$ cells "nonspecifically" by factors secreted by Ia-activated Ly-1 T_H cells. The latter possibility is supported by the finding that mixtures of high doses of purified Ly-1 T_H cells and I-region-incompatible B cells do not exhibit this falloff of activity.

G. Some Implications of These Data

1. Division of Labor among T-Cell Subclasses

These findings extend the developing concept that the regulation of the immune response reflects the different contributions of several distinct T-cell subclasses. A summary of the properties of the several T-cell subclasses that have been defined so far is shown in Table III. These studies clearly indicate that in the mouse, thymus-dependent cell differentiation results in the formation of several distinct sublines of T cells, each programmed to express a characteristic set of immunologic responses. Recent studies of Chess and Schlossman (see Chapter 10) indicate that this concept will soon be extended to man.

Several additional generalizations may be made: T_H cells, which can amplify a number of immune responses, also respond preferentially to I-region determinants. $T_{C/S}$ cells, on the other hand, respond preferentially to H-2 K/D components, and can mediate either killer or suppressor activities. Possibly these

Table III. Properties of Three Major T-Cell Subclasses

Characteristics	T_H	$T_{C/S}$	T_E
Ly expression	1	2, 3	1, 2, 3
Amplifier–helper activity			
B cells–primary antibody response	+		
B cells–secondary antibody response	+		
Ly-2,3 T cells–killer response	+		
Monocytes–macrophages–(DTH)	+		
Suppressor activity			
Primary antibody response		+	+
Secondary antibody response		+	+
After allotype suppression		+	
(T_H target)			
After polyclonal induction		+	
After *H-2* stimulation		+	+
Killer activity			
Allogeneic			
Prekiller		++	±
Killer–effector		++	
TNP-modified self			
Prekiller			++
Killer–effector		++	
MHC reactivity			
I (central) region	+		
K/D (peripheral) region		+	(+)

two subclasses, T_H and $T_{C/S}$, represent two distinct screening systems that can recognize and respond to alterations of cell surface *I*-region or *K/D*-region structures, respectively (or antigen intimately associated with these self-markers). Stimulation of these two screening systems would provoke a series of already-programmed amplifier or cytotoxic/suppressive immune reactions by the respective T-cell subclasses.

The clearest experimental example of the genetic basis for the different immunoregulatory influences of T_H and $T_{C/S}$ cells comes from studies of the regulatory activity of *H-2*-stimulated cells, summarized in part in Fig. 2 and Table III. These studies clearly show that helper and suppressive effects of *H-2*-stimulated T cells on *in vitro* primary antibody responses reflect the separate contribution of T_H and $T_{C/S}$ cells. In addition, we have shown that *I*-region components selectively stimulate *Ly1* T_H activity, resulting in substantially enhanced PFC responses, while *H-2D* or *H-2K* components selectively stimulate

Ly23 $T_{C/S}$ cells to exert powerful suppressive effects on the generation of antibody.

Until recently, cells of the T_E subclass have been the least well characterized of the three major T-cell subpopulations. The findings reported in part here suggest that T_E cells play an essential role in regulating both cellular and humoral immunity to modified autologous cells. First, T_E (*Ly123*) cells are essential, probably as precursors, to the generation of *Ly23* $T_{C/S}$ activity to haptenated-autologous cells. In addition to playing an essential role in the generation of killer cells to "modified-self," T_E cells can also suppress the generation of anti-TNP antibody-forming cells after such stimulation.

The essential contribution of T_E cells in the generation of $T_{C/S}$ killers to "altered-self" stands in contrast to their modest contribution to the generation of *allo*reactive killer cells. Thus, T_E cells in lymph nodes do not contribute significantly to the allogeneic response, and account for only a small portion of the prekiller activity in spleen (perhaps 20–40%). This difference might be explained by the idea that alloreactive T_E cells, sharing properties previously attributed to the "T_1" (Raff and Cantor, 1971; Bach *et al.,* 1976) subclass, give rise to mature alloreactive T_2-like cells in the absence of overt stimulation by antigen. This $T_E \rightarrow T_{C/S}$ maturation step has apparently *not* taken place with respect to reactivity to "modified-self."

Taken as a whole, these findings suggest that cells of the T_E subclass are essential for the regulation of humoral and cellular immunity to "modified-self." This idea also receives support from recent studies of T-cell subclasses present in aging mice, which indicate that by 10–12 months of age, spleen and lymph node T cells contain reduced numbers of *Ly123* T_E cells and increased numbers of T_H and $T_{C/S}$ cells compared with younger 1–3-month-old mice. This reduction of *Ly123* cells is associated with the inability of spleen cells from 8–12-month-old mice to produce killer cells after stimulation with TNP-modified syngeneic spleen cells; at the same time, these spleen cells produce substantial numbers of anti-TNP PFC after such stimulation.

2. Generation of Self-Reactive T cells and T-Cell Diversity: A Tentative Developmental Model

The likelihood that T_E cells can generate cytotoxic effector ($T_{C/S}$) cells after stimulation by haptenated-autologous cells but do not contribute substantially to the formation of alloreactive killer cells has interesting implications concerning the development of T cells expressing recognition units for both histocompatibility (H) components and conventional antigens. It is clearly too early to attempt to build a fully satisfactory working model to explain both the cellular basis and specificity of *H-2*-restricted immune effects. On the other hand, the data presented here have stimulated us to think about *H-2*-restricted immune phenomena along certain lines. The following considerations, therefore, simply represent the frame of reference that we are currently using to account for much recent experimental data of our own and others. They are offered only as an indication of our current thinking and certainly not as a definitive model to account for the complex nature of *H-2*-restricted immune responses.

Two leading models have been proposed to account for the requirement of *H-2* compatibility between immune T cells and TNP or virus-infected target cells. The first holds that this phenomenon reflects recognition by a single receptor of a complex antigen ("neoantigen") formed by juxtaposition of self-*H-2* and the hapten or virus. This model is made less attractive by studies indicating the ubiquitous nature of the *H-2* requirement (Bevan, 1975; Gordon *et al.*, 1975), as well as the difficulty of accounting for this type of receptor diversity at the molecular level. The second model, which is perhaps less popular at the moment, holds that T cells express receptors for self-*H-2K* or -*H-2D* components, in addition to receptors for conventional antigens. One objection to this idea comes from the assumption that prekiller activity to virus-infected or TNP-altered cells and to allogeneic cells resides in the same T-cell population expressing similar recognition mechanisms. The experiments summarized in part here show that this is probably not the case. Indeed, these data suggest that the response to *K/D* alloantigens is "special," and contradict the idea that allogeneic *K/D* components and "altered-self" *K/D* components elicit identical cellular responses. One must therefore again account for the special nature of cellular responses to allogeneic *H-2* components [in this case, their special nature has been extended to *K/D*, in addition to *LAD* (*I*-region), determinants (Wilson and Nowell, 1972)] in the face of the apparent uselessness of alloreactivity in the normal course of biological events in the life of a mouse.

Possibly, *Ly123* T_E cells generated within the thymus may first acquire "V_H"-type chains having low affinity for either allogeneic *H-2* components or specificity for non-*H-2* antigens (Eichmann and Rajewsky, 1975; Binz and Wigzell, 1975). In addition, T_E cells may also express a panel of recognition structures enabling cell interaction to occur among cells expressing autologous or allogeneic *H-2* components. Stimulation of these cells by antigen, e.g., in association with autologous *H-2 K/D* components, would stimulate an appropriate clone(s) of T_E cells to differentiate to $T_{C/S}$ lymphocytes. This differentiation step would be accompanied by the loss of the *Ly-1* cell surface component, the acquistion of killer–suppressor activity, and the ability to recirculate. Such stimulation by a large number of conventional antigens would result in the formation of a "memory pool" of *Ly23* $T_{C/S}$ cells. Reexposure to a given non-*H-2* antigen would result in reactivation of the appropriate antigen-specific $T_{C/S}$ clone. Moreover, since the "V_H" structures on the surfaces, of these cells can also react to at least one of the major *H-2 K/D* allogeneic haplotypes, exposure of the $T_{C/S}$ population to allogeneic cells would result in stimulation of large subsets of this $T_{C/S}$ "memory" pool, resulting in the generation of large amounts of cytotoxic activity. The findings that (1) idiotypes on T cells that recognize allogeneic MHC antigens and those that recognize non-*H-2* antigens have similar structures (Eichmann and Rajewsky, 1975; Binz and Wigzell, 1975) and (2) that cytotoxic/suppressor responses to "modified-self" are generated from the *Ly123* T_E cells, in contrast to generation of cytotoxic/suppressor responses to alloantigens by *Ly23* cells, fits these notions. Although these considerations imply that the generation of mature alloreactive *Ly23* and *Ly1* cells from *Ly123* cells may be driven by exposure to antigen in association with *H-2 K/D-* or *I*-region structures, respectively, it is also likely that a portion of this differentiation may be antigen-independent (Jerne, 1971). In addition, although the "V_H"-type structures directed at allogeneic *H-2* and conventional antigens might be separate from surface structures permitting cell—cell interactions with autologous and allogeneic cells, the two types of receptors might be intimately associated on the cell membrane, perhaps even representing different aspects of single complex T-cell receptor.

The experiments summarized here also indicate that T_H (*Ly1*) activity is preferentially elicited in the presence of *I*-region differences. That T_H cells are selectively activated by *I*-region products is also supported by the finding that *Ly1* cells account for virtually all the MLC reactivity of T cells against *I*-region-incompatible cells and bind specifically to allogeneic *I*-region determinants (manuscript in preparation). The possibility that *Ly1* T_H cells "see" antigen in association with self Ia components fits with the finding that secondary stimulation of T_H cells in the context of either the production of helper activity (Katz *et al.*, 1973) or delayed-type hypersensitivity responses (Miller *et al.*, 1975) requires restimulation in the presence of macrophages (and possibly B cells) expressing *I*-region products identical to those present during priming. Possibly a portion of T_E (*Ly123*) cells may also give rise to T_H (*Ly1*) cells. If so, the mechanism for generation of the T_H population might be similar to the $T_E \rightarrow T_{C/S}$ scheme outlined above, except that in this case, differentiation would be induced by antigen associated with *I*-region components.

Clearly, this model has several difficulties, including the initial requirement for the presence of recognition molecules on immature T_E cells allowing interaction with cells expressing products of any *H-2* haplotype within the species, and the implication that inappropriate *H-2* interaction structures are lost after first exposure to antigen, resulting in *H-2*-restricted immune response phenomena. Nonetheless, these difficulties seem less imposing than those of model-building according to a recognition mechanism based on clones of T cells each expressing single receptors for "neoantigens" formed by the juxtaposition of conventional ("non-*H-2*") antigens and *H-2* molecules.

It should also be clear that (1) much of this developmental model is based on the published work of other investigators (Shevach, 1975; Katz *et al.*, 1973; Shearer *et al.*, 1975; Zinkernagel and Doherty, 1975; Wilson and Nowell, 1972; Eichmann and Rajewsky, 1975; Binz and Wigzell, 1975; Pierce *et al.*, 1976; Katz and Benacerraf, 1975) and (2) in the final analysis, definitive evidence for or against this model will come from a combination of serologic and biochemical analyses of receptor molecules on the surfaces of different T cell subclasses. The contribution of cell-surface *Ly* molecules to these receptors should prove interesting.

III. POSSIBLE MECHANISMS OF $T_{C/S}$ SUPPRESSION

In several different systems, stimulation by conventional antigens, histocompatibility antigens, and mitogens results in the formation of suppressor T cells expressing the *Ly23* phenotype, although in a number of these systems, T_E (*Ly123*) cells may be required for optimal generation of Ly23 suppressive activity. Cells of the *Ly23* subclass also express killer activity against both allogeneic cells and syngeneic cells the surfaces of which have been altered by chemical modification, and therefore this category of T cells has been termed "$T_{C/S}$." If both killer and suppressor activities are mediated by the same *Ly23* cells, one can evisage that *Ly23* T_S activity might be mediated by specific elimination of antigen-reactive T_H or B cells or of antigen-bearing macrophages. At first glance, this hypothesis is in apparent conflict with the finding by Tada, *et al.* (1976) that Ia-containing molecules contained in immune T cells can specifically suppress a subsequent antibody response. It is not clear, however, whether these factors directly suppress helper cells or preferentially stimulate T_E cells to differentiate to $T_{C/S}$ progeny. Activation of the $T_E–T_{C/S}$ system in this fashion would result in an effective cellular mechanism for recognizing and eliminating those cells the surface *H-2 K/D* components of which have been altered by, for example, viruses, as has been suggested previously (Zinkernagel and Doherty, 1975), as well as provide effective control of the generation of antibody-producing cells by the same mechanism of recognition and immune elimination.

IV. DEFINITION OF OTHER (NON-T) LYMPHOCYTE SUBCLASSES EXPRESSING DISTINCTIVE CELL-SURFACE COMPONENTS

The experimental approach described in the preceding sections is based on the notion that the antigenic composition of the plasma membrane of a cell can be related precisely to selective expression of the genome of cells at particular phases in their differentiative histories. This approach has recently been extended in an attempt to serologically define other types of cells that also participate in the immune response. The following accounts describe the serologic identification of two additional types of lymphocytes that play important roles in the immune response.

A. Identification of Natural Killer Cells

Although virtually all forms of cellular immunity have been attributed to T cells, there are two notable exceptions: antibody-dependent cellular cytotoxicity and natural killer activity. The former reaction is apparently mediated by "null" cells or macrophages expressing surface receptors for the Fc portion of immunoglobulin. At the moment, there is no direct evidence that this *in vitro* reaction reflects an important *in vivo* immune mechanism.

"Natural killer" (NK) activity refers to the finding that spleen cells from certain unimmunized mouse strains can kill a variety of C-type MULV$^+$ syngeneic or allogeneic tumor cells (Greenberg and Playfair, 1974; Hanna *et al.*, 1972; Herberman *et al.*, 1975a,b; Ihle *et al.*, 1970; Nowinski and Kaehler, 1974; Oldstone *et al.*, 1972; Sendo *et al.*, 1975; Darling *et al.*, 1975; Kiessling *et al.*, 1975a,b, 1976; Petranyi *et al.*, 1975a,b). This type of NK activity has now been reported in several *in vitro* systems and has been characterized most carefully by Keissling and his colleagues (Kiessling *et al.*, 1975a,b, 1976; Petranyi *et al.*, 1975a,b). These investigators have demonstrated that NK cells have the following properties: (1) they are small lymphocytes; (2) they cannot be classified as T, B, or monocyte macrophage cells using standard cell fractionation procedures (they express neither the Thy-1 antigen nor immunoglobulin, and they are not phagocytic or adherent to nylon wool columns); and (3) they do not express Fc-receptors on their surface and do not mediate antibody-dependent cellular cytotoxicity. Most interestingly, the presence of NK activity is controlled partly by genes within the *H-2* complex, and there is a correlation between the presence of NK activity to a given tumor and *in vivo* resistance to that tumor.

Despite this apparent association between NK activity and resistance to tumor growth, it has not been possible either to directly test the role of NK cells in the prevention of tumor growth or to study their developmental relationships with other lymphoid cell populations. These questions await techniques capable of selectively depleting or purifying the NK-cell lymphocyte subclass from a heterogeneous cell population. The potential importance of NK cells is signified by recent evidence that human peripheral lymphocytes expressing surface properties similar to those of murine NK cells play an important role in the *in vitro* cytotoxic response to autologous leukemia cells (L. Chess, personal communication).

L. Glimcher has investigated the cell-surface phenotype of the NK cell and has found, confirming the work of Kiessling and his colleagues, that NK cells do not express Thy-1, Ig, or Fc receptors (Glimcher et $al.$, 1977). In addition, studies of the Ly phenotype of NK cells have shown them to be $Ly2^-$. We therefore were quite surprised to find that treatment of spleen cells from various mouse strains with "anti-Ly-1.2" sera ($C_3H\alpha CE$) + complement completely eliminated subsequent NK activity against an $MuLV^+$ tumor. Since $Ly-1$ antigens are thought to be expressed exclusively on T cells, and since the NK cell expresses no other T-cell markers (e.g. Thy-1, $Ly-2$), we suspected that the $C_3H\alpha CE$ antiserum contained antibodies to determinants distinct from $Ly-1$ that are expressed on NK cells. To test this idea, we examined the effects of anti-Ly-1.2 + C on the NK activity of spleen cells from two congenic strains of B6 mice, differing only at the relevant $Ly-1$ locus (B6/Ly-1.1$^+$ and B6/Ly-1.2$^+$). NK activity from both congenic strains was equally sensitive to $C_3H\alpha CE$ antiserum, indicating that this antiserum contained anti-NK activity that was distinct from anti-$Ly-1$ activity. Absorption of this serum with B6 Ly-1.2$^+$ thymocytes (which are NK$^-$) completely removed anti-Ly-1.2 activity and left anti-NK activity intact. This absorbed antiserum, provisionally termed $anti$-NK, defines a subclass of lymphocytes that may play an essential role in the immunosurveillance against tumors. Selective removal of NK cells from spleen and bone marrow cells before adoptive transfer to irradiated hosts is now possible and will permit direct testing of this hypothesis.

B. Serologic Definition of a Component on a Subclass of
B Cells That Is Directly Involved in Antigen-Dependent B-Cell
Triggering

The CBA/N mouse, a mutant of CBA/H, expresses an X-linked defect in its ability to respond to type III pneumococcal polysaccharide, a thymus-independent antigen (Amsbaugh, 1972). This defect has been studied mainly by Scher and his colleagues (Scher et $al.$, 1973, 1975a–d; Mosier et $al.$, 1975; Finkelman et $al.$, 1975; Cohn et $al.$, 1976) who have shown that the defective gene is recessive and have confirmed that the defective phenotype is expressed solely in B lymphocytes. The B-cell abnormalities that have been identified in this mutant mouse strain so far include: (1) a reduced response to thymus-dependent antigens compared with that of the CBA/H mouse, possibly reflecting the reduced numbers of Ig$^+$ spleen cells; (2) B cells from CBA/N mice fail to produce high-affinity antibodies after immunization with sheep erythrocytes, fail to develop M-locus determinants, and express abnormally low concentrations of surface C_3 receptors. In addition, all CBA/N T-cell responses that have been examined have been normal, and there is no evidence that abnormal suppressor

T-cell activity accounts for these defective B-cell responses. Taken together, these findings suggest that a subclass of mature B cells is either absent or dysfunctional in the CBA/N mutant strain. We have therefore attempted to immunize mice that express this defect with B cells from normal congenic donors in an attempt to serologically define the missing or defective B-cell subclass (B. Huber, R. Gershon, and H. Cantor).

Since the defective X-linked gene is recessive, the F_1 offspring resulting from a mating between CBA/N female and BALB/c male mice are either defective, if male, or normal, if female. We therefore immunized F_1 (CBA/NX BALB/c) male and female mice with BALB/c spleen cells to produce a test and control serum, respectively. The resulting test serum specifically reacts with a component on the surface of approximately 40–50% of B cells from a panel of normal strains of H-2 different mice. This antiserum, which has provisionally been called αLyb3, does not react with T lymphocytes or thymocytes, and is only weakly reactive against bone marrow cells.

The most interesting property of this antiserum is that inclusion of appropriate amounts of αLyb3 sera in the presence of very low doses of antigen results in substantially enhanced (10–20-fold) specific antibody responses. Since these enhanced PFC responses were specific for the immunizing antigen, and since no PFC response was produced by injection of the antiserum in the absence of antigen, this enhancement is probably due to a second signal produced by a specific interaction between the antiserum and a B-cell surface component. This idea was supported by absorption studies showing that this enhancement was due to a direct interaction between αLyb3 serum and B cells. These findings are consistent with the possibility that this serum defines a component on a subclass of B cells important in B-cell triggering. We are currently investigating the possibility that this component may represent (1) a receptor for one type of T cell product or (2) a component of the "constant-region" portion of the Ig receptor on B cells.

V. REFERENCES

Alter, B.J., Schendel, D.J., Bach, M.L., Bach, F.H., and Klein, J., 1971, *J. Exp. Med.* **137**:1303.

Amsbaugh, D.F., Hansen, C.T., Prescott, B., Stashak, P.W., Barthold, D.R., and Baker, P.J., 1972, *J. Exp. Med.* **136**:931.

Armerding, D., and Katz, D.H., 1974, *J. Exp. Med.* **140**:19.

Bach, J.F., Cantor, H., Roelants, G., and Stutman, O., 1976, in: *Biological Activity of Thymic Hormones* (D.W.V. Bekkum, ed.), Kyooker Publications, Rotterdam.

Bevan, M.J., 1975, *Nature (London)* **256**:419.

Binz, H., and Wigzell, H., 1975, *J. Exp. Med.* **152**:197.

Boyse, E.A., Miyazawa, M., Aoki, T., and Old, L.J., 1968, *Proc. Soc. London Ser. B.* **170**:175.

Boyse, E.A., Itakura, K., Stockert, E., Iritaru, C., and Miura, M., 1971, *Transplantation* **11**:351.

Cantor, H., 1972, *Cell. Immunol.* **3**:461.

Cantor, H., and Boyse, E.A., 1975a, *J. Exp. Med.* **141**:1376.

Cantor, H., and Boyse, E.A., 1975b, *J. Exp. Med.* **141**:1390.

Cantor, H., and Weissman, I., 1976, *Prog. Allergy.* **20**:1.

Cantor, H., Simpson, E., Sato, V., Fathman, G., and Herzenberg, L.A., 1975a, *Cell. Immunol.* **15**: 180.

Cantor, H., Shen, F.W., and Boyse, E.A., 1975b, *J. Exp. Med.* **143**:1391.

Cerottini, J.C., and Brunner, K.T., 1974, *Adv. Immunol.* **19**:67.

Chao, N., Gershon, R.K., and Cantor, H., 1976, manuscript in preparation.

Cohn, P.L., Scher, I., and Mosier, D.E., 1976, *J. Immunol.* **116**:301.

Darling, J.Z., Nowinski, R.C., and Bach, F.H., 1975, *Proc. Natl. Acad. Sci. U.S.A.* **72**:2780.

David, J.R., and David, R.A., 1972, *Prog. Allergy.* **16**:300.

Debre, P., Kapp, J.A., Dorf, M.E., and Benacerraf, B., 1975, *J. Exp. Med.* **142**:1447.

Dutton, R.W., Falkoff, R., Hirst, J., Hoffman, M., Kappler, J.W., Kettman, J.R., Lesley, J.F., and Vann, D., 1971, *Prog. Immunol.* **1**:355.

Eichmann, K., and Rajewsky, J., 1975, *Eur. J. Immunol.* **5**:661.

Finkelman, F.D., Smith, A.H., Sher, I., and Paul, W.E., 1975, *J. Exp. Med.* **142**:1316.

Gershon, R.K., 1974, *Contemp. Top. Immunobiol.* **3**:1.

Glimcher, L., Shen, F.W., and Cantor, H., 1977, *J. Exp. Med.* **145**:1.

Gordon, R.D., Simpson, E., and Samuelson, L., 1975, *J. Exp. Med.* **142**:1108.

Greenberg, A.H., and Playfair, J.H., 1974, *Clin. Exp. Immunol.* **16**:99.

Hanna, M.G., Jr., Tennant, R.W., Yuhas, J.-M., Clapp, N.K., Batzig, B.L., and Snodgrass, M.J., 1972, *Cancer Res.* **32**:2226.

Herberman, R.B., Nunn, M.E., and Lavrin, D.H., 1975a, *Int. J. Cancer* **16**:216.

Herberman, R.B., Nunn, M.F., and Lavrin, D.H., 1975b, *Int. J. Cancer* **16**:230.

Herzenberg, L.A., Okamura, K., Cantor, H., Sato, V., Shen, F.W., Boyse, E.A., and Herzenberg, L.A., 1976, *J. Exp. Med.,* in press.

Huber, B., Devinsky, O., Gershon, R., and Cantor, H., 1976a, *J. Exp. Med.* **143**:1424.

Huber, B., Shen, F.W., Boyse, E.A., and Cantor, H., 1976b, *J. Exp. Med.* **144**:1128.

Ihle, J.N., Yurconic, M., Jr., and Hanna, M.G., Jr., 1970, *J. Exp. Med.* **138**:194.

Itakura, K., Hutton, J.J., Boyse, E.A., and Old, L.K., 1972, *Transplantation* **13**:239.

Jandinski, J., Cantor, H., Tadakuma, T., Peavy, D.L., and Pierce, C.W., 1976, *J. Exp. Med.* **143**:1382.

Jerne, N.K., 1971, *Eur. J. Immunol.* **1**:1.

Kapp, J.A., Pierce, C.W., Schlossman, S., and Benacerraf, B., 1974, (GAT), *J. Exp. Med.* **140**:648.

Katz, D.H., and Benacerraf, B., 1975, *Transplant. Rev.* **22**:175.

Katz, D.H., Hamoaka, T., and Benacerraf, B., 1973, *J. Exp. Med.* **137**:1405.

Kiessling, R., Klein, E., and Wigzell, H., 1975a, *Eur. J. Immunol.* **5**:112.

Kiessling, R., Klein, E., Pross, H., and Wigzell, H., 1975b, *Eur. J. Exp. Med.* **5**:7.

Miller, J.F.A.P., Vadas, M.A., Whitelaw, A., and Gamble, J., 1975, *Proc. Natl. Acad. Sci. U.S.A.* **72**:5095.

Mosier, D.E., Scher, I., Ruhl, H., Cohen, P.L., Zitron, I., and Paul, W.E., 1975, in press.

Nowinski, R.C., and Kaehler, S.L., 1974, *Science* **185**:869.

Oldstone, M.B.A., Aoki, T., and Dixon, F.J., 1972, *Proc. Natl. Acad. Sci. U.S.A.* **69**:134.

Petranyi, G., Kiessling, R., Klein, G., and Wigzell, H., 1975a, *Int. J. Cancer* **15**:935.

Petranyi, G., Kiessling, R., and Klein, G., 1975b, *Immunogenetics* **2**:53.

Pierce, C.W., Kapp, J., and Benacerraf, B., 1976, *J. Exp. Med.,* in press.

Raff, M.C., and Cantor, H., 1971, *Prog. Immunol.* **4**:93.

Scher, I., Frantz, M., and Steinberg, A.D., 1973, *J. Immunol.* **110**:396.

Scher, I., Ahmed, A., Strong, D.M., Steinberg, A.D., and Paul, W.E., 1975a, *J. Exp. Med.* **141**:788.

Scher, I., Steinberg, A.D., Berning, A.K., and Paul, W.E., 1975b, *J. Exp. Med.* **142**:637.

Scher, I., Sharrow, S.O., and Paul, W.E., 1975c, *Fed Proc. Fed. Amer. Soc. Exp. Biol.* **34**:999.

Scher, I., Ahmed, A., Sharrow, S.O., Steinberg, A.D., and Paul, W.E., 1975d, in press.

Sendo, F.T., Aoki, T., Boyse, E.A., and Buafo, C.K., 1975, *J. Natl. Cancer Inst.,* in press.

Shearer, G.M., Rehn, T., and Gabardino, C.A., 1975, *J. Exp. Med.* **141**:1348.

Shen, F.W., Boyse, E.A., and Cantor, H., 1975, *Immunogenetics* **2**:591.

Shevach, E.M., 1976, *J. Immunol.* **116**:1482.

Tada, T., Taniguchi, M., and Takemori, T., 1976, *Transplant. Rev.* **26**:119.

Transplantation Reviews **1**, 1969 (G. Moller, ed.), Williams & Wilkins, Baltimore.

Wilson, D.B., and Nowell, P. C., 1972, *Transplant. Rev.* **12**:3.

Zinkernagel, R.M., and Doherty, P.C., 1975, *J. Exp. Med.* **141**:1427.

Chapter 3

Antigen Receptors of T Helper Cells

Klaus Rajewsky

Institute for Genetics, University of Cologne
Cologne, West Germany

and

Klaus Eichmann

Institute for Immunology and Genetics
Deutsches Krebsforschungszentrum
Heidelberg, West Germany

I. INTRODUCTION

The function of the immune system is based on a large variety of receptor molecules that differ in their binding specificity. These receptors are located in part on the surfaces of the immunocompetent cells, namely, T and B lymphocytes, and in part appear free in the circulation. They mediate the specific recognition of antigens and guarantee the specificity of the immunologic reactions that follow antigen recognition. In addition, since each receptor molecule carries associated with its specific antigen-binding site specific antigenic determinants (so-called *idiotopes*) that distinguish it from, and can be recognized by, other receptor molecules, it appears possible that the immune system regulates itself by internal receptor–receptor interactions (Jerne, 1974).

What is the molecular identity of antigen receptors in the immune system, and what is the genetic basis of their diversity? The classic antigen receptor is the antibody molecule. Antibody molecules consist of heavy and light polypeptide chains that can be classified on the basis of the amino acid sequence of their constant parts. In addition, each chain possesses a variable portion that distinguishes it from the other members of its class. The binding specificity of antibody molecule is defined by the variable portions of its polypeptide chains.

At the structural level, the variable portions represent well-defined structural domains (Edelman and Gall, 1969) that constitute the F_V piece of the antibody molecule (Inbar *et al.*, 1972). The structural subdivision of antibody molecules into variable and constant domains is reflected at the genetic level, since separate genes, called V and C genes, appear to code for the variable and the constant portions of antibody polypeptide chains. These genes are arranged in three unlinked clusters in the genome, namely, the heavy-chain linkage group and linkage groups coding for κ and λ light chains, respectively (reviewed by Gally and Edelman, 1972). Each of these linkage groups consists of a series of V and C genes, and somatic chromosomal rearrangements are required to allow the synthesis of complete antibody polypeptide chains.

We can now ask a few precise and fundamental questions concerning antigen receptors in the immune system. (1) Is the binding specificity of antigen receptors always and exclusively determined by antibody V genes? (2) If so, are all antigen receptors composed of the variable portions of both heavy and light chains? (3) Are all antigen receptors conventional immunoglobulin molecules encoded by both V and C genes of the antibody system?

The structural analysis of antigen receptors is required in order to answer these questions. Strong evidence (not reviewed here) indicates that B lymphocytes, the precursors of antibody-forming cells, carry conventional immunoglobulin molecules as the functional antigen receptors on their surfaces. In contrast, conventional immunoglobulin is not readily detected on the surfaces of T lymphocytes. A long and frustrating debate on this question is documented in the literature over the past six years. Clearly, however, the failure of a number of laboratories to reproduce the positive results of others (reviewed by Vitetta and Uhr, 1975, and Marchalonis, 1976) raises questions concerning the specificity of reagents and suggests that T lymphocytes might carry antigen receptors not identical with, though possibly related to, conventional immunoglobulin. In addition, a large body of evidence suggests that genes in the major histocompatibility complex, which is not linked to any antibody structural gene, specifically affect the recognition of antigens by T lymphocytes (cf. Benacerraf and McDevitt, 1972; Benacerraf and Katz, 1975). In line with these indications, antigen-specific factors produced by murine T cells have been isolated that do not appear to cross-react with conventional immunoglobulin, but carry antigenic determinants encoded by the *I* region of the *H-2* complex (Munro and Taussig, 1975; Takemori and Tada, 1975; Mozes, 1976). Finally, in a number of experimental systems, the specificity of T-cell reactions appears to differ drastically from that expected on the basis of serologic reactions.

The problem of the molecular identity of the T-cell receptor and its genetic coding is thus unresolved. It poses itself with all force, since T cells appear to be of crucial importance for the immune system. T lymphocytes are not only responsible for reactions of cellular immunity, but also, as helper or suppressor cells, regulate lymphocyte activities in both the T- and B-cell compartments.

In this chapter, we review the attempts of this laboratory to characterize and identify antigen receptors on T lymphocytes. Our experiments started from the initial observation that the collaboration of B cells with T helper cells in antibody induction involves the specific recognition of antigen by the helper cells (Mitchison et al., 1970). A detailed study was then carried out in which cross-reactions at the helper-cell level were compared with serologic cross-reactions (Rajewsky and Mohr, 1974). Indistinguishable cross-reaction patterns were found, suggesting that the binding sites of antibody molecules and T-helper-cell receptors are similar if not identical.

This view was at first sight dramatically reinforced when we found that antibody molecules and the functional receptors on T helper cells express identical idiotypic determinants. This result was based on our finding that antiidiotypic antibody could specifically sensitize idiotype-bearing B and T helper lymphocytes (Eichmann and Rajewsky, 1975). In completely unrelated experimental systems, Ramseier and Lindenmann (1972), Binz and Wigzell (Chapter 4), and McKearn et al. (1974a,b) have similarly demonstrated idiotypic cross-reactions between alloantibodies and the receptors on T cells mediating graft-vs.-host and cytotoxic responses. Since idiotypes are markers for the variable portions of antibody molecules and can be used in certain experimental systems, including our own, as genetic markers for antibody V genes in the heavy-chain linkage group (reviewed by Eichmann, 1975a), we were able to provide genetic evidence that the latter genes control the binding sites of both antibody molecules and T-helper-cell receptors (Black et al., 1975; Hämmerling et al., 1976a). It should be stressed, however, that our results relate only to V genes coding for the variable portions of the immunoglobulin *heavy* chains.

Recent results obtained with specifically purified receptor molecules from T lymphocytes suggest that these molecules do not carry any class-specific heavy and light chain determinants (Krawinkel and Rajewsky, 1976), but express, in line with our expectation, variable regions of immunoglobulin heavy chains (Krawinkel et al., 1976, 1977a,b). We shall conclude our chapter with an attempt to visualize the molecular structure of T-cell receptors on the basis of the available experimental evidence including the *Ir* gene phenomenon.

II. FUNCTIONAL SPECIFICITY AND HETEROGENEITY
OF HELPER-T-CELL RECEPTORS

A. The Experimental System

Antibodies as well as helper cells are known to react specifically against a wide variety of antigens. How does the fine specificity of the receptors on these cells compare with that of humoral antibody? Only now can we think of approaching this question directly, i.e., by measuring antigen binding to isolated helper-cell receptors, since methods for the specific isolation of T-cell receptors are becoming available (see Section V). One can also study the problem indirectly, however, namely, by investigating the specificity and heterogeneity of helper cell *function.* Such experiments can provide definitive although limited information on helper-cell-receptor specificity and diversity. They are at the same time essential for the understanding of the physiological role of the helper-cell system.

In our own studies (Rajewsky and Pohlit, 1971; Rajewsky *et al.,* 1972; Rajewsky and Mohr, 1974), we used the cell-transfer system developed by Mitchison (1968), in which a mixture of hapten-primed and carrier-primed cells is transferred to irradiated hosts, which are subsequently challenged by the hapten–carrier conjugates. The secondary antihapten response in this system is taken as a measure of the interaction of carrier determinants with helper-cell receptors (Mitchison *et al.,* 1970). Two sets of experiments were carried out to determine helper-cell specificity and diversity. In the first series of experiments, secondary stimulation in the cell-transfer system was carried out with a series of serologically related carrier molecules to which a hapten (4-hydroxy-5-iodo-3-nitrophenycetyl, NIP) was coupled. We obtained cross-stimulation patterns that were interpreted to reflect carrier cross-reactions at the helper-cell level, and that were shown not to depend on circulating humoral antialbumin antibody in the system. These patterns were compared with the *serologic* cross-reactions of the same carrier molecules, i.e., the cross-reaction patterns at the antibody level. The carrier molecules in our experiments were a series of cross-reacting serum albumins from various animal species.

The cross-stimulation experiments were complemented by a second set of experiments in which helper-cell receptor heterogeneity was assessed in a more direct way and compared with the heterogeneity of humoral antibody. In these experiments, we made use of the same series of cross-reacting albumin carriers and of the possibility to render helper cells specifically tolerant. Consider a pair of cross-reacting serum albumins, BSA and SSA. We paralyze groups of mice with BSA or SSA and immunize them with the cross-reacting albumin. Helper activity for the two carriers is then measured in the cooperating cell-transfer system outlined above. This approach permits one to distinguish cross-reacting from non-cross-reacting helper cells. By extending it to a series of carrier molecules, helper-cell heterogeneity can be assessed in a straightforward way and can also be compared straightforwardly with antibody heterogeneity, since by the help of immunoadsorbents, antibody populations can be similarly classified into cross-reacting and non-cross-reacting subpopulations.

A particular feature of the paralysis experiments deserves special comment. In contrast to the cross-stimulation scheme, it is the virgin (i.e., unprimed) T-cell population that is here classified into subpopulations according to receptor specificities. Note that in addition, conventional humoral antibody cannot obscure the results of this analysis, since low zone paralysis, in particular, is a T-cell phenomenon (Chiller *et al.*, 1971; Mitchison, 1971; Rajewsky, 1971), and the specificity of antibody is indistinguishable in control and paralyzed animals (Rajewsky *et al.*, 1972; Rajewsky and Brenig, 1974).

B. Cross-Reactions at the Helper-Cell Level and at the Level of Humoral Antibody

A summary of our results (Rajewsky and Mohr, 1974) is given in Fig. 1. The figure depicts experiments with four serum albumins, namely, bovine serum albumin (BSA), sheep serum albumin (SSA), deer serum albumin (DSA), and giraffe serum albumin (GSA). Each horizontal series of diagrams represents the cross-reactions of these molecules in antiserum to one of them on the one side (left diagram) and at the level of helper cells induced by the same albumin species on the other (diagrams at right). The serologic cross-reactions are determined in radioactive binding assays, by measuring, over a wide range of antigen concentrations, the ratio of binding of homologous antigen over that of heterologous antigen. Cross-reactions at the helper-cell level are determined in the cooperating cell-transfer system, by measuring, over a wide range of antigen concentrations, the capacity of albumin-specific helper cells to help homologous or heterologous albumins conjugated to the NIP hapten in the induction of a secondary anti-NIP response.

Although the system permits only a qualitative comparison of antibody specificity on the one hand and that of helper-cell function on the other, it is obvious that there is a very striking similarity in the cross-reaction patterns at the antibody and the helper-cell level (Fig. 1). Thus, antibodies and helper cells specific for BSA scarcely distinguish between the four albumins, whereas antibodies and helper cells induced by SSA react preferentially with the homologous albumin (SSA). Antibodies to DSA cross-react strongly with SSA, as do the corresponding helper cells, whereas in both systems, the cross-reaction with BSA is weaker. A detailed discussion of the various data is given in our previous

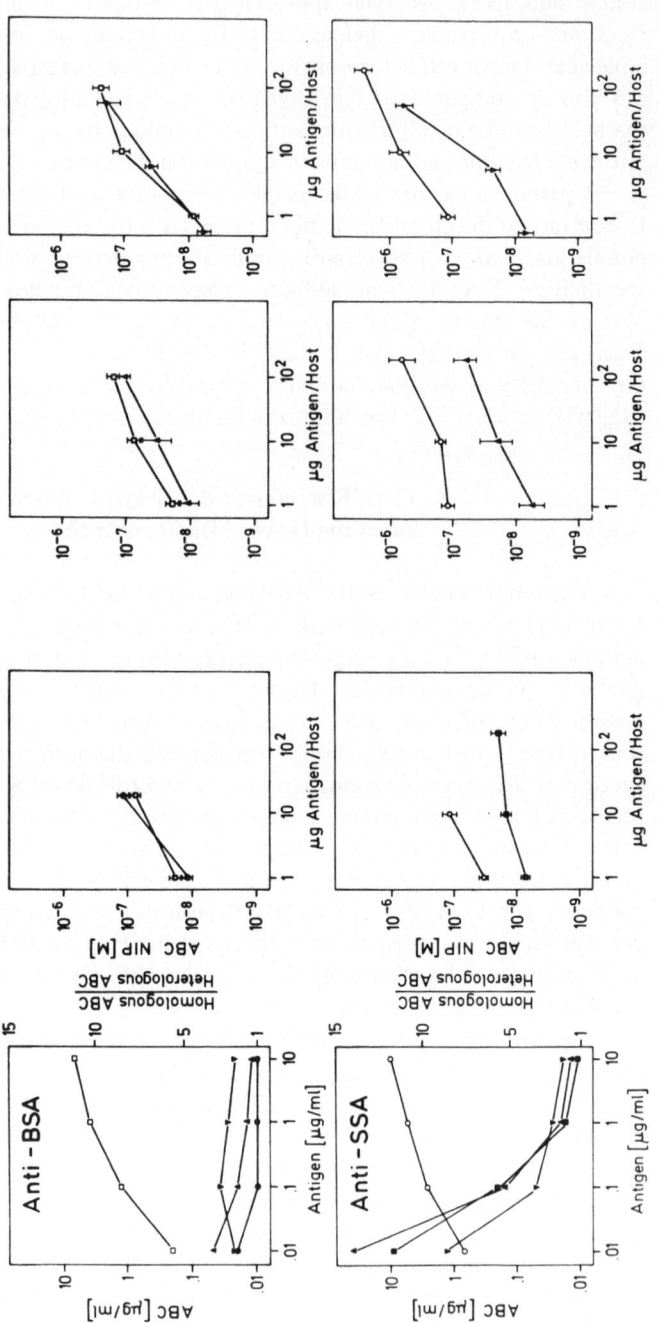

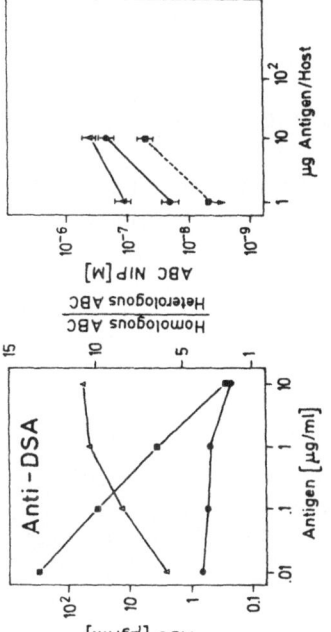

Fig. 1. Cross-reactivity of serum albumins at the helper-cell level and at the level of humoral antibodies. In the *top* horizontal row of diagrams, cross-reactivity is determined with BSA-sensitized helpers and in anti-BSA antiserum. In the *middle* row, helpers and antibodies are induced by SSA; in the *bottom* row, by DSA. In each row, the *left* diagram represents cross-reactions in *antiserum* (which is obtained from the helper-cell donors). Plotted are the homologous antigen-binding capacity (ABC) (e.g., binding of BSA to anti-BSA, anti-SSA to SSA; open symbols, left ordinate) determined at various antigen concentrations (abscissa) and the ratios of homologous to heterologous ABC (e.g., ABC BSA over ABC SSA in anti-BSA; solid symbols, right ordinate), as an expression of cross-reaction. Squares: BSA as homologous (□) and heterologous (■) antigen. Circles: SSA as homologous (○) and heterologous (●) antigen. Triangles: DSA as homologous (△) and heterologous (▲) antigen. Solid inverted triangles (▼): GSA as heterologous antigen. Analogous results were obtained in various pools of antisera. The diagrams at *right* in each horizontal row represent cross-reactions at the *helper-cell level*. BSA-primed (*top* row), SSA-primed (*middle* row), and DSA-primed spleen cells (*bottom* row) were transferred together with NIP-CG-primed cells into irradiated hosts and boosted with graded doses of NIP–serum albumin conjugate (abscissa). The secondary anti-NIP response was determined 10–14 days after boosting (ordinate indicates molar hapten-binding capacity). Each diagram represents a cell-transfer experiment in which T-cell help for the homologous (open symbols) and one heterologous serum albumin carrier (solid symbols) was determined. Each experimental point is the geometric mean of Hapten-binding capacities in 6 individual sera. Symbols correspond to those in the diagrams at left: (□ and ■): NIP-BSA; (○ and ●): NIP-SSA; (△ and ▲): NIP-DSA; (▲): NIP-GSA. Responses in the absence of helper cells were negligible. For further details, see Rajewsky and Mohr (1974).

publications (see Rajewsky and Mohr, 1974), and will not be repeated here. Taken together, the data reveal a strict analogy between the specificity of help and that of humoral antibody, in particular when serologic cross-reactions determined at low antigen concentrations are taken into consideration. At low antigen concentration, the discriminating power of humoral antibody is high due to the specificity of highly avid antibody, and it is the same high discriminating power that helper cells display in the cross-stimulation experiments. The significance of these results is underlined by our finding of the same nonreciprocal cross-reactions at the level both of humoral antibodies and of helper cell function (nonreciprocal cross-reactions appear in the case of SSA/BSA and DSA/BSA (Fig. 1).

C. Heterogeneity of Helper-Cell Receptors and Humoral Antibody

With the use of immunoadsorbents, antibodies against each of our serum albumins can be classified into antibody subpopulations on the basis of their cross-reactivity with related albumins. The results of this analysis were in accord with the serologic analysis depicted in Fig. 1. Thus, as an example, more than 90% of anti-BSA generally cross-reacted with SSA or DSA, whereas approximately 25% of anti-SSA did not react with either BSA or DSA. Paralysis experiments permitted us to carry out a similar analysis of helper-cell receptors, and again the results were strikingly similar to those obtained with humoral antibody. To continue with the example just mentioned, spleen cells from mice tolerant to SSA or DSA and immunized with BSA did not exhibit significant BSA-specific helper function in the adoptive transfer system, although a few BSA (but not SSA or DSA) specific helper cells could still be found in these animals by other methods. In contrast, tolerance to BSA did not prevent the induction of clear-cut SSA or DSA specific helper function by immunization with the latter albumins. The resulting helper cells in these animals were of course unreactive with BSA. Thus, the nonreciprocal cross-reactions found in the previous section reappear in the present analysis, and again similarly at the antibody and helper-cell level.

The body of our experimental data (Rajewsky and Mohr, 1974), which we do not wish to repeat here in any greater detail, shows that within the limits of the experimental system, the antigen-binding heterogeneity of antibodies and helper-cell receptors is similar and of the same order. In addition, the data are in perfect accord with the cross-stimulation data of Fig. 1. This is reassuring, since, as mentioned above, the paralysis experiments almost necessarily relate to *intrinsic* T cell receptors, and not to passively acquired B-cell-derived antibody receptors. The consistency of the paralysis and the cross-stimulation data is therefore in itself an argument against the hypothesis that the receptors on T helper cells are passively acquired cytophilic antibody (Playfair *et al.*, 1974; see also Sections III.B.4 and VI.A).

In addition, the selective modulation of T-cell-receptor specificities in low zone paralysis provides an example of how regulatory processes during ontogeny can differentially modify the specificity distribution in T- and B-cell receptors. Therefore, if such differences are encountered, this does not necessarily imply receptors of a different molecular constitution on the two cell types.

In summary, from our functional analysis, there is no reason to believe that the heterogeneity of helper-cell receptors is restricted as compared with the heterogeneity of antibody combining sites, and in fact, antibodies and helper-cell receptors appear to discriminate among antigens in a similar way. The results described in the next section (see, in particular, Section III.B.2) further support these conclusions.

III. IDIOTYPIC PROPERTIES OF HELPER AND SUPPRESSOR T-CELL RECEPTORS

A. The Experimental System

Our idiotypic analysis of T-cell receptors is based on a series of experiments that made use of the observation that with antiidiotypic antibody to a monoclonal antistreptococcal antibody of strain A/J, we were able to sensitize A/J mice to streptococcal antigens (Eichmann and Rajewsky, 1975). Sensitization occurred not only in the B-cell compartment, but also in the helper-T-cell population. With another class of antiidiotypic antibody, suppressor T cells instead of helpers were specifically sensitized (Eichmann, 1974, 1975b). Hence, our results were most readily interpreted by an interaction of antiidiotypic antibody with receptor molecules on the surfaces of both B and T lymphocytes. This conclusion was further supported by our subsequent observations on the similarity of the antigen-binding specificities of B and T helper cells reactive with antiidiotypic antibody and on their degree of heterogeneity (Black *et al.*, 1975, 1976). Furthermore, the specificity-determining portions of the antigen receptors of both B and T cells appear to be under the control of genes in the same linkage group (Hämmerling *et al.*, 1976a). Experiments supporting each of these points will be reviewed in this section.

The experimental system in which these results were obtained possesses certain properties, some or each of which may be a necessary requirement for demonstrating the findings mentioned above. It is therefore outlined here in some detail.

Most of the experiments employed antibodies to Group A streptococcal carbohydrate (A-CHO), generated in strain A/J mice by immunization with Group A streptococcal vaccine (Strep.A) (Eichmann, 1972). The group-specific polysaccharides of streptococci have long been known to stimulate antibodies of restricted heterogeneity in rabbits (Krause, 1970) and in mice (Briles and Krause, 1972, 1974; Eichmann, 1972; Cramer and Braun, 1975). A major portion of the antibodies to A-CHO in strain A/J represents a single antibody species that is defined by its isoelectric focusing spectrum and by idiotype (Id) (Eichmann, 1973, 1974). The Id is detected by guinea pig antiidiotypic antibody (anti-Id) raised against the anti-A-CHO antibody produced by the AJ/ lymphocyte clone A5A (Eichmann, 1972; Eichmann and Kindt, 1971). The expression of the A5A Id is controlled by a single gene ($A5A^+$) linked to the $Ig-1^e$ allotype locus of A/J mice (Eichmann, 1975a; Eichmann et al., 1974; Eichmann and Berek, 1973, 1974). Anti-Id against the A5A Id can be fractionated into the IgG1 and IgG2 classes of guinea pig IgG (Benacerraf et al., 1963; Eichmann, 1974). Whereas anti-Id belonging to the IgG2 class was shown to stimulate suppressor T cells (Eichmann, 1975b), stimulation of helper T cells was achieved with anti-Id of the IgG1 class (Eichmann and Rajewsky, 1975).

For some experiments, particularly those that were concerned with the genetic control of helper cell responsiveness to ā-Id, we used an additional idiotypic system that employed a myeloma protein rather than an induced antibody for the production of anti-Id. The transplantable BALB/c plasmacytoma S117 secretes an IgA/k immunoglobulin with specificity for N-acetyl-glucosamine (Vicari et al., 1970), the major antigenic determinant of A-CHO (McCarty, 1958). Guinea pig anti-Id against this myeloma protein reacts with the antibodies of Balb/c mice immunized with Strep.A, and genetic analysis demonstrated that the expression of the S117 idiotypic marker is controlled by a gene within the Ig-1 complex of strain BALB/c (Berek et al., 1976). This gene ($S117^+$) segregates in breeding experiments as if it were an allele to the gene $A5A^+$, which controls the expression of the A5A idiotype in association with antibodies to A-CHO in strain A/J and which is linked to the $Ig-1^e$ allotype locus. Another possible allele, linked to the $Ig-1^c$ allotype locus, controls the expression of both S117 and A5A cross-reactive determinants ($S117^{cr}$, $A5A^{cr}$). The distribution of these idiotypic determinants in various lines that carry recombinant Ig-1 haplotype suggests that the A5A and S117 loci are nonallelic and map at different positions in the Ig-1 region (Berek et al., 1976).

The two idiotypic systems provide the opportunity to study linkage relationships of genes that control variable portions and thus the antigen-binding specificity of both T- and B-cell-receptor molecules.

B. Stimulation of Helper T Cells by Antiidiotypic Antibody

1. Detection of B-Precursor and T-Helper-Cell Activity in Mice Treated with Antiidiotypic Antibody

All helper-cell stimulation experiments were done with the IgG1 fractions (āId1) of guinea pig antisera to the idiotype of antibody A5A or to the idiotype of myeloma proteins S117. Quantities corresponding to 0.1 μg idiotype-binding capacity (IBC) (Eichmann, 1974, 1975b) were ultracentrifuged and injected intraperitoneally or intravenously into mice. At 6–8 weeks after this injection, the mice were tested for sensitization to streptococcal antigens and compared with mice that had been injected intraperitoneally or intravenously with 1×10^9 Group A streptococcal particles, as well as with nonimmunized mice (Eichmann and Rajewsky, 1975). Analyses for sensitization were done *in vivo* using cooperative adoptive transfer experiments (Eichman and Rajewsky, 1975) and *in vitro* in a cooperative microculture system (Black *et al.,* 1976). Both types of experiments were designed in such a way that priming in both the B- and the T-cell compartment could be detected. For the *in vivo* experiments, spleen cells from animals that had received either Strep.A or āId 6–8 weeks previously were transferred into sublethally irradiated syngeneic hosts together with spleen cells from syngeneic animals primed with NIP-CG. The animals were then boosted with NIP-conjugated streptococci (NIP-Strep.A) and bled 8–10 days later, and the sera were titrated for antibodies against NIP and A-CHO, respectively, and for A5A idiotype. The induction of a secondary response in such a system relies on the cooperation of antibody-forming-cell precursors and T helper cells (Mitchison *et al.,* 1970). The antihapten (NIP) response thus depends, in the presence of excess hapten-primed precursor cells, entirely on carrier-specific helpers, and can accordingly be used to measure priming to streptococcal antigens in the T-cell compartment. On the other hand, the combined determination of anti-A-CHO and idiotype titers reveals the extent of specific priming in the B-cell compartment (Eichmann and Rajewsky, 1975). The results of a typical experiment appear in Table I.

The antihapten (NIP) responses demonstrate the presence of specific helper function in both Strep.A- and āId1-primed spleen cells. The helper cells induced by āId1 exhibited specificity for streptococci, since they did not help in the response to a conjugate of the hapten with the unrelated carrier guinea pig immunoglobulin. In order to verify that helper function was indeed exerted by T lymphocytes, spleen cell populations were either treated with anti-Thy-1.2 serum in order to eliminate T cells or were passed over Degalan columns (Wigzell and Andersson, 1969; Rajewsky and Mohr, 1974) coated with complexes of mouse Ig and rabbit antibodies to mouse Ig in order to eliminate B cells. Irrespective of whether helper function had been induced by āId1 or Strep.A, the elimination of T cells from the helper cell population led to the elimination of help for the anti-NIP response. The response to A-CHO, however, was only slightly reduced, demonstrating that our antiserum to Thy-1.2 was not toxic for B lymphocytes. In accord with these data are the results obtained with column-passaged cells. The elimination of B cells, verified by the drastic reduction of anti-A-CHO titers, left helper activity untouched (Eichmann and Rajewsky, 1975). Similar results have been obtained *in vitro* (Black *et al.,* 1976). Spleen cells from mice pretreated with Strep.A or with anti-Id1 produced substantial numbers of PFC against TNP when challenged with TNP-Strep.A, whereas cells from normal mice did not. The anti-TNP response could be specifically abolished by treatment of the cells with anti-Thy-1.2 and C'. In other experiments, it was shown that nylon-wool-column-purified T cells (Julius *et al.,* 1973) from anti-Id1-primed mice were fully active as helper cells in this *in vitro* system (Black *et al.,* 1976). Helper function in both the *in vivo* and *in vitro* experimental systems is thus mediated by T cells, and we accordingly conclude that the administration of āId1 confers specific immunity to both the T- and B-cell systems in A/J mice.

2. Specificity and Heterogeneity of Primed Cell Populations

In the experiments summarized in Table I, it was shown that A/J spleen cells primed with anti-A5A Id1 produced exclusively A5A-Id-positive antibodies when transferred into an adoptive host and challenged with Strep.A (Eichmann and Rajewsky, 1975). This result is in contrast to that obtained with cells primed with Strep.A, which produced antibodies of which only about 25% were A5A-Id-positive. This result indicated that anti-A5A-Id1 specifically activated precursor B cells expressing the A5A Id. Using the *in vitro* cooperative system, Black *et al.* (1976) were able to compare the idiotypic and antigen-binding specificities of both B and T lymphocyte populations.

Table II compares the results obtained with B cells to those obtained with T helper cells. For the study of B cells, antigen (A-CHO) or antiidiotypic antibody (ā-A5A) was added to the plaque test in order to inhibit plaque formation. For the study of T cells, A-CHO or āA5A was included in the culture medium to inhibit helper function. In both cases, cells from mice primed with Strep.A were compared with cells from mice primed with āId1 and with unprimed cells. Cells analyzed for B-cell specificity were boosted with Strep.A and plaqued against A-CHO coupled to SRBC (Pavlovskis and Slade, 1969). Cells analyzed for T-cell specificity were boosted with TNP-Strep.A and plaqued against TNP coupled to SRBC (Rittenberg and Pratt, 1969).

It is obvious from the data that B cells primed with Strep.A, although mostly specific for A-CHO, are idiotypically heterogeneous to the extent that about 60% have idiotypes not affected by ā-A5A serum. This finding is in agreement with the *in vivo* results presented in Table I. The population of T cells

Table I. Sensitization of T and B Cells by Antiidiotypic Antibody

Cells analyzed for Strep.A sensitivity[a]	Antigen	Anti-NIP response[b]	Anti-A-CHO response[c]	Idiotype response[d]
–	NIP-CG	74 (1.0)	< 2	ND[e]
–	NIP-Strep.A	5.6 (1.4)	4.1 (1.6)	ND
–	NIP-GPIgG	0.4	< 2	ND
1°āId1	NIP-GPIgG	1.6 (6.3)	< 2	ND
1°āId1	NIP-Strep.A	54.5 (1.2)	89 (1.2)	74 (1.2)
1°āId1, "B cells"	NIP-Strep.A	1.1 (1.2)	36 (1.2)	38 (1.4)
1°āId1, "T cells"	NIP-Strep.A	42.8 (1.4)	6.3 (1.6)	ND
1°Strep.A	NIP-Strep.A	32.8 (1.5)	172 (1.1)	48 (1.2)
1°Strep.A, "B cells"	NIP-Strep.A	2.9 (1.3)	85 (1.3)	18 (1.4)
1°Strep.A, "T cells"	NIP-Strep.A	44.4 (1.8)	10.6 (2.3)	ND

[a]Hosts received 15×10^6 cells primed with NIP-CG and additional cells as indicated in the table. "B cells" stands for spleen cells treated with antiserum to Thy-1.2 and complement. "T cells" stands for spleen cells passaged through Degalan columns coated with MIg–anti-MIg complexes (cell recovery was 10%). In the case of āId1-primed cells, each host received 25×10^6 untreated cells or 9×10^6 "B cells" or 10×10^6 "T cells." In the case of cells primed with A streptococci, the corresponding cell numbers were 20×10^6 untreated cells, 6×10^6 "B cells," and 7.5×10^6 "T cells."
[b]Geometric means of molar serum binding capacities $\times 10^8$ with standard error, determined at 10^{-8} M hapten.
[c]Geometric means of anti-A-CHO serum concentrations (μg/ml) with standard error.
[d]Geometric means of A5A serum concentrations (μg/ml) with standard error.
[e]ND: Not done.
Taken from Eichmann and Rajewsky, 1975.

appears to be even more heterogeneous, to the extent that helper function is only poorly inhibited by A-CHO and almost untouched by anti-A5A serum. This result is expected because of the antigenic complexity of Group A streptococci, which carry a number of antigens in addition to A-CHO (McCarty, 1958). While this complexity is fully expressed at the helper-cell level, it is concealed in the precursor-cell analysis, which employs purified A-CHO as the indicator antigen.

A dramatic reduction of heterogeneity is seen in the cell population primed with āId. Both cell populations are equally well and almost completely inhibited by both A-CHO and āId. This result strongly suggests that the selectivity of lymphocyte activation by antiidiotypic antibody is the same for B precursor and T helper cells.

Black et al. (1976) also used heterogeneous antigens such as C-CHO (Group C streptococcal carbohydrate) or SRBC to analyze the antigen-binding specificity of āId-primed helper cells. In all these experiments, it was clear that T-helper cells activated by āId were essentially specific for the antigen to which the original idiotype was raised. It is an additionally interesting aspect of these studies that the antigen used in our experimental system is a polysaccharide

**Table II. Idiotypic and Antigen-Binding
Specificity of B and T Cells Primed with
Strep.A or with Anti-Id1[a]**

Priming antigen[b]	Inhibitor[c]	PFC-response[d]	
		āA-CHO	āTNP
–	–	0	3
Strep.A	–	100	100
Strep.A	A-CHO	21	65
Strep.A	āId	59	86
āId	–	100	100
āId	A-CHO	23	21
āId	āId	2	2

[a]Data from Black *et al.* (1976).
[b]Mice were primed *in vivo* with 1×10^9 Strep.A particles or with 0.1 μg IBC of anti-A5AId1.
[c]Inhibitors were included in the plaque test agarose for āA-CHO-PFC, and in the culture medium for āTNP-PFC. The concentrations of A-CHO were 20 μg/0.5 ml agarose and 0.1 μg/100 μl culture. The concentration of anti-Id was 0.5 μg IBC/0.5 ml agarose and 0.05 μg IBC/0.1 ml culture medium.
[d]The responses are represented as percentages of controls without inhibitor or with normal guinea pig serum as inhibitor. Geometric means of 8 microcultures with a cell input of 10^6 spleen cells. PFC responses in control cultures ranged from 100 to 500 PFC per culture.

(Coligan *et al.*, 1975). The data in Table II clearly demonstrate that this polysaccharide antigen is recognized by helper T cells.

Taken together, the results of this section are in full accord with those reported in Section II, in that they point to a striking similarity of antigen recognition by B and T helper cells. They extend the previous observations in that they demonstrate functional antigen receptors with similar or identical idiotypic and antigen-binding specificities on antiidiotypically induced B and T helper cells.

3. Genetic Control of Helper-Cell Receptor

As we mentioned above, the A5A idiotype is a strain-specific genetic marker for the gene $A5A^+$ which is linked to the $Ig-1^e$ allotype locus of strain A/J (Eichmann, 1975a). Similarly, Berek *et al.* (1976) described the idiotype of the Balb/c myeloma protein S117 to be a marker for the gene $S117^+$, which is linked to the $Ig-1^a$ allotype locus of this strain. Since both genes encode V_H regions of antibodies with specificity for A-CHO, Hämmerling *et al.* (1976a) investigated

Table III. Strain-Specific Responsiveness
of Helper T Cells to Antiidiotypic Antibody[a]

| Priming antigen[b] | Inhibitor[c] | TNP-PFC response[d] | |
		A/J	BALB/c
–	–	6	8
Strep.A	–	100	100
āA5A	–	96	10
āA5A	āA5A	19	
āA5A	āS117	109	
āS117	–	7	89
āS117	āA5A		91
āS117	āS117		13

[a]Data from Black et al. (1976).
[b]Mice were primed with 1×10^9 Strep.A particles or with 0.1 μg IBC of anti-A5AId1 or anti-S117Id1, respectively.
[c]Inhibitors were 0.01 μg IBC of the respective antisera, included in the culture medium.
[d]The responses are represented as percentages of controls without inhibitor or with normal guinea pig serum as inhibitor. See also Table II.

the question whether the genetic polymorphism that is detected among the idiotypes of antibody molecules would be similarly expressed at the level of T-helper-cell receptors. This question appears particularly important, since the numerous cases of histocompatibility-linked specific controls of immune responsiveness suggest that antigen recognition by helper cells is determined by immune response (Ir) genes (see Section IV) that are located in the *I* region of the *H-2* complex and are thus not linked to the heavy-chain linkage group (Ig-1 complex) (Herzenberg et al., 1968; Eichmann, 1975a). One might speculate, therefore, that the genome of the mouse carries two similar or identical sets of V genes, one located in the Ig-1 complex and expressed in B lymphocytes, the other located in the *I* region of the *H-2* complex and expressed in T lymphocytes.

Table III shows the results of a pilot experiment in which A/J and BALB/c mice were primed in a crisscross fashion with Strep.A, anti-A5A Id1, or anti-S117 Id1. Their spleen cells were challenged in culture with TNP-Strep.A, and 4 days later, the number of TNP-specific PFC in each culture was measured. Some cultures of the homologously primed spleen cells, i.e., anti-A5A Id1-primed A/J spleen cells and anti-S117 Id1-primed BALB/c spleen cells, received anti-A5A or anti-S117 serum to examine the specificity of helper function.

It is apparent from the data that although helper cells were elicited in both strains by priming with Strep.A, only strain A/J produced helper cells in response to priming with anti-A5A Id1, and only BALB/c produced helper cells in response to priming with anti-S117 Id1. Furthermore, the response of anti-A5A Id1-primed A/J cells was inhibited by addition of anti-A5A but not anti-S117 serum to the cultures. Conversely, the response of anti-S117 Id1-primed BALB/c spleen cells could be inhibited by addition of anti-S117 but not anti-A5A serum to the cultures. It is clear from the data that helper-cell priming as well as inhibition of the helper function by āId reveal the same idiotypic polymorphism as has been observed for the corresponding antibodies (Black *et al.*, 1976; Berek *et al.*, 1976).

The genetic basis of helper-cell responsiveness to āId was studied in more detail in a panel of 13 inbred strains of mice that were defined for their *H-2* haplotypes and for the expression of the A5A and S117 idiotypes in their immunoglobulins (Hämmerling *et al.*, 1976a). One group of animals of each strain was immunized with Strep.A, another with anti-A5A Id1, and a third with anti-S117 Id1. In each group, the splenic-helper-cell activity toward Strep.A was measured by *in vitro* challenge with TNP-Strep.A and subsequent determination of TNP-specific PFC. The idiotypic specificity of helper-cell receptors was verified by inhibition experiments in which antiidiotypic antisera were included in the cultures. In all cases, spleen cells of unimmunized animals were also analyzed.

A schematic representation of the overall results is given in Table IV. The detailed experimental data for these strains are not given, because they were strictly analogous to those of strains A/J and BALB/c represented in Table III.

Table IV. Strain Distribution of Helper-Cell Responsiveness to Antiidiotype

Strain	*H-2* complex	Ig-1 complex			Helper-cell stimulation with:		
		Ig-1	A5A	S117	Anti-A5A	A-S117	Strep.A
DBA/2	d	c	cr[a]	cr	+	+	+
RF	k	c	cr	cr	+	+	+
A/J	a	e	+	−	+	−	+
A.SW	s	e	+	−	+	−	+
BALB/c	d	a	−	+	−	+	+
129	b	a	−	+	−	+	+
BAB 14	d	b	−	+	−	+	+
C57B1/10Sn	b	b	−	−	−	−	+
B10.A	a	b	−	−	−	−	+
B10.S(7R)	th	b	−	−	−	−	+
B10.D2	d	b	−	−	−	−	+
B10.BR	k	b	−	−	−	−	+
AKR	k	d	−	−	−	−	+

[a]Strain expresses idiotypes that are cross-reactive but clearly distinct from A5A and S117. From Hämmerling *et al.*, 1976a.

Inspection of Table IV reveals a perfect correlation between helper-cell responsiveness to antiidiotypic stimulation and the presence of the corresponding idiotypic V_H marker at the immunoglobulin level. No such correlation is found between responsiveness and any of the various *H-2* haplotypes. In addition, the *H-2* complexes of three responding strains (A/J, ASW, and DBA/2) do not establish responsiveness when inserted into the genome of a nonresponder (C57B1/10.Sn).

From these studies, it was concluded that helper-cell responsiveness to āId required the presence of the gene that encodes the variable region of the heavy chain of the antibody molecule to which the āId was prepared, but was independent of a particular *H-2* haplotype.

4. Presence of V_H Idiotypes and Absence of V_L Idiotypes on Helper Cell Receptors

Direct evidence for the presence of V_H idiotypes on T helper cells was brought out by the use of antisera that react preferentially with either the V_H or the V_L region of the A5A antibody. These antisera were identified during our attempt to correlate fine specificity behavior of antiidiotypic antisera with pronounced differences in their effectiveness in helper cell sensitization. In these experiments, anti-A5A antisera were screened with respect to the genetic segregation of the idiotypes they detect, and for reactivity with antibody molecules artificially recombined out of heavy and light polypeptide chains from A5A and from pooled mouse IgG (MIgG) (Krawinkel *et al.*, 1976).

Two types of fine specificity behavior observed in these screening studies proved useful for further elucidating the T-cell receptor idiotypes. The first type is characterized by preferential reactivity with recombined molecules containing the A5A H chain (A5AH-MIgGL) and the idiotypes detected by these antisera show an allotype-(C_H)-linked inheritance pattern. The second type shows preferential reactivity with recombined molecules containing the A5A L chain (MIgGH-A5AL) and the idiotypes identified by these antisera segregate unlinked or partially linked to allotype (Krawinkel *et al.*, 1976). These antisera were tested for their capacity to sensitize T helper cells *in vivo* by injecting their IgG1 fractions into mice, and for their capacity to inhibit the helper effect *in vitro* by adding the total antisera to our microculture system (Eichmann, 1977).

Results of representative experiments are summarized in Table V. It is clear from the data that antiidiotypic antibodies with preferential V_L reactivity are rather ineffective in sensitization of T helper cells *in vivo*, and a 10-fold increase of the dose improves the response. In contrast, antiidiotypic antibodies with preferential V_H reactivity are highly effective in helper cell sensitization and a 10-fold increase of the dose impairs the response. Similarly antisera with preferential V_L reactivity do not inhibit helper cells *in vitro* in concentrations at which antisera with preferential V_H reactivity are highly inhibitory.

Table V. Sensitization and Inhibition of T Helper Cells
by Antiidiotypic Antibodies with Preferential
Reactivity Toward V_H or V_L Regions[a]

Antiserum	Sensitization[f] of helper cells ($\bar{a}$ TNP PFC)	Inhibition[g] of helper cells ($\bar{a}$ TNP PFC)
	8	100
NGPS[b]	ND	1:1350 79
		1: 450 72
$\bar{a}$MIg(MIgG abs)[c]	100 μg 6	1:1500 101
		1: 500 89
$\bar{a}$A5A L > H[d]	0.1 μg 21	10 ng 89
	1.0 μg 42	30 ng 85
$\bar{a}$A5A H > L[e]	0.1 μg 90	10 ng 39
	1.0 μg 57	30 ng 13
Strep. A	100	ND

[a]Data from Eichmann, 1977.

[b]Normal guinea pig serum.

[c]Guinea pig antiserum to pooled mouse IgG (MIgG), completely absorbed on a MIgG column, to serve as control for anti-A5A sera which are also absorbed on MIgG columns. 100 μg IgG1 was injected in sensitization experiments.

[d]Anti-A5A antiserum which binds 4.5 times more A5AL-MIgGH molecules than A5AH-MIgGL molecules (for details see Krawinkel et al., 1977). 1.0 μg idiotype binding capacity (IBC) corresponds to about 120 μg IgG1.

[e]Anti-A5A antiserum which binds 13 times more A5AH-MIgGL molecules than A5AL-MIgGH molecules (for details see Krawinkel et al., 1977). 1.0 μg IBC corresponds to about 90 μg IgG1.

[f]Sensitization experiments were carried out by injecting purified IgG1 fractions from the various guinea pig antisera intraperitoneally into A/J mice. Spleen cells were tested for sensitization in our microculture system (Black et al., 1976) using Strep.A-TNP as antigen and testing for anti-TNP plaque-forming cells. The PFC numbers are given as percent of that produced by control cultures of Strep.A-sensitized spleen cells, which vary between 100 and 500 PFC/10^6 input cells.

[g]Inhibition experiments were carried out by adding to the cultures the nonfractionated guinea pig antisera. The antiidiotypic sera are diluted according to their IBC and the control sera were diluted accordingly. The PFC responses are given in percent of responses of cultures that did not contain any inhibitor, which varied between 80 and 300 PFC/10^6 input cells. The spleen cells used in these experiments were presensitized with an anti-A5A antibody with exclusive V_H specificity, whose inhibition data are similar to that with preferential V_H reactivity shown here.

These studies indicate that the receptor of T helper cells sensitized by anti-A5A idiotype antibody does not possess the total complement of the idiotypic determinants of the A5A antibody and is therefore not passively absorbed. The receptor molecule on T cells appears to possess only the V_H region in common with the A5A antibody. The V_L region seems to be either absent or inaccessible to antiidiotypic antibody.

C. Stimulation of Suppressor T Cells by Antiidiotypic Antibody

1. Idiotypic Properties of Suppressor T Cells

Several laboratories have shown that large doses of nonfractionated antiidiotypic antibodies cause the suppression of the production of idiotype on subsequent challenge with antigen (Nisonoff and Bangasser, 1975; Köhler, 1975; Eichmann, 1974). Similarly, guinea pig IgG2 antiidiotypic antibody or unfractionated antiserum against the strain A/J antibody A5A has a suppressive effect on the expression of the A5A idiotype in adult A/J mice immunized with Group A streptococci. High doses of āId2 cause an immediate but transient suppression, whereas low doses of āId2 result in a delayed but chronic suppression that lasted for more than 1 year without any indication of recovery (Eichmann, 1974, 1975b).

Chronic suppression by low doses of unfractionated IgG2 antiidiotypic antibody is the result of the induction of suppressor T cells that appear to be the mirror image of the helper T cells induced by low doses of IgG1 antiidiotypic antibody. Spleen cells from mice that had received low doses of IgG2 antiidiotypic antibody, when transferred into slightly irradiated syngeneic recipients, suppress the idiotypic response in these recipients. Further experiments on these suppressor cells revealed that (1) only about 10^5 spleen cells per recipient are needed for suppression; (2) the suppressor cells can be enriched by adherence to and elution from histamine–rabbit serum albumin Sepharose 2B columns (Eichmann, 1975b); (3) the suppressor cells bear the Ia and presumably also the Ly-2,3 antigens characteristic also of other suppressor cells (Herzenberg et al., 1975; Hämmerling et al., 1976b; Tada et al., 1975); and (4) the suppressor cells can be killed by antiidiotype and C', but not by idiotype and C' (Hämmerling and Eichmann, unpublished data).

The observations that the suppressor T cells are induced as well as eliminated by antiidiotypic antibody suggest that the suppressor cells possess an idiotype-bearing—and thus antigen-recognizing—receptor, as do the helper cells. The differential expression of antigens on helper and suppressor cells indicates that each of the two cell types represents a distinct subclass of T cells with a characteristic effector function.

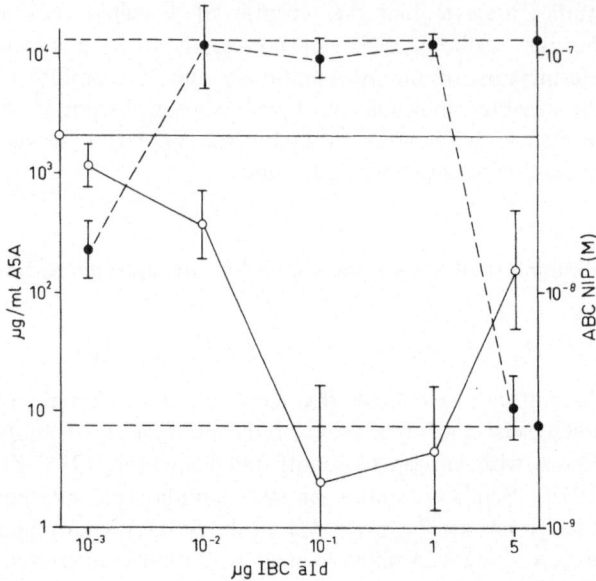

Fig. 2. Dose dependence of the induction of helper cells (●– –●) by anti-A5A Id1, and of the induction of suppressor cells (○——○) by anti-A5A Id2. The antigen-binding capacity for NIP (right ordinate) is a measure of T-helper-cell activity, and was determined in the sera of sublethally irradiated recipient A/J mice that had obtained spleen cells from A/J mice primed with increasing doses of anti-A5A Id1 (abscissa), together with spleen cells from mice primed with NIP-CG. The recipient mice were boosted with NIP-Strep.A to produce an adoptive secondary anti-NIP response. The anti-NIP response without the addition of helper cells and the anti-NIP response of homologously primed and boosted cells are indicated by the lower and upper horizontal dashed lines, respectively. For experimental details, see Eichmann and Rajewsky (1975) and Rajewsky et al. (1976).

The A5A idiotype concentrations (left ordinate) are a measure of suppressor-cell activity, and were determined in the sera of 200-rad-irradiated A/J mice that had received 2.5×10^7 pooled normal spleen cells together with 1×10^5 spleen cells from A/J mice previously treated with increasing doses of anti-A5A Id2 (abscissa). The mice were immunized with Strep.A 6 weeks after cell transfer. The A5A concentration in mice that had received normal spleen cells only is indicated by the solid horizontal line. For experimental details, see Eichmann (1975b).

2. Symmetry of Helper- and Suppressor-Cell Induction

The induction of helper and suppressor T cells by antiidiotypic antibody follows similar dose–response relationships and kinetics.

Figure 2 shows the symmetry of the dose dependences in the induction of helper cells and of suppressor cells by IgG1 and IgG2 antiidiotypic antibodies to A5A in A/J mice. It is clear from the curves that the concentrations of circulating āId antibody needed to induce optimal helper and suppressor cell

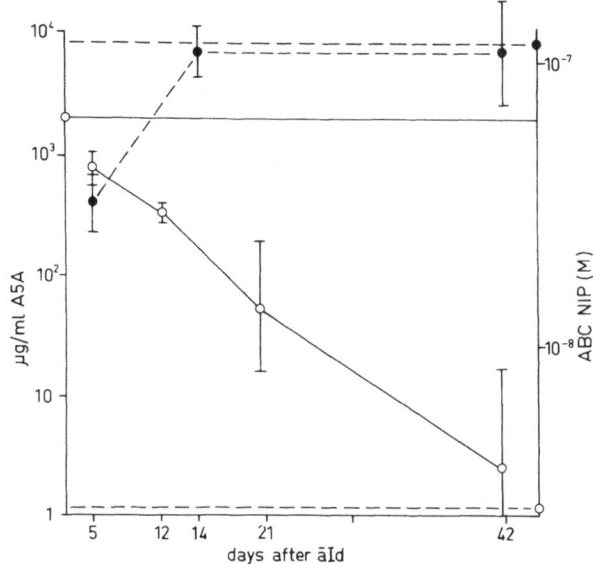

Fig. 3. Time course for the induction of helper cells (●– –●) by anti-A5A Id1 and of the induction of suppressor cells (○——○) by anti-A5A Id2. The antigen-binding capacity for NIP (right ordinate) is a measure of helper-cell activity, and was determined in an adoptive transfer experiment similar to that described for Fig. 2. The recipients received helper cells from mice that had been primed with an optimal dose (0.1 μg IBC) of anti-A5A Id1 at various times before transfer (abscissa). The anti-NIP response without the addition of helper cells and that of homologously primed and boosted cells are indicated by the lower and upper horizontal dashed lines, respectively. For experimental details, see Eichmann and Rajewsky (1975) and Rajewsky *et al.* (1976).

The A5A idiotype concentrations (left ordinate) are a measure of suppressor-cell activity, and were determined in the sera of 200-rad-irradiated recipients that had received 2.5×10^7 pooled normal spleen cells together with 1×10^5 spleen cells from A/J mice treated with an optimal dose (0.1 μg IBV) of anti-A5A Id2 at various times before transfer. The recipients were immunized with Strep.A 6 weeks after transfer. The A5A concentration in the sera of mice that had not received suppressor cells is indicated by the solid horizontal line. For experimental details, see Eichmann (1975b).

functions, respectively, are similar or identical, and that the choice of cell type induced depends solely on the class of antiidiotypic antibody (Rajewsky *et al.,* 1976; Eichmann, 1975b).

A similar symmetry is observed with respect to the time course of induction of helper and suppressor cells by optimal doses of āId. As shown in Fig. 3, both helper and suppressor activity are detected as early as 5 days after injection of āId. Suppressor activity was optimal 6 weeks after injection. The time of optimal helper activity was not determined in the experiment represented in Fig. 3, but in an undocumented experiment, optimal help was also found 6 weeks after injection of āId.

3. The Network Aspect of a Symmetrical Cooperative System
with Similar Idiotypes on T and B Cells

Jerne proposed a network concept of immune regulation the key elements of which are the variable domains of receptor molecules. These domains interact with each other through the recognition of idiotypic determinants (idiotopes) by binding sites (paratopes) (Jerne, 1974, 1976).

This chapter is not the context in which to review the implications of our experiments with respect to the network idea, as has been exhaustively done by Jerne (1976) and others (Richter, 1976; Hoffmann, 1975). Only insofar as the interaction of helper- and suppressor-T-cell receptors with āId is concerned, and in regard to the symmetry of stimulation of those cells, a few points will be mentioned that strongly suggest the participation of antiidiotypic stimulation in the regulation of an immune response: (1) Small quantities of āId may induce the complete set of lymphocytes that participate in a humoral immune response. The quantities (1–100 ng/mouse) are of the same order as the concentration of autogenous āId expected in the circulation (Köhler, 1975). (2) The choice of regulator T cell (suppressor or helper) is made solely by the class of āId. Since suppressor and helper cells are likely to be involved in the majority of immune responses, and since antigens are unlikely to possess the functional properties of Ig subclasses, one can speculate that in most if not all immune responses, the extent of help and suppression is regulated by autogenous āId. It may well be that the true functional significance of Ig classes may be revealed in their role in antiidiotypic regulation. (3) The induction of helpers and suppressors proceeds for a period of at least 6 weeks after a single injection of soluble antiidiotypic antibody. This result can be explained by continuous action of the injected āId throughout this period, but we see as more likely a self-perpetuating idiotype–antiidiotype stimulation process that is merely initiated by the first injection of āId. (4) It may be a necessary prerequisite for a functional idiotypic network that T and B cells recognizing the same determinant can express similar idiotopes. This idiotypic similarity allows for a direct feedback regulation of *all* cells participating in a particular immune response. Only by this means can a network fulfill a physiological function, namely, self-stimulation of a weak and self-suppression of an overwhelming immune response.

IV. Ir GENE CONTROL OF SPECIFIC HELPER FUNCTION

The experimental evidence reported so far is compatible with the simple view that the functional antigen receptors on T helper and suppressor cells are antibody molecules. However, the major histocompatibility complex (MHC), which is of fundamental importance to most T-cell functions, also participates in the control of helper-cell function and thus confuses the picture.

We cannot, in the frame of this chapter, deal in any detail with MHC-linked immune response gene control of immune responsiveness. This has been done in many books and review articles (e.g., Benacerraf and Katz, 1975). Here, we list only those points that are most relevant for the T-cell-receptor problem.

1. Genes in the MHC, which is not linked to any known antibody structural gene, specifically control immune responsiveness to a large variety of antigens. These genes are called *immune response* (Ir) genes (Benacerraf and McDevitt, 1972). In the mouse, they map in the *I* region of the *H-2* complex, and three *Ir* loci have so far been separated by recombination (Schreffler and David, 1975). Ir genes are defined functionally, by the level of the immune response to a given antigen.

2. Ir gene control is exquisitely specific: high-responder animals to one antigen can be low responders to another. Furthermore, it has been possible in the case of two protein antigens, namely, insulin (Keck, 1975) and lysozyme (Hill and Sercarz, 1975), to define single antigenic determinants on the antigenic molecule that appear to be the target of Ir gene control.

3. Ir genes control the overall immune response to multideterminant antigens. Thus, as an example, in the immune response against insulin and lysozymes, a variety of antibodies against various determinants on these antigens are formed. Yet, the overall immune response, which is under Ir gene control, depends on the absence or presence of a single or only a few selected determinants.

4. The Ir gene system appears to be highly polymorphic. This is nicely exemplified by our own investigations on the Ir gene control of responsiveness to porcine lactic dehydrogenase (LDH) in mice (Melchers *et al.,* 1973; Melchers and Rajewsky, 1975). At least five different response levels were found that are controlled by *H-2*-linked Ir genes. Complementation studies and the analysis of mice carrying recombinant *H-2* haplotypes established that responsiveness to LDH is determined by at least two, but probably more than two, distinct and polymorphic interacting loci in the *I* region of the *H-2* complex (Melchers and Rajewsky, 1975; Melchers, unpublished results). Similar results have been obtained in other systems (reviewed by Benacerraf and Dorf, 1976).

5. At the cellular level, Ir genes control regulator (helper or suppressor) T-cell function. It is clear from a large body of experimental evidence, including our own data, that low-responder animals will in general produce a perfectly normal antibody response if one substitutes for helper function by attaching to the antigen a carrier molecule that will be "recognized" by helper cells. In certain systems, however, Ir gene control operates via the induction of antigen-specific suppressor T cells (reviewed by Benacerraf and Dorf, 1976).

6. At the molecular level, the mechanism if Ir gene control is unresolved.

However, the hypothesis that these genes may code for T-cell receptor molecules (Benecerraf and McDevitt, 1972) has recently gained support from the discovery of T-cell-derived antigen-specific factors that specifically enhance or suppress immune responses and carry determinants encoded by the *I* region of *H-2* (Munro and Taussig, 1975; Mozes, 1976; Takemori and Tada, 1975; Tada *et al.*, 1975). Munro and Taussig (1975) and Mozes (1976) have shown in addition that low-responder animals, in contrast to high responders, either fail to produce the specific factor or fail to respond to it. Crosses between these two types of low responders complemented to high responsiveness.

If indeed, as these results suggest, Ir genes participate in the coding of antigen-binding T cell receptors, we have to ask ourselves how the specificity of Ir gene regulation, which suggests a restricted receptor repertoire, can be explained together with our results on the functional specificity (Section II) and idiotypic properties (Section III) of helper-cell receptors.

V. PROPERTIES OF ISOLATED ANTIGEN-BINDING RECEPTORS OF PUTATIVE T-CELL ORIGIN

A. Specific Isolation of Antigen Receptors from T and B Lymphocytes

The structural analysis of T-cell receptors for antigen and a direct determination of their antigen-binding specificity require the chemical isolation of the receptor molecules from the lymphocyte surface. Very recently, we have devised a method by which antigen-binding material can be specifically isolated from antigen-binding T and B lymphocytes (Krawinkel and Rajewsky, 1976; Krawinkel *et al.*, 1976).

In order to achieve this isolation, we made use of the observation by Rutishauser and Edelman (1972) and Kiefer (1973, 1975) and T and B lymphocytes can be specifically adsorbed to hapten-coated nylon at low temperature. The cells can be subsequently released from the nylon mesh by increasing the temperature to 25°C (Kiefer, 1973). We found that after cell release, antigen-binding material can be eluted from the nylon disks with acidic buffer or with buffer containing free hapten. Apparently, the cells leave this material behind when they are released into the medium, and we consider it to represent antigen-binding surface receptors of these cells.

The antigen-binding specificity of the material can be verified by its capacity to inactivate bacteriophage T4 coated with the corresponding hapten, and the haptenated phage inactivation assay (Mäkelä, 1966; Haimovich and Sela,

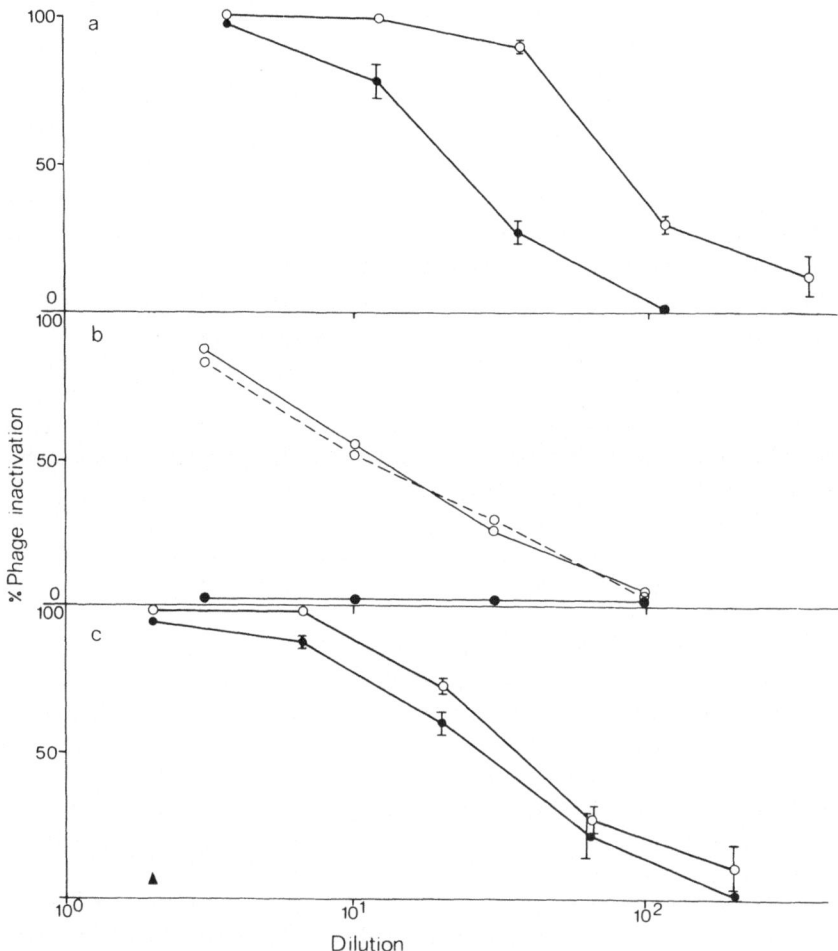

Fig. 4. Inactivation of NIP (4-hydroxy-5-iodo-3-nitrophenacetyl)-T4 phage by NP–nylon-eluted material from various NP_{13}-chicken gammaglobulin primed C57BL/6 lymphocyte populations. (a) Hapten-binding material derived from spleen cells. T-cell content 36%; T-cell input 1.7×10^9 cells; final volume of receptor preparation 6.5 ml. (b) Hapten-binding material derived from B-cell-enriched spleen cells. B-cell content 81%; B-cell input 2.8×10^9 cells; final volume 3 ml. (c) Hapten-binding material derived from T-cell-enriched spleen cells. T-cell content 85%; T-cell input 1.7×10^9 cells; final volume of receptor preparation 6.5 ml. Enrichment of T cells by nylon wool filtration, and of B cells by treatment with antiserum to Thy-1.2 and complement. The fraction of B cells was determined by staining cells with fluorescein-coupled rabbit anti-MIg antiserum and counting stained cells in a fluorescence microscope. NIP-T4 inactivation was measured before (o——o) and after (•——•) absorption of nylon-eluted material by insolubilized polyvalent rabbit anti-MIg serum, and (Fig. 4b) after absorption by insolubilized normal rabbit serum (o– –o). (▲) Inhibition of inactivation by NIP_9-BSA at a concentration of 1.4 mg/ml. None of the receptor preparations inactivated uncoupled T4 phage (not shown). From Krawinkel *et al.*, 1976.

1966; Becker and Mäkelä, 1975) thus provides a convenient method for its titration.

Receptors isolated from splenic lymphocytes by this method fall into two classes. The first class consists of material that binds to insolubilized anti-immunoglobulin antisera. It appears likely that this material is a B-cell product, since more than 95% of the receptors isolated from purified B cells (i.e., splenic lymphocytes treated with antiserum to Thy-1 and complement) carry class-specific immunoglobulin determinants (Fig. 4b).

The second class of antigen-binding material isolated from splenic lymphocytes does not appear to carry class-specific antigenic determinants of immunoglobulin polypeptide chains. Experiments with nylon-wool-purified T lymphocytes (Julius et al., 1973) show that this fraction of antigen-binding material is proportional to the fraction of T lymphocytes in the input cell population (Fig. 4a,c). It is therefore likely to represent antigen-binding receptors of T lymphocytes.

B. Properties of Isolated Receptor Molecules

What are the properties of the fraction of receptor molecules that appears to be T-cell-derived? Our knowledge here is still rather limited.

Extensive experiments have shown that the material does not appear to carry class-specific antigenic determinants of μ, γ, α, δ, k, or λ immunoglobulin polypeptide chains (Krawinkel and Rajewsky, 1976; Cramer et al., 1977). In addition, anti-Ia antisera have so far failed to react detectably with these molecules (Cramer et al., 1977) and in gel filtration and sucrose gradient experiments, antigen-binding activity was found mainly in the region of 7 S IgG, but was not detectable in regions corresponding to the molecular weights reported by others for antigen-specific T-cell-derived factors (Section IV.6).

The variable portion of the receptor molecules has been characterized both in antigen-binding studies and by idiotypic analysis. Whereas in our original study (Krawinkel and Rajewsky, 1976) their average affinity for antigen was found to be distinctly lower than that of B-cell-derived receptors, later experiments have revealed that this result represented an exception rather than the rule, and that the average affinities of both classes of receptor material appear to be in the same range in most instances (Krawinkel et al., 1976, 1977a).

We have recently shown that as expected from our idiotypic analysis of T-cell function (Section III), the receptor material which we consider T-cell-derived carries variable portions of immunoglobulin heavy chains (Krawinkel et al., 1977a). C57BL/6 mice when immunized with NP (4-hydroxy-3-nitrophenacetyl)-carrier conjugates produce rather homogeneous anti-NP antibody in the primary response. This antibody carries a fine specificity marker and an idiotypic marker which are both controlled by a gene or genes in the heavy-chain linkage group (Imanishi and Mäkelä, 1974; Jack et al., 1977). When NP-specific receptor material is isolated from NP-sensitized C57BL/6 lymphocytes, it can be shown that the fraction lacking class- and type-specific immunoglobulin determinants expresses both of these markers. In the case of the idiotype, 60–80% of the receptor material binds specifically to insolubilized antiidiotypic antibody. Genetic experiments indicate that as in the case of humoral antibody, idiotype and fine specificity of the receptor material are controlled by a gene or genes in the heavy-chain linkage group. Finally, our preliminary indication that receptor material derived from rabbit T-lymphocytes carries the a locus allotypic specificities (though again lacking class-specific immunoglobulin determinants) (Krawinkel et al., 1976) has been confirmed in more recent experiments (Krawinkel et al., 1977b). The a locus allotypic specificities are genetic markers of variable portions of immunoglobulin heavy chains.

VI. DISCUSSION

A. General Considerations: One Class or Several Classes of T-Cell Receptors?

In this chapter, we have dealt with four different pieces of information concerning antigen recognition by T lymphocytes:

1. The specificity and heterogeneity of helper-cell receptors as compared with that of humoral antibody.
2. The idiotypic specificity of helper- and suppressor-cell receptors.
3. Biochemical and serological properties of isolated antigen-binding receptors of putative T-cell origin.
4. Ir gene control of immune responsiveness at the (T) helper-cell level.

Does all this information relate to a single class of receptor molecules? This question will turn up again and again in this discussion. The reason is that the problem of antigen recognition by T cells has been approached from a variety of angles, and a number of apparently conflicting phenomena have been discovered. Thus, T-cell receptors exhibit a tremendous discriminatory capacity toward antigens (Section II), yet a large proportion, probably the majority of the T-cell population, is specific for products of the major histocompatibility locus (Wilson et al., 1968; Nisbet et al., 1969; Ford et al., 1975; Chapter 4). Functional T-cell receptors bear idiotypes of immunoglobulin heavy chains (Section II), yet antigen-specific T-cell factors have been isolated that carry antigenic determinants coded for by the MHC (see Section IV), and these factors, as well as antigen-binding material specifically isolated from T cells, do not react with class-specific antiimmunoglobulin antisera (Section V). In addition, Ir genes in the MHC control antigen recognition by T cells in a seemingly specific way (Section IV), and T cells appear to see antigen in association with products of the MHC (Chapters 5 and 6).

The easiest way to resolve these discrepancies is to assume two distinct classes of T cell receptors, one related to conventional immunoglobulin, the other coded for in the MHC. These two classes of receptors could be expressed either in all T cells or in distinct T-cell subpopulations that have indeed been very distinctly defined functionally and on the basis of their surface antigens (see Chapter 2).

A special form of this general idea is the view that helper or suppressor T cells or both recognize antigen via passively adsorbed B-cell-derived antibody (Crone *et al.*, 1972; Playfair *et al.*, 1974). One might imagine, for example (Crone *et al.*, 1972), that antigen could primarily bind to the "intrinsic" surface receptors of these cells, and then in turn bind humoral antibody from the circulation. This second layer of receptor molecules could then determine helper- and suppressor-cell specificities in the secondary response. Antigen-mediated arming of T lymphocytes by humoral antibody has indeed been observed (Hudson *et al.*, 1974; Krammer *et al.*, 1975), although its functional significance remains obscure.

We shall still make an attempt in the discussion that follows to incorporate all our experimental evidence and that of other authors into the picture of only one kind of receptor molecule. The concept of two unlinked genetic loci such as the *Ig-1* and the *H-2* complex participating in the construction of single receptor molecule is in fact no more than an extension of a principle already encountered in the classic antibody molecule.

In particular, we see no good reason at this stage to seriously consider the "arming" hypothesis outlined above. The arguments for this do not come only from the general agreement of many laboratories that little conventional immunoglobulin is present on T lymphocytes under physiological conditions (reviewed by Viretta and Uhr (1975), whereas antigen receptors *not* carrying class-specific immunoglobulin determinants can be isolated from these cells (Section V and Chapter 4). In addition, our data in Section II.C suggest pronounced binding heterogeneity at the level of the intrinsic receptors of virgin T helper cells, and the results are in good accord with those obtained for the specificity of sensitized T helper cells (Section II.B). Furthermore, our own attempts (Rajewsky and Rottländer, 1967; Rajewsky *et al.*, 1969), as well as those of many other authors (reviewed by Katz and Benacerraf, 1972, and Janeway *et al.*, 1975), to substitute helper function by passive administration of antibody have entirely failed. Janeway *et al.* (1975) listed the various systems in which antibody-mediated enhancement of immune responses has been observed, and we share entirely their view that these effects are likely to be based on mechanisms other than classic T—B collaboration. As an example, the enhancement of the immune response by IgM antibodies (Henry and Jerne, 1968) may relate to the gross distribution of antigen in the body (Dennert *et al.*, 1971). Finally, immuno-globulin idiotypes have been discovered on T-cell receptors in our system (Section III), as well as in other systems (Ramseier, 1973, 1974; McKearn *et al.*, 1974a,b; Binz *et al.*, 1975; Binz and Wigzell, Chapter 4), and in one of them, there is evidence that the idiotypic receptors are indeed synthesized by the T cells that carry them (Chapter 4). Our own experiments which show that T-cell receptors and antibodies share indeed only the variable region of the heavy chain almost formally disprove the arming hypothesis. Although it could still be argued that only free heavy chain V regions are absorbed to and serve as receptors on T cells, it seems more reasonable to assume that the idiotypic determinants are indeed a product of the T cells that express them. We consider it justified therefore to continue our discussion on the basis that these deter-minants are part of the intrinsic T-cell-receptor molecules.

B. Variable Portion of T-Cell Receptors

1. Antigen-Binding Properties of T-Cell Receptors

Our functional analysis of the antigen-binding properties of T-helper-cell receptors indicates that these receptors and humoral antibodies exhibit similar heterogeneity and discriminate antigens similarly. This conclusion is in accord with a large body of evidence from many laboratories (including the work of Weinbaum *et al.*, 1974, in a very similar system), but also disagrees at first sight with results obtained in a variety of experimental systems in which pronounced differences between antibody specificity and the specificity of T-cell function have been observed (reviewed by Paul, 1970; Schlossman, 1972; Rajewsky and Mohr, 1974; and Janeway, 1976).

It is clear, however, that this discrepancy does not necessarily relate to the molecular identity of the T-cell receptor. First of all, the functional analysis of T-cell-receptor specificity suffers *a priori* from the fact that the functional activation of a T cell by antigen must be expected to depend not only on the receptor—determinant interaction, but also on many other properties of the antigen, such as charge, state of aggregation, gross distribution in and elimination from the body, and so on. This problem which was carefully avoided in our experiments, poses itself most severely when cross-reactions of native and chemically modified antigens are compared at the T- and B-cell levels, and it appears significant to us that perhaps the most striking example of differences in T- and B-cell "recognition" has arisen in such systems.

Second, it is well established that the repertoire of specificities is differentially modulated in the T- and B-cell system during ontogeny. An example of this is selective T-cell paralysis induced by low doses of antigens (Chiller *et al.*, 1971; Mitchison, 1971; Rajewsky, 1971) leading to a severe restriction of helper-cell heterogeneity as compared with that of antibody-forming cell percursors (Rajewsky and Brenig, 1974; Section II.C). Again, this problem was eliminated in our cross-stimulation experiments. It is relevant in this context to mention the problem of carbohydrate-specific receptors in the T-helper-cell system. Carbohydrate-specific helper cells have to our knowledge not so far been detected in animals sensitized with carbohydrate antigens. However, the experiments reported in Section III.B.2 clearly demonstrate that helper cells, if sensitized with antiidiotypic antibody instead of the corresponding carbohydrate antigen, can very well express receptors with specificity for carbohydrate antigens.

Taking the various data together, the functional analysis of the antigen-binding properties of T-helper-cell receptors suggests that the repertoire of binding sites in this system is large, potentially as large as that of antibody-combining sites. In addition, the similarity of antigen discrimination by helper-cell receptors and humoral antibodies found under appropriate conditions suggests that the binding sites on these two classes of molecules may be structurally related. This view is reinforced by the finding of the same idiotypic determinants on the antigen-binding portions of both molecules.

However, there is also experimental evidence from which serious objections to this simple interpretation can be derived.

One such piece of evidence was obtained in experiments in which the binding of antigens to the T- and B-cell surface was compared (Hämmerling and McDevitt, 1974). Striking differences in the specificity of binding were observed that could be explained either by a lower density or, more likely, a lower affinity of T-cell receptors as compared with the receptors on B cells. Our initial data on the affinity for antigen of isolated receptor molecules were in accord with the latter interpretation (Krawinkel and Rajewsky, 1976). However, as mentioned in Section V.B, later, more systematic experiments again support the notion that in general, the affinities of T- and B-cell receptors for antigen are rather similar (Krawinkel *et al.*, 1977a).

Directly relevant for helper T cells, though only indirectly related to helper cell receptor specificity, is the Ir gene phenomenon (Section IV). Ir genes in the MHC specifically control T-helper-cell function in specific immune responses. The possibility that these genes participate in the coding for T-cell-receptor molecules is supported by the discovery of antigen-specific T-cell factors carrying antigenic determinants encoded by genes in the same region of the *H-2* complex in which the Ir genes are also located (discussed below). Apparently, the specificity of Ir gene control is profoundly different from the specificity of humoral antibodies, since it concerns the overall immune response to multideterminant antigens. Thus, if Ir genes do indeed code for T-cell receptors, the diversity of these receptors must be severely restricted at least in a functional sense.

We shall have to examine at the end of our discussion whether and how these conflicting findings can be incorporated into the picture of a single class of T-cell-receptor molecule.

2. Idiotypic Properties of T-Cell Receptors

There is no doubt that āId reacts with T cells in our experimental systems. This reaction is demonstrated in various ways: (1) āId stimulates helper cells *in vivo*. (2) āId stimulates suppressor cells *in vivo*. (3) āId inhibits helper function *in vitro*. (4) Preliminary evidence indicates that āId and C′ kill suppressor cells *in vitro*. The questions that must be discussed in this connection are: (1) Does this interaction occur with the antigen-receptor of T cells? (2) What is the significance of this serologic cross-reaction and that of the other results that relate to the idiotypic properties of T cells, such as the comparison of B- and T-cell-receptor specificity and heterogeneity? (3) If we accept the experimental data as meaningful, what is the part of the antibody that is shared between B- and T-cell receptor molecules?

We have good reason to believe that the molecule on T cells that reacts with āId is indeed the functional receptor molecule. This is brought out, first, by the specificity of āId for binding-site-related antigenic determinants of antibodies (Brient *et al.,* 1971; Hopper and Nisonoff, 1971), which makes it very unlikely that the same āId would react with a molecule not possessing an antigen-binding site on T cells. Second, the stimulatory effect of āId together with the antigen specificity of the activated cell population can be explained only by an interaction of the stimulating agent with the antigen-recognizing molecule on the cell. Third, the inhibition of helper function by āId *in vitro* strongly indicates that the idiotype-bearing molecule on T helper cells represents the functional antigen receptor of these cells. We therefore conclude that āId reacts with the antigen receptors of T helper and, by analogy, suppressor cells. Similar results have been obtained by Binz and Wigzell (Chapter 4), McKearn *et al.* (1974a,b), and Ramseier (1973, 1974) in unrelated experimental systems.

All these experiments, however, merely demonstrate that an interaction between āId and T-cell receptors occurs. With respect to the molecular identity of T-cell receptors, this demonstration has no greater significance than has any serologic cross-reactivity. Therefore, two additional parameters of B/T similarity have been established that made use of our previous observations that (1) B cells or antibodies reactive with A-CHO are idiotypically heterogeneous and (2) B cells or antibodies possess strain-specific idiotypes that are controlled by polymorphic genes that can be identified with the respective āId reagents.

For both these parameters, experiments were designed to investigate whether or not they apply to T-cell receptors as well. With respect to hetero-geneity, it was found that helper cells stimulated with antigen (Group A streptococci) contained few idiotype-positive cells, whereas all the helper cells stimulated with āId were idiotype-positive. Furthermore, helper cells stimulated with streptococci, a complex assembly of antigens, were only in part specific for A-CHO, which is but one of the streptococcal antigens. This finding was in contrast to that with helper cells stimulated with āId, all of which has specificity for A-CHO. These results are essentially in accord with the notion that T-cell receptors are identical to antibodies with respect to the clonal distribution and heterogeneity of specificities and of idiotypes.

A number of more technical objections that concern the nature of our antiidiotypic reagents should be discussed here. One concerns the possibility that these reagents are contaminated by antiidiotypic antibody against T-cell receptor that was copurified with the idiotype. In this case, two types of āId would coexist within our āId sera, one directed against T-cell-receptor idiotypes and stimulating T lymphocytes. It was particularly for this reason that we attempted to achieve helper-cell stimulation with āId to the S117 myeloma protein. This protein is produced in the absence of antigenic stimulation, and is therefore unlikely to contain any T-cell-derived receptor molecule. However, anti-S117 stimulates helper cells as well as does anti-A5A.

Other possible sources of error are the possible contamination of our antiidiotypic reagents with antigen, as well as the ubiquitous occurrence of Group A streptococci, which leads to the possibility of previous exposure in any experiment. Apart from the reasons discussed elsewhere (Eichmann and Rajew-sky, 1975) that argue against antigen contamination of our antisera, we consider the pronounced differences in the heterogeneity of antigen-primed and of āId-primed cell populations the most convincing evidence in favor of the notion that antigen exposure plays no role in our idiotype stimulation experiments (Black et al., 1975, 1976; Hämmerling et al., 1976b; Eichmann and Rajewsky, 1975).

After having accepted the conclusion that the antigen receptor of T cells possesses idiotypic determinants in common with B-cell receptors and anti-bodies, let us now consider the structural basis for this sharing of idiotypic determinants. Our antiidiotypic reagents are produced against intact antibody molecules, and the notion of idiotypic specificity comes from their lack of reactivity with normal mouse immunoglobulin or antibodies of other speci-ficities, and from the partial inhibition of their interaction with the idiotype by the immundominant sugar of A-CHO, N-acetyl-D-glucosamine (Eichmann, 1972; Berek et al., 1976; Berek, unpublished data). Thus, the shared idiotypic deter-minants of B- and T-cell receptors are in all likelihood located in the variable region of the receptor molecule.

The further identification of the shared region is based on genetic as well as

immunochemical evidence. In the early work on helper cell stimulation (Eichmann and Rajewsky, 1975) only such antisera were used that were preselected in
genetic experiments to reveal an allotype-linked inheritance pattern (Eichmann,
1975a). Thus, the antisera used were reactive with products of genes in the Ig-1
complex which is believed to contain the structural genes for the immunoglobulin heavy chains (Potter and Lieberman, 1967; Herzenberg et al., 1968;
Eichmann, 1975a). Five distinct idiotypic phenotypes of antibodies to A-CHO
correspond to five different pseudoallelic haplotypes, each containing a C_H gene
defined by the allotype and one or two V_H genes defined by idiotypes (Berek et
al., 1976). Each of these idiotypic phenotypes is inherited as a single linkage
group such that the Ig-1 complex alone determines the idiotypic phenotype.
Although the variable region of an antibody is composed of the variable regions
of both heavy and light polypeptide chains, our antiidiotypic reagents were
specific for heavy-chain variable regions alone.

The genetic evidence is based on our analysis of the polymorphism of
the genes that control T-helper-cell responsiveness to aId (Hämmerling et al.,
1976a). The rationale of this analysis was that a T cell can respond to āId only if
it carries the corresponding Id on its surface. Therefore, if the same genetic
polymorphism is expressed in helper-cell responsiveness to āId and the idiotypic
specificity of serum antibody, it becomes very likely that the idiotypic determinants on antibody molecules and T-cell surface receptors are controlled by the
same genes. Our analysis suffered from the lack of strains that were congenic for
the appropriate Ig-1 complexes. In all cases without exception, however, helper-
cell responsiveness to antiidiotypic stimulation correlated with the presence of
the corresponding Id or a cross-reacting one in the antibody population. When-
ever helper cells could be induced by āId, their function could be specifically
inhibited by the same and only the same antiidiotype.

This finding clearly indicates that both B- and T-cell idiotypes are under the
control of the Ig-1 complex. Furthermore, the data virtually rule out the
possible participation of genes in the H-2 complex in the control of T-cell
responsiveness to antiidiotypic stimulation for two reasons. The first is the
evidence in favor of the control of responsiveness by the Ig-1 complex. The
second is the apparent irrelevance of the H-2 haplotype for helper-cell sensitization by āId. When the I regions of three different strains that are responsive to
antiidiotypic stimulation (DBA/2, A/J, and S.SW) are crossed into the genome
of a nonresponder strain (C57B/10), responsiveness is not established. The
argument hinges on the assumptions that (1) the A5A and S117 idiotypes can be
expressed on the C57B1/10 genetic background and (2) the C57B1/10 strain is
not a low responder to antiidiotypic stimulation in general. Both assumptions
appear reasonable, although we cannot so far prove them to be correct. We have
shown, however, that the unresponsiveness of the various H-2 congenic strains
with the B10 background cannot be explained on the basis of a possible general

control of nonresponsiveness to antiidiotypic stimulation by Ir genes in the *H-2* complex, because the responding strains A/J, A.SW, and DBA/2 carry the same *I* regions of *H-2* in their genome as do the nonresponding strains B10.A, B10.S(7R), and B10.D2, respectively.

There is thus good reason to believe that the idiotype-bearing molecules on T cells are encoded by the same genes that control the antibody idiotypes. As was discussed above, these genes are variable-region genes for the immuno-globulin heavy chain. From these considerations, we have to conclude not only that idiotypic determinants are shared between T-cell receptors and antibodies, but that the total gene product of the V_H gene is the same for both molecules.

The identification by immunochemical and genetic means of antiidiotypic antisera that possess preferential V_L reactivity and their functional comparison to antisera that possess preferential V_H reactivity lends further support to the notion of V_H regions on T cells. A very clear correlation was found between the specificity of an antiidiotypic antibody for determinants in the V_H region and its capacity to interact with T-cell receptors. The obvious inability of antiidio-typic antibodies with V_L specificity to interact with T cells is strongly suggestive but not formal proof for the absence of V_L regions from T cells (Krawinkel *et al.*, 1976; Eichmann, 1977).

As discussed in Section V.B, variable portions of immunoglobulin heavy chains have also been identified with the help of idiotypic and fine specificity markers on our isolated receptor molecules (Krawinkel *et al.*, 1976, 1977a,b). It is reassuring to see that two entirely different experimental approaches thus lead to consistent results.

C. Constant Part of T-Cell Receptor

Very little is known about the structure of those parts of T-cell-receptor molecules that are not concerned with antigen binding. From our own experi-ments isolated receptor molecules appear to have a molecular weight in the range of $1-2 \times 10^5$ daltons and do not carry any class-specific antigenic determinants of immunoglobulin light and heavy chains (Krawinkel and Rajewsky, 1976; Section V). We have not been able so far to detect Ia determinants on those molecules (Cramer *et al.*, 1977), but the evidence here is preliminary. Our results are in good accord with those obtained by Binz and Wigzell (Chapter 4), who have detected T-cell-derived molecules with similar properties in the serum. At the present state, the constant part of these molecules can largely be defined only negatively in that serologically, it does not resemble the constant part of any conventional immunoglobulin polypeptide chain.

A second group of antigen-specific factors produced by T cells has been defined on the basis of functional activity, namely, suppressive or enhancing effects on specific immune responses (Mozes, 1976; Munro and Taussig, 1975; Tada *et al.*, 1975; Kapp *et al.*, 1976). These factors appear to have molecular weights in the order of 45,000 daltons, not to react with antiimmunoglobulin antisera, and to carry antigenic determinants encoded in the *I* region of the *H-2* complex. The *I* region of *H-2* may also determine the effector function of such factors, since factors controlled by the *I-A* subregion enhanced the B-cell responses (Munro and Taussig, 1975; Mozes, 1976), whereas the suppressive factor of Tada *et al.* (1975) is controlled by a locus between the *I-B* and *I-C* subregions (Tada, personal communication).

Thus, the dilemma already encountered at the functional level, namely, how to reconcile the exquisite specificity of T cell functions with the Ir gene phenomenon, reappears at the molecular level. Do the two kinds of antigen-binding T-cell-derived molecules represent two distinct classes of antigen receptors, or can we still interpret the results in the sense of a unifying picture of the T-cell receptor?

D. Possible Structure of the Complete T-Cell-Receptor Molecule

We will now consider various possibilities for the structure of a T-cell-receptor molecule, taking into account the following facts that appear to be either firmly established or at least very likely: (1) The V_H gene product is part of the specificity-determining region of the T-cell receptor. (2) The constant part is not a conventional C_H gene product. (3) Products of genes in the *I* region of *H-2* constitute constant parts of the molecule, and are also involved in specificity-determining portions. (4) A conventional immunoglobulin light chain does not appear to be a part of the T-cell receptor.

There are two models for the genetic control of the variable regions of immunoglobulin polypeptide chains including heavy chains. A simple model, based on the existence of a variable and a constant part of each chain and on the sharing of the same V_H region among different classes of rabbit heavy chains (reviewed by Kindt, 1975), proposes a V gene that encodes the entire variable region of each polypeptide chain. A more complex model, based on the discovery of the hypervariable regions in L-chains (Wu and Kabat, 1970) and subsequently in H-chains (Capra and Kehoe, 1975) proposes that the subgroup specific residues of the V region are coded for by genes separate from those encoding the hypervariable regions. The latter are translocated and inserted into the more constant parts as episomes, thus allowing for a great deal of diversity by scrambling the positions of hypervariable episomes (Wu and Kabat, 1970; Capra and Kindt, 1975).

Depending on which of these alternatives is correct, our genetic evidence suggests that either the total V_H region or only the hypervariable parts of it are shared between antibodies and T-cell receptors. We will, however, not differentiate between these possibilities in this discussion, since the problem of translocation (Gally and Edelman, 1972) is similar in either model. The question can be approached, however, by analyzing rabbit T-cell receptors for the presence of *a* locus allotypes, which presumably are specific for the more constant parts of the V_H region (Mole *et al.*, 1971). Recent experiments indeed suggest that these allotypic markers are expressed in receptor molecules isolated from rabbit T cells (Krawinkel *et al.*, 1976, 1977b).

How does a V_H region get connected with a C region that is not the product of a C_H gene? It would be tempting to speculate that V_H genes from the *Ig-1* complex translocate into the *H-2* complex to encode a single polypeptide chain that has antibody–idiotypic determinants together with Ia antigenic determinants. Although such a mechanism is by no means excluded, we do not favor this possibility simply because of our difficulties in imagining a reliable translocation between nonhomologous chromosomes.

For the construction of a heavy-chain analogue of the T-cell receptor, we prefer the translocation of the V_H gene onto a C_H gene in the *Ig-1* complex the product of which is not expressed in humoral antibodies. The difficulty of this model is the lack of serologic cross-reactivity with anti-Ig antisera described earlier. If the T-cell-receptor C_H gene is situated in the *Ig-1* complex, it would be the product of gene duplication and thus have structural elements in common with antibody C_H genes. We have to assume, then, that this gene is so highly conserved in evolution that those species that are commonly used for the production of antisera (mostly the rabbit) against mouse or human Ig cannot recognize this molecule. There are a number of observations in favor of this assumption. U. Hämmerling *et al.* (1976) obtained a chicken anti-mouse-IgM serum that reacts strongly with T cells, and they interpret this finding as a consequence of a greater evolutionary distance between the species involved. The reaction of this antiserum with mouse IgM could be absorbed only incompletely with T cells, suggesting partial cross-reactivity between the T-cell-surface molecule and IgM. Furthermore, the numerous cases in which various investigators have observed immunoglobulin-like molecules on T cells could be explained by occasional antisera that react with this hitherto unknown C_H region (reviewed by Marchalonis, 1976).

In addition, we have to consider the possibility that there is not one C_H gene and its product coding for a single T-cell-receptor C_H region, but that there are several such genes. T-cell-receptor heavy chains would then show a class heterogeneity similar to that shown by B-cell receptors, and their analysis would be even more complicated. This class heterogeneity could be connected with the various T-cell effector functions and classes of T cells already known (Chapter 2).

How do we account, then, for the presence of I-region-encoded antigenic determinants on T-cell-derived antigen-recognizing molecules? We will consider primarily two different molecular models for a T-cell recognition system without favoring one over the other. In both models, the heavy chain of the T-cell receptor described above will be the same. In model A, this heavy chain is associated, either through disulfide links or noncovalently, with an I-region gene product that directly modulates the binding site of the V_H region and thus contributes to specific recognition. In model B, the heavy chain, possibly in combination with an unknown light-chain analogue, and the I-region product are separate molecules. The latter permits or prevents antigen-mediated activation or suppression of immunocompetent cells on the basis of a hitherto unknown discriminatory mechanism

In model A, the I-region-encoded light-chain analogue consists either of a constant part only or of a constant and a variable part. In the latter case, there would exist in the H-2 complex a fourth V-gene cluster the products of which would combine with V_H regions to produce the V region of T-cell-receptor molecules. In the former case, the light-chain analogue of the T-cell receptor is essentially restricted to a limited choice of constant parts. A few major classes, each encoded by one of the major subregions of the I region, would confer the main effector function to the molecules, such as the ability to be accepted by B cells as well as the ability to function as an enhancing or suppressive molecule (Munro and Taussig, 1975; Takemori and Tada, 1975; Tada et al., 1975). In addition, each major class would possess a limited number of subclasses, each of which in combination with the variable regions of various heavy chains would produce the V regions of the T-cell receptor. These would maintain the idiotypes of antibodies bearing the same V_H region and would possess specificities related but not identical to that of antibody molecules. This could explain a number of observations on specificity differences between T and B cells reviewed above, such as the preferential recognition by T cells of structures coded for by the MHC, which could be mediated by the I-region-encoded polypeptide chains. The model would also be compatible with the notion that T cells recognize antigen in association with products of the MHC (Chapters 5 and 6). Finally, model A could accommodate the various molecular weights of antigen-specific T-cell factors as compared with that of our own isolated receptor molecules if we allow fragmentation of the molecule similar to that in the case of antibody molecules.

There are difficulties with the model, on the other hand, in explaining the Ir gene phenomenon, particularly as far as complex antigens are concerned. How can a diverse receptor repertoire acquire a defect for a series of antigenic determinants that have nothing more in common than being together on one complex protein?

We can construct ways in which this could happen, particularly if we assume that the *I*-region-encoded light-chain analogue occurs only in a limited set of subclasses. Genetic lack of a subclass could cause lack of recognition of a whole group of antigens. Recognition can be restored by addition of new determinants that can be recognized by T cells bearing other, nondefect, subclasses as light-chain analogues of their receptor. Antigen-specific Ir gene control is a false interpretation based on our inability to recognize the groups of antigens that are controlled by one subclass of L-chain analogues.

Model B avoids such rather difficult constructions in assuming a regulatory role for the *I*-region product in the ability of the cell to become activated by antigen. In this model, all T cells possess in principle the same receptor repertoire as B cells, and can also recognize the same antigens. This recognition, however, leads to a response (in the sense of sensitization or suppression) of the virgin cell only when the antigen can also interact with the *I*-region product. There may be a limited diversity of these products, so that genetic polymorphism could easily lead to lack of reaction to even complex antigens. In this way, we can for instance easily explain that polysaccharide-specific T cells are difficult to demonstrate by immunization with polysaccharide, but are readily demonstrable by immunization with the proper antiidiotypic antibody. We simply have to assume that polysaccharides commonly cannot successfully interact with the *I*-region product, whereas antiidiotypic antibodies can. Model B would also be in accord with our failure to detect Ia determinants on our isolated T-cell receptor, but these data are still preliminary.

It should also be pointed out, however, that if indeed double recognition of antigen is required in T-cell sensitization, one would not necessarily have to invoke a restricted spectrum of receptor specificities in order to explain the Ir gene phenomenon. The overall response would then also depend on the spatial arrangement of antigenic determinants on the antigenic molecule. Limitations of immune responses on this basis have been observed not only in T–B collaboration (Cecka *et al.*, 1976), which represents a well-established system of double recognition (Mitchison *et al.*, 1970), but also in the process of T-cell activation (Goodman *et al.*, 1974). The recent results of Erb *et al.* (1976) would fit nicely into this scheme. These authors have found that the recruitment of helper T cells *in vitro* depends on an *I*-region-coded antigen-binding factor that has a molecular weight similar to those of the Ia-bearing factors described above and is in the hands of Erb and his colleagues macrophage-derived.

To reiterate, we do not favor any of these models for the molecular nature of the T-cell recognition system over the other. It appears to us, however, that the question of the molecular nature of the T-cell receptor is no longer a matter of theoretical models. The discovery of antiidiotypic antibodies as probes for T-cell receptors, as well as the availability of methods for receptor isolation, shifts this question to the level of direct experimentation.

ACKNOWLEDGEMENTS

This chapter is based on experimental work and discussions to which many collaborators in the laboratory in Cologne have contributed, among them C. Berek-Jack, S. J. Black, C. Brenig, M. Cramer, G. J. Hämmerling, G. von Hesberg, Th. Imanishi-Kari, R. S. Jack, U. Krawinkel, I. Melchers, R. Mohr and H. Wirges-Koch. The work on isolated lymphocyte receptors would have been impossible without the help of Dr. O. Mäkelä, who kindly provided hapten-coated bacteriophages prepared by M. Becker and himself. We should also like to thank Ms. Åsa Böhm for typing this manuscript.

Our work was generously supported by the Deutsche Forschungsgemeinschaft through SFB 74.

VII. REFERENCES

Becker, M., and Mäkelä, O., 1975, Modification of bacteriophage with hapten-Σ-amino-caproyl-N-hydroxysuccinimide esters: Increased sensitivity for immunoassay, *Immunochemistry* 12:329.

Benacerraf, B., and Dorf, M., 1976, The nature and function of specific H-linked immune response genes and immune suppression genes, in: *The Role of Products of the Histocompatibility Gene Complex in Immune Responses*, p. 225 (D.H. Katz and B. Benacerraf, eds.), Academic Press, New York.

Benacerraf, B., and Katz, D.H., 1975, The histocompatibility-linked immune response genes, *Adv. Cancer Res.* 21:121.

Benacerraf, B., and McDevitt, H.O., 1972, Histocompatibility-linked immune response genes, *Science* 175:273.

Benacerraf, B., Ovary, Z., Bloch, K.J., and Franklin, E.C., 1963, Properties of guinea pig 7S antibodies. I. Electrophoretic separation of two types of guinea pig 7S antibodies, *J. Exp. Med.* 117:937.

Berek, C., Taylor, B., and Eichmann, K., 1976, Genetics of the idiotype of Balb/c myeloma S117: Multiple chromosomal loci for V_H genes encoding specificity for Group A streptococcal carbohydrate, *J. Exp. Med.* 144:1164.

Binz, H., Kimura, A., and Wigzell, H., 1975, Idiotype-positive T lymphocytes, *Scand. J. Immunol.* 4:413.

Black, S.J., Eichmann, K., Hämmerling, G.J., and Rajewsky, K., 1975, Stimulation and inhibition of T cell helper function by anti-idiotypic antibody, in: *Membrane Receptors of Lymphocytes*, p. 117 (M. Seligmann, J.L., Preud'homme, and F.M. Kourilsky, eds.), North-Holland Publishing Co., Amsterdam and New York.

Black, S.J., Hämmerling, G.J., Berek, C., Rajewsky, K., and Eichmann, K., 1976, Idiotypic analysis of lymphocytes *in vitro*. I. Specificity and heterogeneity of B and T lymphocytes reactive with anti-idiotypic antibody, *J. Exp. Med.* 143:846.

Brient, B.W., Haimovich, J., and Nisonoff, A., 1971, Reaction of anti-idiotypic antibody with the hapten binding site of a myeloma protein, *Proc. Natl. Acad. Sci. U.S.A.* 68:3136.

Briles, D.E., and Krause, R.M., 1972, Mouse antibodies to Group A streptococcal carbohydrate: Use of idiotypy to detect inbred strain specificity and to monitor spleen cell
transfer in syngeneic mice, *J. Immunol.* 109:1311.

Briles, D.E., and Krause, R.M., 1974, Mouse strain specific idiotypes and interstrain
idiotypic cross-reactions, *J. Immunol.* 113:522.

Capra, J.D., and Kehoe, J.M., 1975, Hypervariable regions, idiotypy and the antibody
combining site, *Adv. Immunol.* 20:1.

Capra, J.D., and Kindt, T.J., 1975, Antibody diversity: Can more than one gene encode
each variable region?, *Immunogenetics* 1:417.

Cecka, J.M., Stratton, J.A., Miller, A., and Sercarz, E., 1976, Structural aspects of immune
recognition of the lyzozymes. III. T-cell specificity restriction and its consequences for
antibody specificity, *Eur. J. Immunol.,* in press.

Chiller, J.M., Habicht, G.S., and Weigle, W.O., 1971, Kinetic differences in unresponsiveness
of thymus and bone marrow cells, *Science* 171:813.

Coligan, J.E., Schnute, W.C., and Kindt, T.J., 1975, Immunochemical and chemical studies
on streptococcal group-specific carbohydrates, *J. Immunol.* 114:1654.

Cramer, M., and Braun, D.G., 1975, Genetics of restricted antibodies to streptococcal group
polysaccharides in mice, *Eur. J. Immunol.* 5:823.

Cramer, M., Krawinkel, U., Hämmerling, G., Black, S.J., Berek, C., Eichmann, K., and
Rajewsky, K., 1977, Antigen receptors on mouse T-lymphocytes, in: *Proc. 3rd Ir Gene
Workshop* (W.E. Paul, H.O. McDevitt, and B. Benacerraf, eds.), Academic Press, New
York, in press.

Crone, M.M., Koch, C., and Simonsen, M., 1972, The elusive T cell receptor, *Transplant.
Rev.* 10:36.

Dennert, G., Pohlit, H., and Rajewsky, K., 1971, Cooperative antibody: A concentrating
device, in: *Cell Interactions and Receptor Antibodies in Immune Responses,* p. 3 (O.
Mäkelä, A. Cross, and T.U. Kosunen, eds.), Academic Press, New York.

Edelman, G.M., and Gall, W.E., 1969, The antibody problem, *Annu. Rev. Biochem.* 38:415.

Eichmann, K., 1972, Idiotypic identity of antibodies to streptococcal carbohydrate in
inbred mice, *Eur. J. Immunol.* 2:301.

Eichmann, K., 1973, Idiotype expression and the inheritance of mouse antibody clones, *J.
Exp. Med.* 137:603.

Eichmann, K., 1974, Idiotype suppression. I. Influence of the dose and of the effector
functions of anti-idiotypic antibody on the production of an idiotype, *Eur. J.
Immunol.* 4:296.

Eichmann, K., 1975a, Genetic control of antibody specificity in the mouse, *Immunogenetics* 2:491.

Eichmann, K., 1975b, Idiotype suppression. II. Amplification of a suppressor T cell with
anti-idiotypic activity, *Eur. J. Immunol.* 5:511.

Eichmann, K., 1977, manuscript in preparation.

Eichmann, K., and Berek, C., 1973, Mendelian segregation of a mouse antibody idiotype,
Eur. J. Immunol. 3:599.

Eichmann, K., and Berek, C., 1974, Genetically controlled idiotype expression in inbred
mice, *Ann. Immunol. (Inst. Pasteur)* 125c:359.

Eichmann, K., and Kindt, T.J., 1971, The inheritance of individual antigenic specificities of
rabbit antibodies to streptococcal carbohydrates, *J. Exp. Med.* 134:532.

Eichmann, K., and Rajewsky, K., 1975, Induction of T and B cell immunity by antiidiotypic antibody, *Eur. J. Immunol.* 5:661.

Eichmann, K., Tung, A.S., and Nisonoff, A., 1974, Linkage and rearrangement of genes
encoding mouse immunoglobulin heavy chains, *Nature (London)* 250:509.

Erb, P., Feldmann, M., and Hogg, N., 1976, The role of macrophages in the generation of T helper cells. IV. Nature of a genetically related factor derived from macrophages incubated with soluble antigens, *Eur. J. Immunol.*, in press.

Ford, W.L., Simmonds, S.I., and Alkins, R.C., 1975, Early events in a systematic graft-versus-host reaction. II. Autoradiographic estimation of the frequency of donor lymphocytes which respond to each Ag-B determined antigenic complex, *J. Exp. Med.* 141:681.

Gally, J.A., and Edelman, G.M., 1972, The genetic control of immunoglobulin synthesis, *Annu. Rev. Genet.* 6:1.

Goodman, J.W., Bellone, C.J., Hanes, D., and Nitecki, D.E., 1974, in: *Progress in Immunology II*, p. 27 (L. Brent and J. Holborow, eds.), North-Holland Publishing Co., Amsterdam and New York.

Haimovich, J., and Sela, M., 1966, Inactivation of poly-DL-alanyl bacteriophage T4 with antisera specific toward poly-DL-alanine, *J. Immunol.* 97:338.

Hämmerling, G.J., and McDevitt, H.O., 1974, Antigen binding T and B lymphocytes. I. Differences in cellular specificity and influence of metabolic activity on interaction of antigen with T and B cells, *J. Immunol.* 112:1726.

Hämmerling, G.J., Black, S.J., Berek, C., Eichmann, K., and Rajewsky, K., 1976a, Idiotypic analysis of lymphocytes *in vitro*. II. Genetic control of T helper cell responsiveness to anti-idiotypic antibody, *J. Exp. Med.* 143:861.

Hämmerling, G.J., Eichmann, K., and Sorg, C., 1976b, Differential expression of Ia antigens on suppressor T cells, helper T cells and B precursor cells, in: *The Role of Products of the Histocompatibility Gene Complex in Immune Responses,* p. 417 (D.H. Katz and B. Benacerraf, eds.), Academic Press, New York.

Hämmerling, U., Mack, C., and Pickel, H.-G., 1976, Immunofluorescence studies of Ig determinants of mouse thymocytes and T cells, *Immunochemistry* 13:525.

Henry, C., and Jerne, N.K., 1968, Competition of 19S and 7S antigen receptors in the regulation of the primary immune response, *J. Exp. Med.* 128:133.

Herzenberg, L.A., McDevitt, H.O., and Herzenberg, L.A., 1968, Genetics of antibodies, *Annu. Rev. Genet.* 2:209.

Herzenberg, L.A., Okumura, K., and Metzler, M., 1975, Regulation of immunoglobulin and antibody production by allotype suppressor T cells in mice, *Transplant. Rev.* 27:57.

Hill, S.W., and Sercarz, E.E., 1975, Fine specificity of the *H-2* linked immune response gene for the gallinaceosus lysozymes, *Eur. J. Immunol.* 5:317.

Hoffman, G.W., 1975, A theory of regulation and self–nonself discrimination in an immune network, *Eur. J. Immunol.* 5:638.

Hopper, J.E., and Nisonoff, A., 1971, Individual antigenic specificity of immunoglobulin, *Adv. Immunol.* 13:58.

Hudson, L., Sprent, J., Miller, J.F.A.P., and Playfair, J.H.L., 1974, B-cell derived immunoglobulin on activated mouse T lymphocytes, *Nature (London)* 251:60.

Imanishi, T., and Mäkelä, O., 1973, Strain differences in the specificity of mouse antihapten antibodies, *Eur. J. Immunol.* 2:323.

Imanishi, T., and Mäkelä, O., 1974, Inheritance of antibody specificity. I. Anti-(4-hydroxy-3-nitrophenyl)acetyl of the mouse primary response, *J. Exp. Med.* 140:1498.

Inbar, D., Hochmann, J., and Givol, D., 1972, Localization of antibody-combining sites within the variable portions of heavy and light chains, *Proc. Natl. Acad. Sci. U.S.A.* 69:2659.

Jack, R.S., Imanishi-Kari, T., and Rajewsky, K., 1977, manuscript in preparation.

Janeway, C.A., Jr., 1976, The specificity of T lymphocyte responses to chemically defined antigens, *Transplant. Rev.* 29:164.

Janeway, C.A., Jr., Koren, H.S., and Paul, W.E., 1975, The role of thymus-derived lymphocytes in an antibody-mediated, hapten-specific helper effect, *Eur. J. Immunol.* **5**:17.

Jerne, N.K., 1974, Towards a network theory of the immune system, *Ann. Immunol. (Inst. Pasteur)* **125c**:373.

Jerne, N.K., 1976, The immune system. A web of V-domains, *Harvey Lect.* **70**, in press.

Julius, M.H., Simpson, E., and Herzenberg, L.A., 1973, A rapid method for the isolation of functional thymus-derived murine lymphocytes, *Eur. J. Immunol.* **3**:645.

Kapp, J.A., Pierce, C.W., De La Croix, F., and Benacerraf, B., 1976, Immunosuppressive factor(s) extracted from lymphoid cells in nonresponder mice primed with L-glutamine acid^{60}-2-allonine^{30}-L-tyrosine^{10} (GAT), *J. Immunol.* **116**:305.

Katz, D.H., and Benecerraf, B., 1972, The regulatory influence of activated T cells on B cell responses to antigen, *Adv. Immunol.* **15**:2.

Keck, K., 1975, Ir-gene control of immunogenicity of insulin and A-chain loop as a carrier determinant, *Nature (London)* **254**:78.

Kiefer, H., 1973, Binding and release of lymphocytes by hapten-derivatized nylon fibers, *Eur. J. Immunol.* **3**:181.

Kiefer, H., 1975, Separation of antigen-specific lymphocytes. A new general method of releasing cells bound to nylon mesh, *Eur. J. Immunol.* **5**:624.

Kindt, T.J., 1975, Rabbit immunoglobulin allotypes, *Adv. Immunol.* **20**:57.

Köhler, H., 1975, The response to phosphorylcholine: Dissecting an immune response, *Transplant. Rev.* **27**:24.

Krammer, P.H., Hudson, L., and Sprent, J., 1975, Fc receptors, Ia-antigens, and immunoglobulin on normal and activated mouse T lymphocytes, *J. Exp. Med.* **142**:1403.

Krause, R.M., 1970, The search for antibodies with molecular uniformity, *Adv. Immunol.* **12**:1.

Krawinkel, U., and Rajewsky, K., 1976, Specific enrichment of antigen-binding T and B lymphocyte surface receptors, *Eur. J. Immunol.* **6**:529.

Krawinkel, U., Cramer, M., Berek, C., Hämmerling, G., Black, S.J., Rajewsky, K., and Eichmann, K., 1976, On the structure of the T cell receptor for antigen, *Cold Spring Harbor Symp. Quant. Biol.* **41**, in press.

Krawinkel, U., Cramer, M., Imanishi-Kari, T., Jack, R.S., Mäkelä, O., and Rajewsky, K., 1977a, manuscript in preparation.

Krawinkel, U., Cramer, M., Mage, R., Kelus, A.S., and Rajewsky, K., 1977b, manuscript in preparation.

Mäkelä, O., 1966, Assay of anti-hapten antibody with the aid of hapten-coupled bacteriophage, *Immunology* **10**:81.

Marchalonis, J.J., 1976, Surface immunoglobulin of B and T lymphocytes. Molecular properties, association with the cell membrane and a unified model of antigen recognition, in: *Contemporary Topics in Molecular Immunology,* Vol. 5 (H.N. Eisen and R.A. Reisfeld, eds.), pp. 125–160, Plenum Press, New York.

McCarty, M., 1958, Further studies on the chemical basis for serological specificity of Group A carbohydrate, *J. Exp. Med.* **108**:311.

McKearn, T.J., Stuart, F.P., and Firch, F.W., 1974a, Anti-idiotypic antibodies in rat transplantation immunity. I. Production of anti-idiotypic antibodies in animals repeatedly immunized with alloantigens, *J. Immunol.* **113**:1876.

McKearn, T.J., Hamada, Y., Stuart, F.P., and Fitch, F.W., 1974b, Antireceptor antibody and resistance to graft-versus-host disease, *Nature (London)* **251**:648.

Melchers, I., and Rajewsky, K., 1975, Specific control of responsiveness by two complementing *Ir* loci in the *H-2* complex, *Eur. J. Immunol.* **5**:753.

Melchers, I., Rajewsky, K., and Shreffler, D.C., 1973, Ir-LDH$_B$: Map position and functional analysis, *Eur. J. Immunol.* **3**:754.

Mitchison, N.A., 1968, Recognition of antigen, in: *Differentiation and Immunology,* Vol. 7, p. 29 (K.B. Warren, ed.), Academic Press, New York.

Mitchison, N.A., 1971, The relative ability of T and B lymphocytes to see protein antigen, in: *Cell Interactions and Receptor Antibodies in Immune Responses,* p. 249 (O. Mäkelä, A. Cross, and T.U. Kosunen, eds.), Academic Press, London.

Mitchison, N.A., Rajewsky, K., and Taylor, R.B., 1970, Cooperation of antigenic determinants and of cells in the induction of antibodies, in: *Developmental Aspects of Antibody Formation and Structure,* Vol. II, p. 547 (J. Sterzl and I. Riha, eds.), Publishing House of the Czechoslovak Academy of Science, Prague.

Mole, L.E., Jackson, S.A., Porter, R.R., and Wilkinson, J.M., 1971, Allotypically related sequences in the Fd fragment of rabbit immunoglobulin heavy chains, *Biochem. J.* **124**:301.

Mozes, E., 1976, The nature of antigen specific T cell factors involved in the genetic regulation of immune responses, in: *The Role of Products of the Histocompatibility Gene Complex in Immune Responses,* p. 485 (D.H. Katz and B. Benacerraf, eds.), Academic Press, New York.

Munro, A.J., and Taussig, M., 1975, Two genes in the major histocompatibility complex control immune response, *Nature (London)* **256**:103.

Nisbet, H.W., Simonsen, M., and Zaleski, M., 1969, The frequency of antigen-sensitive cells in tissue transplantation, *J. Exp. Med.* **129**:459.

Nisonoff, A., and Bangasser, S.A., 1975, Immunological suppression of idiotypic specificities, *Transplant. Rev.* **27**:100.

Paul, W.E., 1970, Functional specificity of antigen-binding receptors of lymphocytes, *Transplant. Rev.* **5**:130.

Pavlovskis, O., and Slade, H.D., 1969, Adsorption of ^{3}H-fatty acid esters of streptococcal groups A and E cell wall polysaccharide antigens by red blood cells, *J. Bacteriol.* **100**:641.

Playfair, J.H.L., Marshall-Clarke, S., and Hudson, L., 1974, Cooperation by mouse T lymphocytes: The role of antibody in T cell specificity, *Eur. J. Immunol.* **4**:54.

Potter, M., and Lieberman, R., 1967, Genetics of immunoglobulins in mice, *Adv. Immunol.* **7**:91.

Rajewsky, K., 1971, The carrier effect and cellular cooperation in the induction of antibodies, *Proc. R. Soc., London Ser. B.* **176**:385.

Rajewsky, K., and Brenig, C., 1974, Paralysis to serum albumins in T and B lymphocytes in mice. Dose dependence, specificity and kinetics of escape, *Eur. J. Immunol.* **4**:120.

Rajewsky, K., and Mohr, R., 1974, Specificity and heterogeneity of helper T cells in the response to serum albumins in mice, *Eur. J. Immunol.* **4**:111.

Rajewsky, K., and Pohlit, H., 1971, Specificity of helper function, *Prog. Immunol.* **1**:337.

Rajewsky, K., and Rottländer, E., 1967, Tolerance specificity and the immune response to lactic dehydrogenase isoenzymes, *Cold Spring Harbor Symp. Quant. Biol.* **32**:547.

Rajewsky, K., Schirrmacher, V., Nase, S., and Jerne, N.K., 1969, The requirement of more than one antigenic determinant for immunogenicity, *J. Exp. Med.* **126**:1131.

Rajewsky, K., Brenig, C., and Melchers, I., 1972, Specificity and suppression in the helper system, in: *Cell Interactions, 3rd Lepetit Colloquium,* p. 196 (L. Silvestri, ed.), North-Holland Publishing Co., Amsterdam.

Rajewsky, K., Hämmerling, G.J., Black, S.J., Berek, C., and Eichmann, K., 1976, T lymphocyte receptor analysis by anti-idiotypic stimulation, in: *The Role of Products*

of the Histocompatibility Gene Complex in Immune Responses, p. 445 (D.H. Katz and
    B. Benacerraf, eds.), Academic Press, New York.
Ramseier, H., 1973, Antibodies to receptors recognizing histocompatibility antigens, Curr.
    Top. Microbiol. and Immunol. 60:31.
Ramseier, H., 1974, Antibodies to T cell receptors and to histocompatibility antigens, Cell.
    Immunol. 8:177.
Ramseier, H., and Lindenmann, J., 1972, Aliotypic antibodies, Transplant. Rev. 10:57.
Richter, P.H., 1976, The network idea and the immune system, in: Theoretical Immunol-
    ogy (G.B.A. Perelson and G. Pimbley, eds.), Marcel Dekker, New York, in press.
Rittenberg, M.B., and Pratt, K.L., 1969, Anti-TNP plaque assay—Primary response of Balb/c
    mice to soluble and particulate immunogen, Proc. Soc. Exp. Biol. Med. 132:575.
Rutishauser, U., and Edelman, G.M., 1972, Binding of thymus- and bone marrow-derived
    lymphoid cells to antigen-derivatized fibers, Proc. Natl. Acad. Sci. U.S.A. 69:3774.
Schlossman, S.F., 1972, Antigen recognition: The specificity of T cells involved in the
    cellular immune response, Transplant. Rev. 10:97.
Schreffler, D.C., and David, C.S., 1975, The H-2 major histocompatibility complex and the I
    immune response region: Genetic variation, function and organization, Adv. Immunol.
    20:125.
Tada, T., Taniguchi, M., and Takemori, T., 1975, Properties of primed suppressor T cells
    and their products, Transplant. Rev. 26:106.
Takemori, T., and Tada, T., 1975, Properties of antigen-specific suppressive T cell factor in
    the regulation of antibody response of the mouse. I. In vivo activity and immuno-
    chemical characterization, J. Exp. Med. 142:1241.
Vicari, G., Sher, A., Cohn, M., and Kabat, E.A., 1970, Immunochemical studies on a mouse
    myeloma protein with specificity to certain β-linked terminal residues of N-acetyl-
    glucosamine, Immunochemistry 7:829.
Vitetta, E.A., and Uhr, J.W., 1975, Immunoglobulin receptors revisited, Science 189:964.
Weinbaum F.I., Butchko, G.M., Lerman, S., Thorbecke, G.J., and Nisonoff, A., 1974,
    Comparison of cross-reactivities between albumins of various species at the level of
    antibody and helper T cells—Studies in mice, J. Immunol. 113:257.
Wigzell, H., and Andersson, B., 1969, Cell separation on antigen coated columns. Elimina-
    tion of high rate antibody forming cells and immunological memory cells, J. Exp. Med.
    129:23.
Wilson, D.B., Blyth, I.L., and Nowell, P.C., 1968, Quantitative studies on the mixed lym-
    phocyte interaction in rats. Kinetics of the response, J. Exp. Med. 128:1157.
Wu, T., and Kabat, E.A., 1970, An analysis of the sequence of the variable regions of Bence
    Jones proteins and myeloma light chains and their implications for antibody comple-
    mentarity, J. Exp. Med. 132:211.

Chapter 4

Antigen-Binding, Idiotypic T-Lymphocyte Receptors

Hans Binz and Hans Wigzell

Department of Immunology
Uppsala University Biomedical Center
Uppsala, Sweden

I. INTRODUCTION

Specific immune cognition and recognition are intrinsic capacities of mature, immunocompetent lymphocytes. B and T lymphocyte populations can both be shown to display this ability with high discriminatory power. At the single-cell level, however, both B and T lymphocytes express antigen-binding receptors with extreme restriction (Raff *et al.*, 1973; Binz and Wigzell, 1975a). It would seem likely that in fact all receptors for antigen on a single B (Raff *et al.*, 1973) or T (Binz and Wigzell, 1975a) lymphocyte express the same antigen-binding specificity. When T and B lymphocytes are compared with respect to their capacity to react against various epitopes, largely overlapping recognition spectra of antigenic specificities are found (Rajewsky and Mohr, 1974). Comparable mechanisms for the generation of diversity at the single-cell level of T and B cells would thus seem logical and economical. Whereas the biochemistry and underlying genetics of the B-cell receptors for antigen are by now relatively well understood, considerably less is known of the T-cell system.

Starting with the B lymphocytes, the cell-bound antigen-specific receptors would seem comparatively conventional immunoglobulin molecules, skewed as to class distribution in comparison to the serum immunoglobulins (Wigzell, 1973), but otherwise of very similar biochemical setup. The genes coding for B-cell immunoglobulins are known to be located in three gene clusters, one for the heavy chain and two for the respective light chains. No evidence exists that any of these loci are genetically linked to the genes coding for the major histocompatibility antigens of the various species.

T lymphocytes, on the other hand, do normally fail to express on their outer surface endogeneous, conventional immunoglobulin molecules (Vitetta *et al.*, 1972; Grey *et al.*, 1972; Lisowska-Bernstein *et al.*, 1973; Abney and Parkhouse, 1974; Fröland and Natvig, 1971; Crone *et al.*, 1972; Mond *et al.*, 1972). Exceptions to this rule have been published indicating the presence of a molecule on T cells carrying κ light chains and with a heavy chain similar to that of IgM (Marchalonis *et al.*, 1972a,b; Feldmann, 1974; Hämmerling and Rajewsky, 1971). We have so far been unable to find such IgM-like or light-chain molecules as participants in the creation of antigen-binding receptors on T lymphocytes. Adding to the confusion concerning the structure of the T-cell receptors are the recent findings from several groups (Benacerraf and McDevitt, 1972; Shevach *et al.*, 1974; Katz and Benacerraf, 1975) that at least in the mouse, antigen-binding specific factors produced by T lymphocytes would seem to carry Ia antigenic markers while being devoid of serologic characteristics associated with immunoglobulins. These Ia genes are located within the same chromosomal region as the immune response genes known to determine whether an individual will or will not express T-lymphocyte reactivity against several antigens (Katz and Benacerraf, 1975). Thus, it has been proposed that the products of the Ia genes are directly involved in the creation of the antigen-binding receptors on T lymphocytes (Benacerraf and McDevitt, 1972).

The present approach to the study of the T-cell receptors is based on the knowledge that the striking, unique characteristics of the immunoglobulin molecules do reside in their variable polypeptide parts. Since these variable regions are known to be directly involved in the creation of the antigen-binding sites, preservation of genes governing their production would have great survival value. In agreement with such reasonings are the findings that the stretches between the hypervariable sequences in the variable regions have been preserved during phylogeny to a much greater extent than the constant regions of the immunoglobulins (Wu and Kabat, 1970). It would thus seem likely that the B- and T-lymphocyte receptors for antigen may use the same (or at least partly the same) genes for the creation of the actual antigen-binding sites of their receptors. As for the constant regions, a similar demand for sharing would not prevail, and thus different genes may here contribute to the creation of receptors in the two lymphocyte groups.

Using such reasoning, we have taken advantage of the fact that the antigen-binding regions of immunoglobulins can themselves be used as immunogens, leading to the production of antiidiotypic antibodies (Hopper and Nisonoff, 1971). We have thus attempted to make antiidiotypic antibodies against B- or T-cell receptors or both with specificity for the same antigenic specificitites. Successful production of anti-T idiotypic antibodies has been demonstrated

(Binz and Wigzell, 1975b). This chapter will deal with the use of such antiidiotypic antibodies in the fine analysis of structure and function of the T-cell receptors for antigen.

Our experimental systems have involved the use of mice or rat strains differing at their major histocompatibility complex genes in an attempt to produce antibodies against the receptors or antibodies reactive with these transplantation antigens. We have followed the design of Ramseier and Lindenmann 1969, in which antibodies produced in one strain against the alloantigens of the other parental strain, if inoculated into F_1 hybrids between the two strains, should lead to induction of antialloantibody synthesis in the recipients. Alternatively, lymphocytes from one parental strain can be used analogously as the alloantibodies. The underlying theory behind this design is that F_1 hybrid animals would recognize as foreign only those antigen-binding areas with specific reactivity against the other parental alloantigens, but would share the rest with the inoculum. Thus, the F_1 hybrids would be able to make highly specific antiidiotypic antibodies without absorptions. In this review, we will only present and discuss our own data on the analysis of the antigen-binding T-cell receptors using the design described above and similar designs. It should be stressed, however, that important pioneering work using the antireceptor approach has been carried out using an assay of complicated nature but yielding in essence results very similar to those to be presented in this article (Ramseier and Lindenmann, 1972a,b; Ramseier, 1973, 1974a,b, 1975, 1976). Also, other researchers have contributed essential information using similar approaches (McKearn, 1974; McKearn et al., 1974a,b).

II. METHODS AND MATERIALS USED IN THE INDUCTION AND ANALYSIS OF ANTIIDIOTYPIC ANTIBODIES

Animals

Inbred rats or mice of our own breeding colony were used unless otherwise stated. Strains will be indicated in the description of experimental data.

Lymphocyte Preparations

Single-cell suspensions were prepared using standard procedures (Binz and Wigzell, 1975b; Billingham and Silvers, 1961).

T Lymphocytes. Mouse or rat T lymphocytes were prepared from spleen and lymph node cell suspensions via filtration through Degalan or glass-bead columns coated with anti-Ig antibodies (Wigzell and Andersson, 1969). B-cell contamination averaged less than 2%.

B Lymphocytes. Anti-T specific sera (Binz and Wigzell, 1975b) in the presence of complement were used to lyse away the T cells. Cells were then filtered through sterile gauze and washed thrice. Such cells prepared from spleen and lymph node suspensions averaged more than 90% B lymphocytes as judged by surface Ig markers. In some experiments involving *in vitro* culture, the cell suspensions were treated with trypsin after the cytotoxic experiment to further remove dead cells and debris.

Tests

Indirect Hemagglutination. This test for the detection of antiidiotypic antibodies was carried out using sheep erythrocytes coated with rat IgG molecules using chromic chloride techniques (Wells *et al.*, 1973).

Graft vs.-Host Reactions. These reactions were done using the local popliteal lymph node assays (Ford *et al.*, 1970).

Mixed Leukocyte Cultures. These were performed as previously described for mouse (Binz and Askonas, 1975) and rat (Binz and Wigzell, 1975b) lymphocytes.

Radioimmunoassays. These were carried out on idiotype-positive or -negative lymphocytes according to one of three principles. First, IgG from antiidiotypic antiserum was labeled directly with ^{125}I (Hunter and Greenwood, 1962). Second, IgG from rabbit–anti-rat-Ig antisera was iodinated and used as secondary reagent in an indirect assay for the detection of cell bound antiidiotypic antibodies (Binz and Wigzell, 1975b). Third, protein A from *Staphylococcus aureus* with specific binding to the Fc region of most mammalian IgGs (Forsgren and Sjöqvist, 1966) was used in ^{125}I-labeled form as indicator of cell-bound IgG molecules (Dorval *et al.*, 1974).

III. INDUCTION AND CHARACTERISTICS OF ANTIIDIOTYPIC ANTIBODIES RAISED AGAINST T- OR B-CELL RECEPTORS FOR ANTIGEN

A. Induction of Antiidiotypic Antibodies

Two principal approaches to induce antiidiotypic antibodies have been used:

(1) Inoculation of immunocompetent lymphocytes of one parental strain into F_1 hybrids between the donor strain and another strain of animals. The underlying principle as outlined above (Ramseier and Lindenmann, 1969) is that such F_1 hybrid animals will recognize as foreign only the idiotypic receptors on those lymphocytes that carry specific reactivity against the alloantigens of the

other parental strain. This would then direct the immune response of the F_1 hybrid exclusively against the relevant idiotypes and would largely exclude requirements of extensive absorption of the antiidiotypic antisera to make these specific.

(2) Immunization of animals with alloantibodies or purified idiotypic receptor molecules with the same antigen-binding specificity as the conventional antibodies. These immunization procedures can be carried out using either the same parent–F_1 hybrid combinations as outlined above or animals of another species as recipients (Binz and Wigzell, 1975c). In the latter case, however, stringent controls or absorptions or both are necessary to make sure that the antisera induced in the recipient are true antiidiotypic and do not contain additional "disturbing" antibodies directed against other constant-region markers of the inoculated molecules.

Starting with the use of inoculation of immunocompetent lymphocytes from parental strain donors into F_1 hybrid animals as a means to produce F_1-antiparental idiotypic antibodies, the following conclusions can be drawn: It is possible to use this approach to induce the synthesis of specific antiidiotypic antibodies *if the inoculum contains T lymphocytes* or a mixture of T and B cells, but not with normal B lymphocytes alone (Binz and Wigzell, 1975b; Binz, 1975). Purified T lymphocytes are significantly better than a mixture of T and B lymphocytes to induce relevant antiidiotypic antibodies, as exemplified in Table I. In fact, we have reason to believe that the presence of B cells in the inoculum might cause an active suppression of the induction of antiidiotypic antibodies, superseding their functioning as a physical dilution factor of the T cells. Whether this B-cell inhibitory activity is taking place via tolerance-inducing means by confronting the immune system of the F_1 hybrid with the idiotype-positive molecules in a nonimmunogenic form is unknown but plausible.

Table I. Superiority of Parental T Lymphocytes to a Mixture of T Plus B Lymphocytes in Provoking Antialloantibody Production in F_1 Hybrids[a]

Immunizing cells	Target cells	Day postimmunization 5[b]
DA, T + B, 2.5×10^7	SRBC, DA anti-Lewis IgG	2.0 ± 0.0
DA, T 2.5×10^7	SRBC, DA anti-Lewis IgG	3.0 ± 0.4
Lewis, T + B, 2.5×10^7	SRBC, Lewis anti-DA IgG	2.4 ± 0.5
Lewis, T 2.5×10^7	SRBC, Lewis anti-DA IgG	7.0 ± 1.1

[a]All sera were tested against SRBC coated with IgG from DA, Lewis, or (DA×Lewis)F_1 normal sera, as well as against SRBC coated with IgG from DA anti-Lewis or Lewis anti-DA immune sera. All sera were preadsorbed with SRBC before testing. Only groups in which agglutination occurred are listed in the table.
[b]Mean ± S.E. of $\log_2$ titers.

Table II. Time Kinetics of Antialloantibody Production in F_1 Hybrid Rats Inoculated with Parental Lymphocytes[a]

Immunizing cells	Target cells	Days postimmunization			
		4	7	10	15
DA, T + B, 5×10^7	SRBC, DA anti-Lewis IgG	3.5±0.3	5.8±0.5	6.5±1.0	6.3±1.0
Lewis, T + B, 5×10^7	SRBC, Lewis anti-DA IgG	3.0±1.0	2.7±0.9	4.0±1.5	3.5±0.5

[a]All sera were tested against SRBC coated with IgG from DA, Lewis, or (DA × Lewis)F_1 normal sera, as well as against SRBC coated with IgG from DA anti-Lewis or Lewis anti-DA immune sera. All sera were preadsorbed with SRBC before testing. Only groups in which agglutination occurred are listed in the table.

Even though parental B lymphocytes alone are unable to induce antiidiotypic antibodies, they are quite able to specifically remove such antibodies, thereby demonstrating the presence of idiotype-positive receptors on the surfaces of these cells (Binz, 1975; Binz and Wigzell, 1975b; Binz and Askonas, 1975). The reason for the superior immunogenic ability of the parental T lymphocytes in comparison to the B cells is unknown, but we believe it most likely involves the enhancing allogeneic effect known to exist in experimental systems involving GvH reactions (Katz and Osborne, 1972). One would thus assume that normal B lymphocytes, *if presented in an immunogenic form,* would be able to function as inducers of antiidiotypic antibodies in the same manner as their soluble products, the immunoglobulin molecules, can be made to do in the present system (Binz and Lindenmann, 1974; McKearn, 1974).

Induction of antiidiotypic antibodies in F_1 hybrid recipients via inoculation of parental lymphocytes is a swift process, as indicated in Table II, and such antibodies can be detected within a few days. Direct proof that these antibodies are indeed produced by the F_1 hybrids has come from analysis of allotype markers present on the antiidiotypic antibodies (Binz and Lindenmann, 1974). Our routine procedure for induction of anti-T-cell-receptor idiotypic antibodies has been to use repeated administration of purified parental T lymphocytes into adult F_1 hybrid recipients (Binz and Wigzell, 1975b), but several procedures are known to function (Binz and Wigzell, 1975b; Binz, 1975; McKearn, 1974; Elves, 1973). Whereas virtually all F_1 hybrid rats respond by demonstrable production of antiidiotypic antibodies in these experiments when assayed via sensitive indirect hemagglutination techniques, few antisera reach titers high enough to make them useful in direct radioimmunoassays for detection of idiotypic receptors on lymphocytes (Binz and Wigzell, 1975b). It would seem quite clear that it is easier to get useful, high-titered antiidiotypic antisera in the present systems in rats than in mice (Binz and Wigzell, 1975b; Binz and Askonas, 1975), but there also exist sizable variations among strains of the same species. We have no simple explanation for these differences.

The second approach to inducing antiidiotypic antibodies against receptors with specificity for the major histocompatibility complex determined antigens consists in the immunization of animals using soluble alloantibodies of relevant specificity. This approach has been shown to lead to production of antialloantibodies in the F_1 hybrid animals as detected by direct or indirect radioimmunoassays using lymphocytes of donor genotype as targets (Binz and Lindenmann, 1972a, 1974; Binz and Wigzell, 1975b). Immunizations were carried out using either multiple intradermal injections of alloantisera into the F_1 hybrid recipients or administering the alloantisera in a polymerized form with adjuvants (Binz et al., 1974a; McKearn, 1974). This immunization procedure does frequently lead to production of antiidiotypic antibodies in the F_1 hybrids with a preferential reactivity with parental idiotype-positive B lymphocytes (see Binz et al., 1974a, and Section III.C).

Extensions of the use of naturally occurring soluble idiotypic molecules in normal serum as immunogen have recently been applied (Binz and Wigzell, 1975c). Here, using antiidiotype antibody immunosorbants, we have produced highly purified idiotype-positive, antigen-binding molecules. These "pure" reagents have then been used as immunogens either across species barriers (Binz and Wigzell, 1975c) or within the species (see Section VIII). Successful synthesis of antiidiotypic antibodies reactive with both T and B lymphocytes carrying relevant idiotype-positive receptors has thus been produced.

B. Demonstration of the Antiidiotypic Nature of the Present Antisera

The present antisera, i.e., the antisera produced in F_1 hybrid animals, are true antiidiotypic antisera by a variety of criteria. For example, if (Lewis X DA)F_1 hybrid rats are inoculated with Lewis T lymphocytes and anti-(Lewis-anti-DA) antibodies are produced in the F_1 hybrids, such antisera will agglutinate only with sheep erythrocytes coated with Lewis-anti-DA alloantibodies, and not red cells coated with Lewis-anti-BN alloantibodies (Binz and Wigzell, 1975b). Lewis, BN, and DA do all differ with regard to the Ag-B locus, the major histocompatibility locus of the rat (Festing and Staats, 1973). Furthermore, in the presence of complement, these antisera will selectively destroy the capacity of Lewis T cells to react against DA as measured by GvH or MLC reactions without reducing activity against BN alloantigens (Binz and Wigzell, 1975b and Section III). Similar results proving the antiidiotypic nature of these sera have been obtained in the mouse system as well (Binz and Askonas, 1975), and have also been found in the analysis of antiidiotypic antisera produced across the species barrier (Binz and Wigzell, 1975c).

C. Relationships Between Idiotypic Determinants Present on B- or T-Cell Receptors with Specificity for the Same Antigen

A major aim in the present experiments has been to analyze the genetic relationships between B- and T-cell receptors with specificity for the same antigen as reflected by their sharing of idiotypes. Some early experiments using alloantiserum inoculated into F_1 hybrid recipients as immunogen followed by an analysis of the specificity of the antiidiotypic antibodies produced revealed the following (Binz and Lindenmann, 1972a): *Using radioimmunoassay techniques on purified lymphocyte populations, it could be shown that these "early" antisera showed preferential reactivity with the parental B lymphocytes,* with no detectable ability to bind to the T cells from the same individual (Binz *et al.,* 1974a). Using other assays, however, the very same antiserum could be shown to indeed contain anti-T-cell reactive antibodies. This was demonstrated by their capacity to block the relevant immunocompetent T cells by either binding to the relevant allogeneic monolayer cells *in vitro* (Binz *et al.,* 1974b) or inhibiting their GvH activity *in vivo* (Binz, Lindenmann, and Wigzell, 1973).

We have recently used an additional antiidiotypic antiserum induced via immunization with alloantiserum to analyze this question further. This anti-

Table III. Evidence That B Lymphocytes Carry Idiotypic Determinants That Are Not Expressed on Corresponding T Cells

Cells[a]	Incubated with[b]:	Antiserum absorbed with[c]:	Uptake of ^{125}I Protein A (mean cpm of triplicates ±S.E.)
Lewis S	Anti-(Lewis anti-DA)	–	4528±132
Lewis T	Anti-(Lewis anti-DA)	–	3103±290
Lewis S	Anti-(Lewis anti-DA)	Lewis T cells	2221±245
Lewis T	Anti-(Lewis anti-DA)	Lewis T cells	1050±131
Lewis S	Anti-(Lewis anti-DA)	Lewis S cells	1136±126
Lewis T	Anti-(Lewis anti-DA)	Lewis S cells	1010± 35
Lewis S	F_1 normal serum	–	822±110
Lewis T	F_1 normal serum	–	810±112
DA S	F_1 normal serum	–	808± 94
DA T	F_1 normal serum	–	943± 24
DA S	Anti-(Lewis anti-DA)	–	835± 96
DA T	Anti-(Lewis anti-DA)	–	822±177

[a] 10×10^6 cells/well. S denotes a mixture of spleen plus lymph node cells; T denotes anti-Ig column purified T lymphocytes.
[b] Anti-(Lewis anti-DA) was raised in $(L \times DA)F_1$ animals against specific L anti-DA alloantibodies absorbed on F_1 spleen cells. The antisera or normal F_1 serum was used 1:2 diluted.
[c] Antiserum, 1 ml, was absorbed twice for 30 min at 4°C with either 2×10^8 spleen plus lymph node cells or purified T cells.
For other details of this kind of test system, see Binz and Wigzell (1975b).

serum reached high enough antiidiotypic titer to be useful in radioimmunoassays on lymphocytes, and, like the earlier ones, could be shown to react with preferential activity toward B lymphocytes. This antiserum, however, also displayed significant reactivity with T cells (see Table III). When this antiserum was absorbed with excess parental T lymphocytes, all antiidiotype activity against the T lymphocytes was removed, but considerable activity against the B cells remained. If, however, the B lymphocytes were incubated when absorbing the antiserum, this incubation removed all activity against both B and T lymphocytes. These data strongly suggest that T- and B-lymphocyte receptors for alloantigens share idiotypic determinants. Antisera *induced against B-cell idiotypic immunoglobulin molecules* may, however, contain two types of antiidiotypic antibodies: one kind reacting with both T- and B-cell idiotypes, one with exclusive ability to react with some B-cell receptor unique idiotypes.

Our major effort, however, has been to prove shared or identical idiotypes on T- and B-cell receptors for antigen *using as immunogen highly purified peripheral T lymphocytes* (Binz and Wigzell, 1975b). Antisera induced in F_1 hybrid animals via inoculation of parental T lymphocytes frequently contain antiidiotypic antibodies reacting with relevant T cells (see Tables IV–VI) or with

Table IV. Removal by Lewis Anti-DA IgG Alloantibodies of Antiidiotypic Antibodies Directed Toward T-Cell Idiotypes

Lymphoid cells[a]	Incubated with:	Uptake of [^{125}I] rabbit anti-rat Ig (mean cpm of triplicates ± S.E.)[b]
LT	(L×DA)F$_1$ anti-LT (serum 1003)	70.074±2.119
LT	(L×DA)F$_1$ normal serum	22.367±2.026
LT	Serum 1003 absorbed on L anti-DA IgG	24.505±0.787
LT	Serum 1003 absorbed on L normal IgG	51.545±6.648
LT	Serum 1003 absorbed on (L×DA)F$_1$ normal IgG	56.551±3.355
LT	Serum 1003 bound and eluted from L anti-DA IgG	64.931±9.626
LT	Serum 1003 bound and eluted from L normal IgG	19.542±0.469
LT	Serum 1003 bound and eluted from (L×DA)F$_1$ normal IgG	21.618±2.401
DA T	Serum 1003	29.271±2.819
DA T	(L×DA)F$_1$ normal serum	25.444±0.384
DA T	Serum 1003 absorbed on L anti-DA IgG	32.788±2.350
DA T	Serum 1003 absorbed on L normal IgG	28.713±1.164
DA T	Serum 1003 absorbed on (L×DA)f$_1$ normal IgG	27.542±1.037
DA T	Serum 1003 bound and eluted from L anti-DA IgG	25.659±0.304
DA T	Serum 1003 bound and eluted from L normal IgG	28.245±2.537
DA T	Serum 1003 bound and eluted from (L×DA)F$_1$ normal IgG	25.786±2.829

[a]LT: Lewis T lymphocytes.
[b]Input per well: 2×10^6 cpm of [^{125}I] rabbit anti-rat Ig.

Table V. Removal by Lewis Anti-DA IgG Alloantibodies of Antiidiotypic Antibodies Directed Toward T-cell Idiotypes: MLC Reactivity[a]

Responding cells	Stimulator cells (2000-rad-irradiated)	Responding cells treated with:	[³H]TdR incorporated (mean cpm ± S.E.)	
			Mixture[b]	Parental cells[c]
L	(L×DA)F$_1$		32.933±0.245	1.017±0.084
L	(L×DA)F$_1$	(L×DA)F$_1$, normal serum + C′	32.112±0.145	1.566±0.352
L	(L×DA)F$_1$	Antiserum + C′	1.938±0.029	1.133±0.043
L	(L×DA)F$_1$	Antiserum abs. on (L anti-DA)-IgG + C′	30.929±0.292	1.006±0.048
L	(L×DA)F$_1$	Antiserum abs. on L normal IgG + C′	1.680±0.419	1.040±0.062
L	(L×DA)F$_1$	Antiserum abs. on (L×DA)F$_1$, normal IgG + C′	1.609±0.113	1.015±0.057
L	(L×DA)F$_1$	Antiserum bound and eluted from L anti-DA IgG + C′	3.013±0.273	1.087±0.072
L	(L×DA)F$_1$	Antiserum bound and eluted from L normal IgG + C′	31.525±0.743	2.037±0.741
L	(L×DA)F$_1$	Antiserum bound and eluted from (L×DA)F$_1$, normal IgG + C′	30.987±1.155	1.777±0.373
L	(L×BN)F$_1$		22.857±0.891	1.814±0.799
L	(L×BN)F$_1$	(L×DA)F$_1$, normal serum + C′	21.844±1.091	1.007±0.154
DA	(L×DA)F$_1$	(L×DA)F$_1$, normal serum + C′	30.294±0.528	1.134±0.061
DA	(L×DA)F$_1$	Antiserum + C′	29.915±0.257	1.227±0.081

[a]MLC was performed in round-bottom microtiter plates using 1.5×10⁶ responder cells and 0.75×10⁶ stimulator cells in a total volume of 0.2 ml RPMI 1640 and 5% fresh normal rat serum. 16 hr pulse on day 3 with 2 μCi [³H]TdR. Stimulator cells alone gave 100–400 cpm.
[b]Mean of triplicate wells.
[c]Mean of duplicate wells.

Table VI. Removal by Lewis Anti-DA IgG Alloantibodies of Antiidiotypic Antibodies Directed Toward T-Cell Idiotypes: GvH Reactivity

Host	Cells injected[a]	Injected cells treated with:	Mean of "Lewis" lymph node weight (mg ± S.E.)[b]	Mean of "DA" lymph node weights (mg ± S.E.)[b]	Mean log ratio ± S.E.
(L×DA)F$_1$	L, DA	(L×DA)F$_1$ normal serum + C'	28.5±3.3	26.4±2.9	−0.02±0.02
(L×DA)F$_1$	L, DA	Aid.[c] + C'	6.1±1.0	32.6±5.6	0.73±0.06
(L×DA)F$_1$	L, DA	Aid. abs. on L anti-DA IgG + C'	27.7±1.6	25.0±0.3	−0.04±0.02
(L×DA)F$_1$	L, DA	Aid. abs. on L normal IgG + C'	6.2±0.6	33.6±3.5	0.70±0.07
(L×DA)F$_1$	L, DA	Aid. abs. on (L×DA)F$_1$ normal IgG + C'	4.1±0.4	33.0±2.2	0.89±0.01
(L×DA)F$_1$	L, DA	Aid. abs. and eluted from L anti-DA IgG + C'	5.1±1.0	29.7±2.7	0.78±0.09
(L×DA)F$_1$	L, DA	Aid. abs. and eluted from Lewis normal IgG + C'	21.8±1.0	22.9±0.7	0.02±0.01
(L×DA)F$_1$	L, DA	Aid. abs. and eluted from (L×DA)F$_1$ normal IgG + C'	26.2±1.2	23.5±1.4	0.05±0.05

[a]$3×10^6$ spleen and lymph node cells were injected into each footpad.
[b]Mean of 4–7 lymph nodes.
[c]Aid: antiidiotypic antiserum of specificity anti-(Lewis anti-DA) raised in (L×DA)F$_1$ rats against purified Lewis T cells.

highly purified IgG alloantibodies specific for the same alloantigens as the T receptors (see Tables I and II).

Thus, although the antisera was induced by supposedly pure, normal T lymphocytes, they could be shown to react with high titer against a typical B-cell product in a highly specific manner. This could mean that T and B lymphocytes express shared idiotypic determinants on their receptors with similar antigen-binding specificity. Alternatively, contaminating B cells or B-cell products were present in the inoculated T-cell suspension in great enough amounts to allow the induction of anti-T and anti-B idiotypic antibodies, respectively. The essential issue was then to prove that the antiidiotypic antibodies reactive against T-cell receptors and those that reacted with the IgG alloantibodies were the very same antibody molecules. This could be shown in two ways (Binz and Wigzell, 1975b). In the first approach, highly purified IgG alloantibodies of relevant specificity were covalently attached to Sepharose. Anti-T-cell idiotypic antisera were then filtered through such immunosorbant columns (and control columns). The passed or the bound and acid-eluted antibodies were then analyzed for their capacity to bind to T lymphocytes or inhibit T-cell function. The examples of these experiments shown in Table IV (see also Tables V and VI) demonstrate that the relevant IgG alloantibody columns could remove all antibodies reactive with the idiotypic T-cell receptors. These antibodies were recovered in the acid eluates. Control columns had no effect. Similar results, although using less purified Ig alloantiserum as immunosorbant, were produced in the mouse (Binz and Askonas, 1975). We could thus conclude that *using anti-T cell idiotypic antibodies, IgG molecules with the same antigen-binding specificity as the T-cell receptors do express the full repertoire of idiotypic determinants found on these T-cell receptors.*

In view of the previous results (see Table III) using alloantibodies as immunogens for the induction of antiidiotypic antibodies, which resulted in induction of some seemingly exclusive anti-B-cell idiotype-reactive antibodies, we also asked a converse question: Using anti-T-cell idiotypic antisera, will purified T lymphocytes be able to remove all antibodies reactive with idiotypes present on the relevant idiotypic IgG molecules? Using rat-IgG-alloantibody-coated sheep erythrocytes in the indirect hemagglutination assay, it was found possible to completely remove all agglutinating antiidiotypic antibodies with pure parental T lymphocytes, as shown in Table VII. Here, purified T lymphocytes were at least equal in absorbing ability to a 1:1 mixture of T and B lymphocytes, thereby excluding any responsibility of B-cell contamination for the results. This proved that the present antiidiotypic antisera raised against T-cell idiotypic receptors do not contain any exclusive anti-B-cell idiotype-reactive antibodies and do further certify the purity of the T-cell suspensions used as immunogen.

From the present data, it would thus seem quite clear that the antigen-

Table VII. Capacity of Normal Lewis T
Lymphocytes to Adsorb Away (Lewis × DA)F$_1$
Anti-Lewis T-Cell Antibodies

Inhibitory cells[a]	Agglutination titers[b]
Lewis T + B	2^7
Lewis, T	2^5
(Lewis × DA)F$_1$, T+B	2^{11}
(Lewis × DA)F$_1$, T	2^{12}
0	2^{13}

[a]10^7 cells of the indicated type were added to each hole in the microplate, after which twofold dilutions of (L×DA)F$_1$ anti-L T serum were added. The purity of T cells with regard to B-cell contamination was 98% or more. B-cell contamination in T+B cell populations was 50–60%. T+B: spleen and lymph node cell mixture; T: T cells purified out of the T+B population via passage through anti-Ig columns.
[b]Agglutination as assessed against SRBC coated with Lewis-anti-DA IgG antibodies. Controls including SRBC coated with IgG from normal Lewis, DA, or F$_1$ sera, as well as IgG from Da-anti-Lewis immune sera, were negative.

binding receptors on T and B lymphocytes at least in part use similar if not identical genes in their buildup of their respective antigen-binding areas. Analysis of the T-cell receptor in physically isolated form would be necessary to further explore this genetic relationship in biochemical terms. Further aspects of this relationship will be elaborated on in Section IX.

IV. INHIBITION OF T-CELL FUNCTIONS BY ANTIIDIOTYPIC ANTIBODIES

A. Inhibition of T-Cell Function *in Vivo* (Graft-vs.-Host Reaction)

It is of obvious importance to establish a highly specific, selective immunosuppression of transplantation reactions *in vivo*. Antiidiotypic antibodies directed against the variable part of alloantibodies or the variable part of T-cell receptors for alloantigens of corresponding specificity can be used as a tool for such a selective immunologic disarmament (Binz *et al.,* 1973, 1974b; Binz and Wigzell, 1975b; McKearn, 1974; McKearn *et al.,* 1974b). The aim of this section is to describe different approaches and mechanisms for the suppression of the graft-vs.-host (GvH) reaction *in vivo*.

1. Test System

In order to study the suppressive effect of antiidiotypic antibodies in transplantation reactions, we have chosen the GvH reaction as an experimental model for an allograft reaction. This reaction in mice as measured by the spleen weight assay has been shown to depend mainly on T-cell function (Cantor, 1972). On the other hand, it has been claimed that in certain GvH reactions, B lymphocytes may also participate (Barchilon and Gershon, 1970). It was therefore important to demonstrate that our test system, the local GvH reaction in mice and rats as measured in the popliteal lymph node assay measures mainly T-cell function.

In mice, a high dose of parental mouse lymphocytes is needed to elicit a significant GvH reaction. The dose of 1.5×10^7 parental spleen cells per footpad is much higher than the dose needed to elicit a significant reaction in rats. Anyway, in rats as well as in mice, the mean lymph node weights were found to be linearly related to the dose of cells injected when plotted on a double-log scale (Ford et al., 1970). The T cell is the main type of cell involved in the local popliteal lymph node assay in rats as well as in mice. Treatment of the parental cells with an anti-T-cell serum and complement almost completely abolished the GvH reactivity, whereas treatment of the cells with anti-Ig and complement or passage through an anti-Ig column had no such effect (Binz and Askonas, 1975).

2. Active Immunization

Having established the T-cell involvement in our test system, we tried to suppress the GvH reactivity of parental cells in F_1 rats that had been immunized with alloantibodies raised in one inbred strain of rats against a single skin graft from the other inbred strain. It has been shown previously that alloantibodies against the major histocompatibility locus of another inbred strain of rats can provoke antiidiotypic antibodies when injected into F_1 hybrid animals between these two strains (Binz and Lindenmann, 1974). Although it was found that some of these antiidiotypic antisera react mainly with parental B lymphocytes (Binz et al., 1974a), the present test system requires an antiserum that also contains antibodies directed toward the idiotype(s) present on parental T-lymphocyte receptors.

(Lewis × DA)F_1 rats were immunized twice at 2-week intervals with Lewis anti-DA alloantiserum obtained from Lewis rats that had rejected DA skin (Binz et al., 1973). In the same way, (Lewis × DA)F_1 rats were immunized with DA anti-Lewis alloantiserum. One week after the last injection, a GvH reaction was induced in the popliteal lymph nodes by injecting 5×10^6 parental lymphocytes into the footpads of these actively immunized F_1 rats. Seven days later, the

Table VIII. Suppression of GvH Reactivity in Actively
Immunized $(L \times DA)F_1$ Rats

Host	Actively immunized with:	Mean of "Lewis" node weights (mg ± S.E.)	Mean of "DA" node weights (mg ± S.E.)	Mean log ratio ± S.E.
$(L \times DA)F_1$	$L \rightarrow DA$	38.74±3.08	86.05∓4.64	−0.361±0.041[a]
$(L \times DA)F_1$	$DA \rightarrow L$	71.78±3.53	43.63±3.82	0.240±0.047[b]

[a]Mean of 20 lymph nodes. 5×10^6 viable parental lymphocytes were injected into each footpad. The popliteal lymph nodes were removed 7 days later. Significantly different from 0 $(P \ll 0.01)$.
[b]Mean of 19 lymph nodes. Significantly different from 0 $(P \ll 0.01)$.

lymph nodes were removed and weighed. Table VIII shows the result of such an experiment. (Lewis X DA)F_1 rats immunized with Lewis anti-DA alloantiserum suppressed the GvH reactivity of Lewis parental lymphocytes, but not the reactivity of DA parental cells. On the other hand, (Lewis X DA)F_1 rats immunized with DA anti-Lewis alloantiserum suppressed only the GvH reaction of DA lymphocytes, but not the reaction of Lewis cells. Lymph nodes from normal F_1 animals of the same age showed an average weight of around 7 mg, and are therefore even smaller than the nodes of F_1 animals in Table VIII in which suppression occurred. We can therefore conclude that the suppression of the GvH reaction induced by parental lymphocytes in F_1 rats actively immunized with alloantisera of corresponding specificity was specifically inhibited. This inhibition was partial rather than complete.

3. Passive Immunization

Different mechanisms may be involved in this specific suppression. Most likely, antiidiotypic antibodies directed against parental T-cell receptors for alloantigens of corresponding specificity were responsible for this suppression. Such antiidiotypic antibodies were indeed found in such animals, and a close relationship could be found between the titer of the antiidiotypic antisera and protection against lethal GvH reactivity (McKearn et al., 1974b; see below). An alternative explanation, however, would be that Lewis anti-DA or DA anti-Lewis alloantibodies may cause the suppression by covering certain antigenic DA or Lewis sites in the F_1 hosts. To exclude such an assumption, passive immunization studies were done, and the specificity of the antisera was established by absorption procedures.

Serum from (Lewis X DA)F_1 rats actively immunized with Lewis anti-DA alloantiserum was taken 1 week after the last injection and was absorbed with

Table IX. Suppression of GvH Reactivity in Passively Immunized (L×DA)F$_1$ Rats[a]

Host	Passively immunized with serum:	Serum adsorbed with spleen cells from:	Mean of "Lewis" lymph node weights (mg ± S.E.)	Mean of "DA" lymph node weights (mg ± S.E.)	Mean log ratio ± S.E.
(L×DA)F$_1$	Anti-(L→DA)	(L×DA)F$_1$	41.81±14.65	107.70±5.91	−0.508±0.184[b]
(L×DA)F$_1$	Anti-(L→DA)	(L×DA)F$_1$ + Lewis	94.50± 9.08	86.60±6.66	0.035±0.003[c]
(L×DA)F$_1$	Anti-(L→DA)	(L×DA)F$_1$ + DA	62.41± 6.54	96.30±9.54	−0.187±0.084[b]

[a]Means of a few lymph nodes. Conditions are the same as described in Table II. Serum was absorbed twice with (L×DA)F$_1$ cells, and some of it three times with either Lewis or DA spleen cells.

[b]Significantly different from 0 ($P < 0.05$). Not significantly different from Table II, upper line.

[c]Not significantly different from 0.

(Lewis X DA)F_1 spleen cells; part was also absorbed with either Lewis of DA spleen cells. Such absorbed antiserum was not injected into normal (Lewis X DA)F_1 rats, and parental GvH reactions were induced in these passively immunized animals as described for the actively immunized rats. Table IX gives an example of such an experiment. The inhibition of the GvH reaction of parental lymphocytes could be passively transferred with serum from (Lewis X DA)F_1 rats actively immunized with Lewis anti-DA alloantibodies. The suppressive character of this antiserum was kept after absorption with (Lewis X DA)F_1 or DA spleen cells, but not after the absorption with Lewis spleen cells. The same type of experiment was done with antiserum of reverse specificity, and essentially the same results were obtained. These experiments exclude the possibility that remaining alloantibodies injected into F_1 rats play a major role in the suppression of the parental GvH reactions. Traces of the original injected Lewis anti-DA alloantibodies would have been absorbed out with (Lewis X DA)F_1 or DA spleen cells. On the other hand, the suppressive factor found in the F_1 antiserum could be removed only by Lewis lymphocytes, indicating clearly that the factor was directed toward Lewis cells, whereas the original alloantibody used for immunization was directed toward DA.

An alternative explanation involving inhibition of GvH reactions by a complex of alloantibodies and histocompatibility antigens will be discussed below.

In conclusion, we can say that it is possible to suppress the local GvH reaction of parental lymphocytes in F_1 animals by active immunization with alloantibodies of corresponding specificity. Passive transfer and adsorption studies indicate that one factor involved in the suppression is humoral antibodies of antiidiotypic nature directed toward receptors for alloantigens of T cells. These findings were confirmed by McKearn (1974), McKearn et al. (1974b), Elves (1973), and Joller (1972).

4. Induction by Parental T Lymphocytes of Protection Against GvH Reaction

Similar experiments were done in mice, and essentially the same results were obtained. (CBAXC57B1/6)F_1 mice repeatedly injected with CBA spleen cells suppressed GvH reaction of CBA lymphocytes but not the reactivity of C57B1/6 lymphocytes. So far, however, the F_1 animals were always immunized by injecting alloantibodies (a B-cell product) or by injecting parental spleen cells (Binz et al., 1973, 1974b; Binz 1975; McKearn, 1974) containing both parental T and B lymphocytes. It was therefore important to establish which cell type causes the induction of the protection against parental lymphocytes of corresponding specificity. (CBAXC57B1/6)F_1 mice were therefore immunized with either CBA spleen cells, purified CBA T lymphocytes, or purified CBA B cells. F_1 mice got at least four injections of 5×10^6 parental cells of either type at

Table X. Induction of Specific Immunity in F_1 Hybrids
by Parental T Lymphocytes[a]

Hosts	Immunized with:	Mean of "CBA" lymph node weights (mg)	Mean of "C57BL/6" lymph node weights (mg)	Mean log ratio ± S.E.
(CBA×C57BL/6)F_1	CBA spleen cells	1.3	3.5	0.440±0.062[b]
(CBA×C57BL/6)F_1	CBA T cells	1.7	4.1	0.391±0.039[b]
(CBA×C57BL/6)F_1	CBA B cells	4.3	4.2	−0.014±0.021[c]

[a]Five hosts were injected four times with $5×10^6$ CBA cells of the indicated type at weekly intervals. The GvH reaction was induced in popliteal lymph nodes 10 days after the last injection with $1.5×10^7$ CBA or C57BL/6 lymphocytes. Popliteal lymph nodes were removed 7 days later and weighed. For details, see Binz (1975).
[b]Significantly different from 0 ($P < 0.01$).
[c]Not significantly different from 0.

weekly intervals. GvH reactions were induced 10 days after the last injection by injecting $1.5×10^7$ CBA or C57B1/6 spleen cells into the footpads of the actively immunized hosts. Popliteal lymph nodes were removed 7 days later and weighed. Table X shows a summary of such experiments. It was found that purified parental CBA T lymphocytes were able to induce a protective response in (CBA×C57B1/6)F_1 mice against the GvH reactivity of CBA spleen cells. F_1 mice immunized with purified parental B lymphocytes could not suppress the same GvH reactivity.

5. Removal of Suppressive Activity from F_1 Antisera by the Corresponding Parental T and B Lymphocytes

The findings described above are somewhat contradictory to earlier findings in which the product of B lymphocytes of corresponding specificity, the alloantibodies, could provoke antibodies of antiidiotypic nature and induce protection against parental GvH reactions (see Table VIII). In order to sort out these conflicting findings, the experiments described below were done. As already shown in rats, the protective immunity of F_1 rats could be passively transferred by serum (see above). In addition, these blocking antibodies could be removed only by absorption with the corresponding parental cells. The same was found to be true in mice (Binz, 1975). Serum from (CBA×C57B1/6)F1 mice that had been repeatedly immunized with purified CBA T lymphocytes was absorbed, before injection into normal (CBA×C57B1/6)F_1 mice, with either CBA T or CBA B lymphocytes. Each normal (CBA×C57B1/6)F_1 host received 0.8 ml of either unabsorbed or absorbed serum. GvH reactions were induced with CBA and C57B1/6 parental cells. Table XI shows such an experiment.

Table XI. Adsorption of the Inhibitory Activity of F_1 Sera by the Corresponding Parental T and B Cells[a]

Host	Host passively immunized with:	Serum absorbed with:	Mean of "CBA" lymph node weights (μg)	Mean of "C57BL/6" lymph node weights (μg)	Mean log ratio ± S.E.
(CBA×C57BL/6)F$_1$	(CBA×C57BL/6)F$_1$	_[b]	0.9	3.7	0.629±0.043[c]
(CBA×C57BL/6)F$_1$	(CBA×C57BL/6)F$_1$	CBA T cells	3.7	4.2	0.054±0.017[d]
(CBA×C57BL/6)F$_1$	Anti-CBA T	CBA B cells	3.7	4.1	0.015±0.030[d]
(CBA×C57BL/6)F$_1$	Anti-CBA T	C57BL/6 B cells	1.6	4.0	0.407±0.022[c]

[a]Five hosts were passively immunized intraperitoneally with 0.9 ml antiserum (produced in the same way as described in Table II). Four ml serum was adsorbed three times with 5×10^7 cells for 30 min at 4°C.
[b]The serum was not absorbed.
[c]Significantly different from 0 ($P < 0.01$).
[d]Not significantly different from 0.

Antibodies to CBA T lymphocytes raised in $(CBA \times C57B1/6)F_1$ mice could no longer suppress the GvH activity of CBA lymphocytes in F_1 mice after absorption with CBA T or CBA B lymphocytes. On the other hand, absorption of the same antiserum with C57B1/6 lymphocytes did not remove the suppressive activity that was found in unabsorbed antiserum. Thus, CBA purified B lymphocytes could remove the inhibitory activity of F_1 antisera provoked in F_1 mice against CBA T lymphocytes.

In conclusion, we can say that the inhibition of GvH reactions of parental lymphocytes as measured in the popliteal lymph node assay in F_1 hybrid animals can be induced by parental T lymphocytes, but not with parental B cells, under the conditions used. On the other hand, the protective capacity of F_1 antisera raised against parental T lymphocytes can be fully absorbed by parental B lymphocytes of corresponding specificity, reinforcing again the concept that T and B lymphocytes that have the capacity to react against the same antigenic determinants share similar or identical idiotypes.

6. Transfer of Protection Against GvH Reactions by T Lymphocytes from Immune F_1 Animals

It must be stressed that not all F_1 antisera (either rat or mouse) show the capacity to transfer the inhibition of GvH reaction into normal F_1 animals. On the other hand, the parental GvH reactions in actively immunized animals is in most cases suppressed. Passive transfer of serum could reveal only the humoral part of the F_1 response, in which cellular effector mechanisms may also be involved. To test this assumption, F_1 lymphocytes from $(CBA \times C57B1/6)F_1$ mice actively immunized with CBA T lymphocytes were transferred into normal F_1 mice 10 days after the last injection, and a GvH reaction was provoked 24 hr later. It was found that the GvH reaction of parental lymphocytes of corresponding specificity could specifically be inhibited.

To eliminate the possibility that humoral antibodies produced by the transferred B lymphocytes caused the inhibition, purified F_1 T lymphocytes from actively immunized F_1 mice were transferred into normal F_1 animals. Again, a specific suppression could be detected (see Table XII). It was found that 10^7 or more F_1 T lymphocytes were necessary to transfer significant protection. Later, it was found that such a suppressive effect of immune F_1 cells passively transferred into normal F_1 mice could be detected close to 1 year after the last injection of 2×10^7 immune F_1 T cells.

7. Cytoxicity of F_1 Antisera to GvH-Reactive T Lymphocytes

It was found in previous experiments that antiidiotypic antibodies in the presence of complement were cytotoxic for the corresponding idiotype-positive

Table XII. Specific Suppression of GvH Reactions Caused by Passive Transfer of Immune F_1 T Lymphocytes

Host	Passively immunized intraperitoneally with[a]:	Mean of "CBA" lymph node weights (mg)	Mean of "C57BL/6" lymph node weights (mg)	Mean log ratio ± S.E.
(CBA×C57BL/6)F_1	5×10^7 F_1 immune T cells	2.3	4.5	0.29±0.09
(CBA×C57BL/6)F_1	1×10^8 F_1 immune T cells	2.5	5.0	0.33±0.06
(CBA×C57BL/6)F_1	1×10^8 F_1 immune spleen cells	2.4	3.9	0.20±0.06
(CBA×C57BL/6)F_1	1×10^8 F_1 normal spleen cells	4.6	4.7	0.01±0.02

[a](CBA×C57BL/6)F_1 immune cells were removed from F_1 animals 10 days after 4 injections of 1×10^7 CBA T cells at weekly intervals. F_1 immune T cells were purified via anti-Ig columns. GvH reactions were induced 24 hr later as described in Table X.

Table XIII. Cytotoxic Effect of F_1 Antisera on GvH-Reactive Lymphocytes

Hosts	Cells injected[a]	Injected cells treated with:	Mean lymph node weights (mg ± S.E.)[b],[c]	Mean log ratio ± S.E.[b]
(DA×BN)F_1	DA	Anti-(DA anti-BN) + complement	17.7±0.1	−0.327±0.038[d]
		Anti-(DA anti-BN) alone	37.8±2.4	
		Anti-(DA anti-BN) + complement	18.3±1.1	−0.209±0.031[d]
		Complement alone	30.5±3.2	
(Lewis × BN)F_1	Lewis	Anti (L anti-BN) + complement	15.7±0.8	−0.208±0.027[d]
		Anti (L anti-BN) alone	25.3±1.2	
		Anti (L anti-BN) + complement	13.6±0.9	−0.238±0.024[d]
		Complement alone	23.5±1.0	

[a]5×10^6 parental lymphocytes were injected into each footpad.
[b]Means of 16–22 lymph nodes.
[c]Normal lymph nodes weigh 3–9 mg.
[d]Significantly different from 0.

B lymphocytes (Binz *et al.,* 1974a). The sera were later tested for their cytotoxic effect on GvH-reactive lymphocytes. Parental lymphocytes to be injected into the footpads of F_1 hosts were treated with either antiserum and complement or antiserum or complement alone. In the earlier experiments, the treated cell suspensions were then trypsinized and allowed to recover and then tested for GvH reactivity. This procedure was later found not to be necessary, and the parental lymphocytes were injected directly after the treatment with the antiserum and complement. As shown in Table XIII, DA lymphocytes treated with F_1-anti-(DA anti-BN) and complement and injected into (DA×BN)F_1 hosts showed a marked reduction in GvH activity, whereas DA lymphocytes treated with either antiserum or complement alone showed normal activity. The same pattern of reactions was found when Lewis lymphocytes were treated with F_1-anti-(Lewis anti-BN). These experiments suggest that the inhibition of the GvH activity of parental lymphocytes was most likely due to killing, rather than to blocking of the reactive cells. It is somewhat surprising that the antiidiotypic antisera themselves could not block any reactivity even in short-term *in vitro* cultures such as MLC and CML (see below). The reason is probably that the receptors are shed together with the antibodies within a very short time and new receptors are generated that give full reactivity back to the cells.

To demonstrate specificity, antiidiotypic antibodies were tested for their cytotoxic effect on T lymphocytes GvH-reactive toward third-party alloantigens. Table XIV shows such an experiment. Lewis lymphocytes treated with anti-(Lewis anti-DA) and complement and injected into either (Lewis × DA)F_1 or (Lewis × BN)F_1 hosts could no longer provoke a GvH reaction in (Lewis × DA)F_1 animals, but showed normal reactivity in (Lewis × BN)F_1 hosts toward BN antigens. This finding demonstrates clearly that the antiidiotypic antiserum contained antibodies specific for receptors on those Lewis lymphocytes that have the capacity to react against DA alloantigens. Similar experiments were established in mice, and essentially the same results were obtained (Binz, 1975).

8. Removal of Activity of F_1 Antisera Directed Against Parental T Lymphocytes by Alloantibodies of Corresponding Specificity

As pointed out in Section III, antiidiotypic antibodies of specificity Anti-(Lewis anti-DA) raised in (Lewis × DA)F_1 animals against purified Lewis T cells do react with highly purified Lewis anti-DA alloantibodies, a B-cell product. It was important to prove similarity or identity of idiotypic determinants on receptor molecules on the surfaces of Lewis T lymphocytes and humoral alloantibodies, of corresponding specificity. IgG from Lewis anti-DA alloantibodies or normal Lewis serum or normal (Lewis × DA)F_1 serum (controls) was linked to activated Sepharose and used as an immunoabsorbent. Anti-(Lewis

Table XIV. Elimination of Specifically Lewis Anti-DA GvH-Reactive Lymphocytes by Anti-(Lewis Anti-DA) Antibodies

Host	Cells injected[a]	Injected cells treated with[b]:	Mean of "Lewis" lymph node weights (mg ± S.E.)[c]	Mean of "DA" lymph node weights (mg ± S. E.)[c]	Mean of "BN" lymph node weights (mg ± S.E.)[c]	Mean log ratio ± S.E.
(L×DA)F$_1$	L	(L×DA)F$_1$ normal serum + C'	70.7±8.6	—	—	-0.01±0.02[d]
	DA	(L×DA)F$_1$ normal serum + C'	—	70.2±7.6	—	-0.81±0.02[e]
(L×DA)F$_1$	L	Anti-(L anti-DA) + C'	11.2±0.9	—	—	
	DA	Anti-(L anti-DA) + C'	—	73.2±5.03	—	
(L×BN)F$_1$	L	(L×DA)F$_1$ normal serum + C'	33.7±5.3	—	—	-0.01±0.05[d]
	BN	(L×DA)F$_1$ normal serum + C'	—	—	32.2±2.5	
(L×BN)F$_1$	L	Anti-(L anti-DA) + C'	31.5±3.7	—	—	-0.00±0.07[d]
	BN	Anti-(L anti-DA) + C'	—	—	31.9±4.3	

[a] 5×10^6 spleen and lymph node cells of the respective strain were injected into each footpad. The nodes were removed 7 days later and weighed.
[b] C': Complement.
[c] Mean weights of 4 nodes.
[d] Not significantly different from 0.
[e] Significantly different from 0 ($P<0.01$).

anti-DA) serum, which has been shown to specifically eliminate anti-DA-reactive Lewis T lymphocytes in the presence of complement (see Table V), was absorbed on either immunoabsorbent and subsequently analyzed for elimination of GvH-reactive Lewis T lymphocytes. In addition, material absorbed and eluted from the immunoabsorbent was tested for its inhibitory capacity.

Lewis anti-DA IgG immunoabsorbents removed the antiidiotypic antibodies with capacity to react with normal anti-DA-reactive Lewis T lymphocytes. Moreover, the bound material could be removed from the immunoabsorbents by low-pH and high-ionic-strength treatment, and the eluted material showed full capacity to eliminate, in the presence of complement, anti-DA-reactive Lewis T lymphocytes as measured in the GvH reaction. Lewis normal IgG or IgG from (Lewis × DA)F_1 normal serum did not influence the suppressive capacity of antiidiotypic antibodies. These data strongly suggest very similar or identical idiotypes on IgG molecules produced by Lewis B cells against DA alloantigens, and on antigen-binding receptors on normal Lewis T lymphocytes, which have the capacity to react against DA alloantigens.

B. Inhibition of T-Cell Function *in Vitro* (Mixed Leukocyte Culture)

1. Inhibition of Mixed Leukocyte Culture

Another reaction that is thought to depend mainly on T lymphocytes is the mixed leukocyte culture (MLC) (Wilson *et al.*, 1967; L. C. Andersson *et al.*, 1973; Alm and Peterson, 1970). Since there is evidence that the same subpopulation of T lymphocytes is responsible for reactivity in GvH reactions and MLC, the obvious step was to test the effect of antiidiotypic antibodies on the response in the MLC (Bach *et al.*, 1972; Klein and Park, 1973).

In a first series of experiments, several different antiidiotypic antisera raised in (CBA×C57B1/6)F_1 mice by various immunization schedules were tested for their capacity to block the GvH reaction and the response in MLC of corresponding parental T lymphocytes (Binz and Askonas, 1975). A close correlation was found between the inhibition of GvH reactions and MLC. Some of these sera were analyzed in a more detailed form, and their specificity was tested. It was shown, first, that the activity of such F_1 antisera could be absorbed away only by absorption with the appropriate parental genotype. Second, it was found that the inhibition of the response in the MLC, as found earlier in GvH reactions, could be demonstrated only when responder cells were treated with the antiserum and complement prior to the culture. Addition of antiserum alone to

Table XV. Inhibition of Specific Mixed Leukocyte Culture Reactions by Treatment of Responder Lymphocytes with Antiidiotypic Antibodies and Complement[a]

Responding cells	Stimulator cells	Responding cells treated with:	[³H]TdR incorporated (cpm ± S.E.)	
			Mixture[b]	Parental cells[c]
CBA	(CBA×C57BL/6)F$_1$	Normal (CBA×C57BL/6)F$_1$ serum + C'	35.712±0.964	3.327±0.127
CBA	(CBA×C57BL/6)F$_1$	Antiserum (10%) present in culture	33.207±0.777	3.760±0.345
CBA	(CBA×C57BL/6)F$_1$	Antiserum + C'	5.143±0.564	2.979±1.524
C57BL/6	(CBA×C57BL/6)F$_1$	Normal (CBA×C57BL/6)F$_1$ serum + C'	23.992±0.561	3.554±0.204
C57BL/6	(CBA×C57BL/6)F$_1$	Antiserum (10%) present in culture	25.212±0.723	3.302±0.057
C57BL/6	(CBA×C57BL/6)F$_1$	Antiserum + C'	26.239±0.685	3.510±0.230
CBA	(CBA×DBA/2)F$_1$	Normal (CBA×C57BL/6)R serum + C'	51.569±1.088	5.098±1.173
CBA	(CBA×DBA/2)F$_1$	Antiserum + C'	53.027±1.487	4.675±0.647

[a]MLC was performed in microtiter plates using RPMI 1640 complemented with 5% FCS and 5% normal (CBA×C57BL/6)F$_1$ serum previously absorbed with F$_1$ erythrocytes as a medium and 0.75×10⁶ responder cells and 1.5×10⁶ 1500-rad-irradiated stimulator cells per well. The culture was pulsed for 16 hr on day 2 with 2 µCi [³H]TdR.
[b]Mean of triplicate wells.
[c]Mean of duplicate wells. Irradiated stimulator cells alone gave 100–1000 cpm.

culture caused no reduction in MLC activity. Table XV gives an example of such an experiment. With the aid of complement, (CBA×C57B1/6)F_1 anti-(CBA anti-C57B1/6) antiserum did block, in a highly specific way, the response of CBA responder cells to C57B1/6 antigens. F_1 normal serum had no such effect. F_1 antiserum present during the entire culture period in a concentration up to 10% had no suppressive effect, confirming the earlier findings in GvH reactions.

2. Removal of Suppressive Effect of F_1 Antiserum by Absorption on Alloantibody Immunoabsorbents As Measured in Mixed Leukocyte Culture

Antiidiotypic antibodies of specificity anti-(Lewis anti-DA) were absorbed on either Lewis anti-DA IgG, Lewis normal IgG, or (Lewis × DA)F_1 immunoabsorbents. The absorbed antisera and the material bound and eluted from the immunoabsorbents by low-pH and high-ionic-strength treatment were subsequently tested for inhibition of the MLC response. The results obtained are shown in Table V. They are essentially the same as already shown in GvH reactions (see Table 6). It was possible to remove the antiidiotypic antibodies responsible for the suppression of the MLC response by Lewis anti-DA IgG immunoabsorbents. Lewis normal IgG or IgG from (Lewis × DA)F_1 normal serum did not remove any relevant antibodies. The bound material could be eluted and showed a high activity in suppression. These experiments again support the concept that T and B lymphocytes that have the capactiy to react against the same alloantigens share idiotypic determinants.

3. Inhibition of Secondary Mixed Leukocyte Culture Responses

In the last experiment of this series, we tried to inhibit a secondary response in MLC by antiidiotypic antibodies. Lewis T lymphocytes were primed *in vivo* with a DA skin graft. Three months later, spleen and lymph node cells from these animals were removed and used for a secondary MLC. As a control, lymphocytes from normal Lewis animals were used. Figure 1 shows such an experiment. The peak of the primary response of Lewis normal lymphocytes responding against either irradiated DA or irradiated BN lymphocytes was found around 120 hr. The responses were about the same regardless whether the responder cells were untreated or treated with F_1 normal serum and complement. The primary response against DA could be abolished by treating the responder cells with the antiidiotypic antiserum of specificity anti-(Lewis anti-DA). On the other hand, the primary response to BN antigens was not affected. The peak of the secondary response was found between 24 and 48 hr, and this response was not affected when treated with normal F_1 serum and complement. The secondary response was almost completely abolished by treating the responding cells with antiidiotypic antiserum and complement. Thus, no differ-

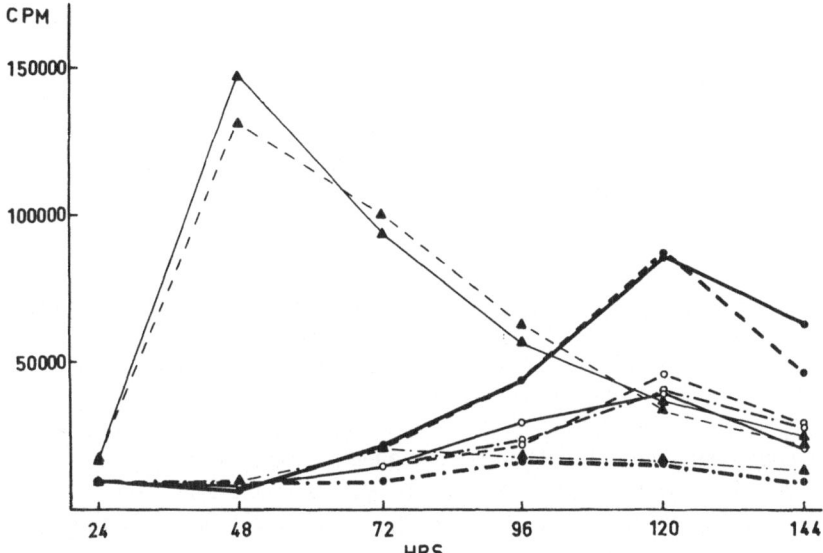

Fig. 1. Inhibition of primary and secondary MLC by the use of antiidiotypic antibodies. MLCs were performed in microtiter plates using 0.25×10^6 responder cells and 0.5×10^6 2000-rad-irradiated stimulator cells per well in EHAA medium (Click et al., 1972) complemented with 5% fresh normal rat serum. Triplicate cultures were pulsed for 6 hr with 1 μCi [^{3}H]TdR. (●) Primary culture of Lewis lymphocytes against DA; (○) primary culture of Lewis lymphocytes against BN; (▲) secondary culture of Lewis lymphocytes, primed 3 months before *in vivo* with DA lymphocytes, against DA. (———) Nontreated responder cells; (– – –) responder cells treated prior to the culture with normal (Lewis × DA)F$_1$ serum and complement; (–·–·–·) responder cells treated prior to the culture with antiidiotypic antiserum and complement. Control cultures (responder cells alone) gave 4000–6000 cpm; irradiated stimulator cells, 200–400 cpm.

ences in T-cell idiotypes were found on cells participating in primary or secondary MLCs.

4. Elimination of Killer T Cells with Antiidiotypic Antibodies and Complement

In the mouse, MLC reactivity and killer-T-cell activity are directed to a major extent against different antigenic determinants of the major histocompatibility complex locus (Peck *et al.*, 1976). It is likely that this is also the case for the rat. In the present rat systems, two experiments have been carried out in an attempt to test whether *in vitro* activated killer T cells are blocked by the relevant antiidiotypic antibodies. The results were analogous to those obtained in the MLC reaction. In the presence of antiserum and complement, there was a specific elimination of killer activity. In the absence of complement, however, antiidiotypic serum in the killer test failed to interfere with the cytolytic reactions. These data, although preliminary, thus suggest that it is indeed possible to induce antiidiotypic antibodies directed against the antigen-binding receptors of rat T killer cells. Whether these idiotypes are distinct from those present on the T lymphocytes responding in MLC against the same Ag–B complex is unknown.

V. DIRECT VISUALIZATION OF IDIOTYPE-POSITIVE T LYMPHOCYTES USING FLUORESCENT ANTIBODY TECHNIQUES, AUTORADIOGRAPHY, OR ELECTRONMICROSCOPY MEASUREMENTS

Our present antiidiotypic antisera frequently react with idiotypic receptors on relevant T lymphocytes with such strength as to allow detection by direct radioimmunoassay techniques. It would thus seem quite possible that idiotype-

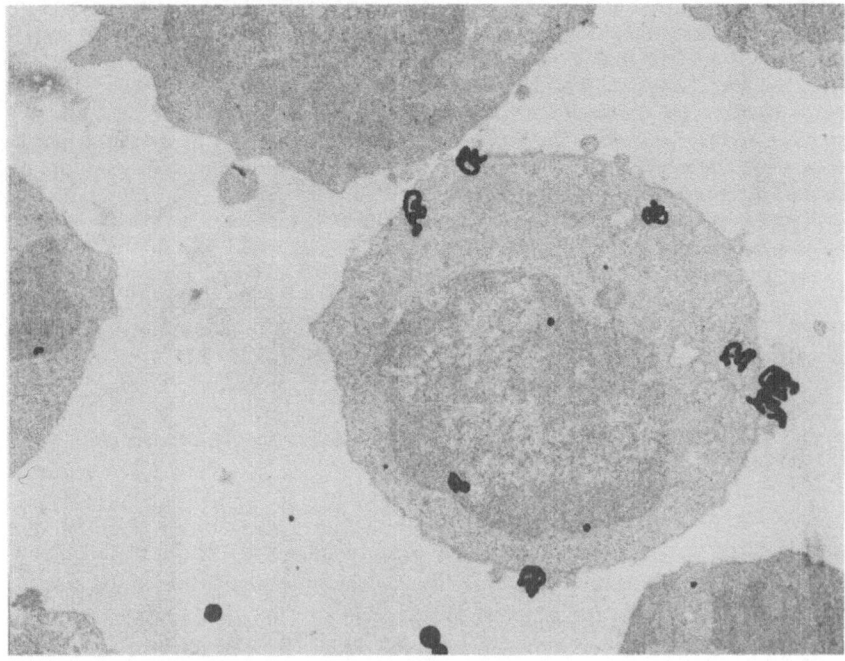

Fig. 2. CBA T lymphocytes reacted with anti-(CBA anti-C57B1/6) serum and ^{125}I-labeled rabbit anti-mouse IgG. Autoradiography after 10 weeks of exposure. ×13,000.

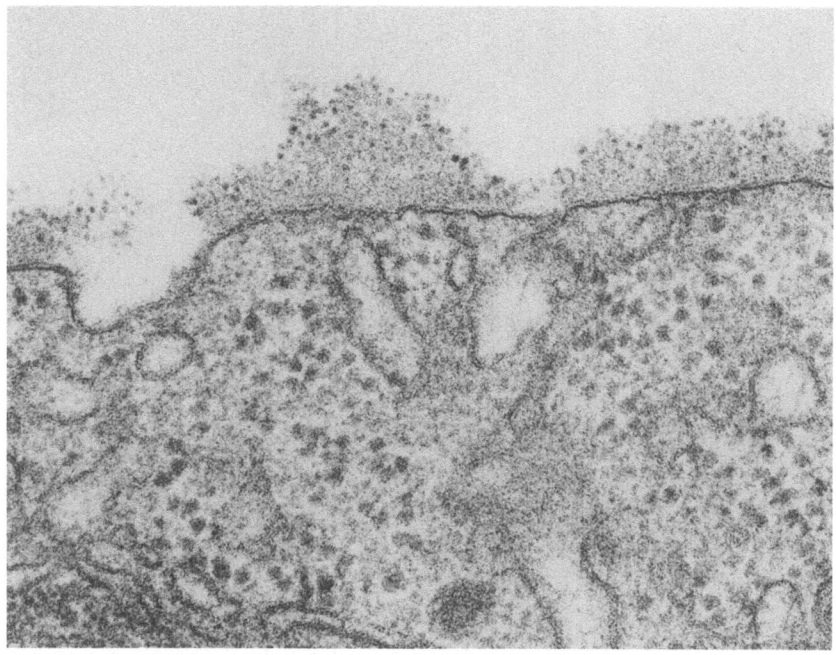

Fig. 3. CBA T lymphocyte reacted with anti-(CBA anti-C57B1/6) serum, rabbit anti-mouse IgG, and ferritin-conjugated guinea pig anti-rabbit IgG. ×95,000.

positive T lymphocytes could be visualized using such antireceptor antibodies. Using purified T lymphocytes from normal CBA mice and F_1-anti-(CBA-anti-C57BL/6) antibodies followed by a second layer of [^{125}I] rabbit-anti-mouse immunoglobulin antibodies, this was indeed found possible (Binz *et al.*, 1975a). The cells were screened for bound radiolabeled anti-Ig antibodies using auto-radiography techniques for light or electron microscopy. Control experiments using normal F_1 serum as the first layer demonstrated that less than 1% of the cells demonstrated high binding (30 grains or more), with the great majority being negative. We believe these background cells to represent contaminating B lymphocytes being detected by the second anti-Ig reaction. However, using the F_1-anti-(CBA-anti-C57BL/6) antiserum (the same serum that suppressed CBA T cells from reacting against C57BL/6 in MLC; see Table XV), about 5% of the CBA T lymphocytes were heavily stained [(CBA×C57BL/6)F_1 T cells were stained only to background 1% levels]. This finding would thus suggest that a quite sizable proportion of the CBA T lymphocytes do carry idiotypic receptors denoting reactivity against C57BL/6 alloantigens. Experiments suggesting such figures of T lymphocytes predetermined to react across the major histocompatibility complex locus using entirely different approaches have previously been

Table XVI. Grain Counts of Lewis and (Lewis × DA)F$_1$ T Lymphocytes Incubated with (Lewis × DA)F$_1$ Anti-Lewis T Cell Serum and (Lewis × DA)F$_1$ Normal Serum[a]

Cells[a]	Serum	Grain count distribution (% of total population)									
		0–4	5–9	10–19	20–29	30–39	40–49	50–59	60–69	70–79	80 or more
Lewis T	F$_1$ anti-Lewis T	88	3	0.7	0	0.3	0	0	0.3	0	7.0
Lewis T	F$_1$ normal serum	93	6	0.2	0.5	0.2	0	0	0	0	0.5
(Lewis × DA)F$_1$ T	F$_1$ anti-Lewis T	96	3	0	0.4	0	0	0	0	0	0.7
(Lewis × DA)F$_1$ T	F$_1$ normal serum	90	8	1.1	0	0	0	0	0	0	1.4

[a]T lymphocytes were prepared from normal spleen and lymph node cells, filtered through an anti-Ig column. A total of 300–400 cells per group was counted. The cells were incubated at 4°C for 1 hr with F$_1$ normal or F$_1$ anti-Lewis T cell serum, followed by radiolabeled rabbit anti-rat Ig. Smears were dried and fixed for 24 hr in 100% methanol. Ilford G-5 emulsion was used. Autoradiographs were exposed at 4°C for 5 days in the dark and developed with Kodak ID-19. Cells were stained with Giemsa. Reproduced from *Journal of Experimental Medicine* 142:1218 (1975).

reported (Ford *et al.,* 1975; Howard and Wilson, 1974; Nisbet *et al.,* 1969; Wilson *et al.,* 1968), and the present experiments would thus be entirely in agreement with these earlier observations. Similar results as to frequency of idiotypic CBA T lymphocytes were obtained using electron-microscopic examinations after 10 weeks' autoradiography. Figure 2 shows an example of such a cell using the procedures described above. In other experiments, triple-layer techniques were used, with "cold" rabbit-anti-mouse Ig antibodies as the second layer and ferritin-conjugated guinea pig-anti-rabbit Ig antibodies as the third layer. A large surface area of the idiotypic CBA T lymphocytes could be shown by these procedures to be covered with ferritin, indicating a high density of idiotypic receptors on these cells (see Fig. 3).

We then carried out similar but more extensive studies in the rat idiotypic system using light-microscope autoradiography. As can be seen from Table XVI, again we found a strikingly high frequency of normal T lymphocytes carrying idiotypic markers of a given specificity. Pooling several experiments by using cells heavily labeled with silver grains and subtracting the contamination with B lymphocytes, we found 6.3% T lymphocytes with idiotypic markers of anti-DA specificity to be present in a normal Lewis T cell population. This figure is

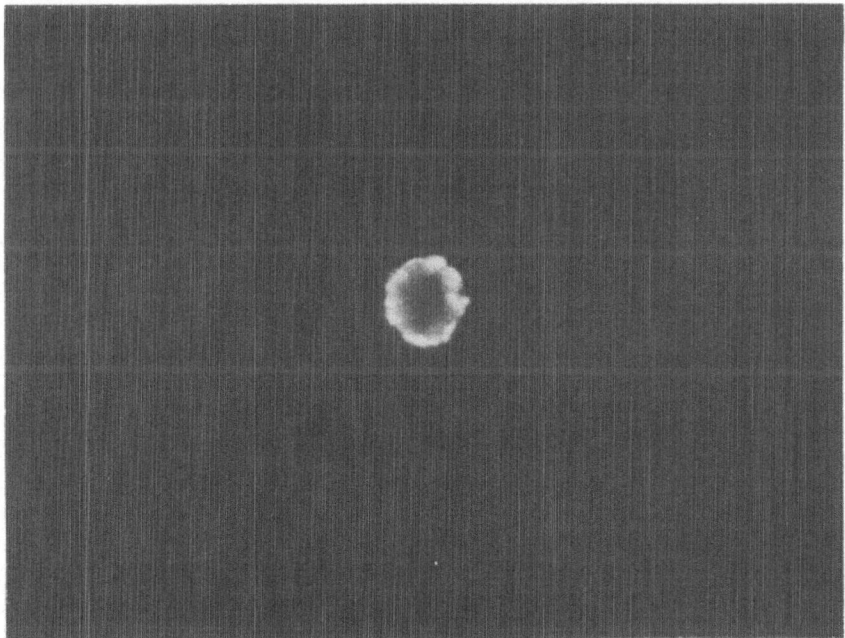

Fig. 4. Idiotype-positive Lewis T lymphocyte reacted with FITC-conjugated anti-(Lewis anti-DA).

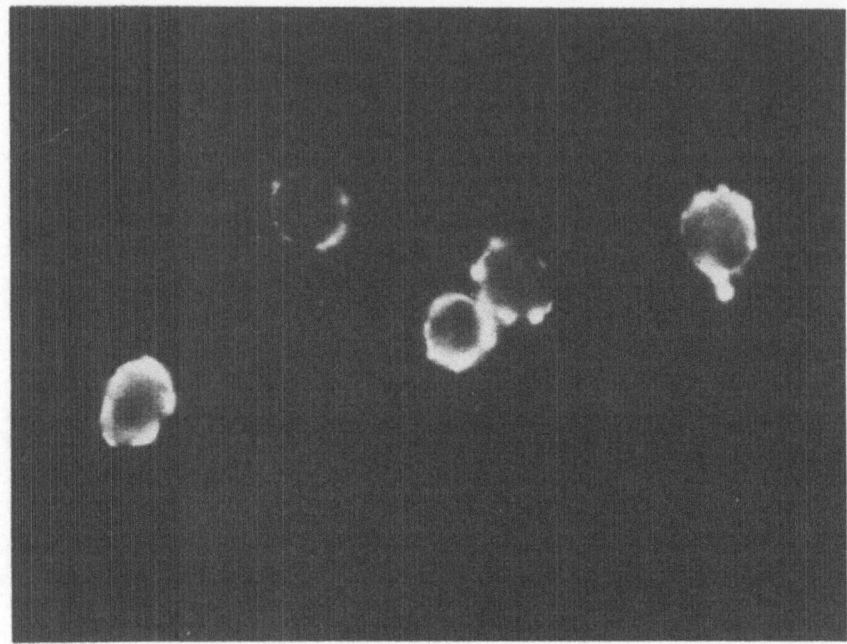

Fig. 5. Purified idiotype-positive Lewis T lymphocytes (see the text) stained with FITC-labeled anti-(Lewis anti-DA).

Table XVII. Percentage of Anti-DA Idiotype-Positive Lewis T and B Lymphocytes

Cells[a]	Incubated for 1 hr at 4°C with:	Total cells counted	Positive cells	
			Number	% of total cell population
Lewis T	FITC anti-(Lewis anti-DA) diluted 1:2	2361	147	6.23
DA	FITC anti-(Lewis anti-DA) diluted 1:2	516	0	0
Lewis B	FITC anti-(Lewis anti-DA) diluted 1:2	3210	33	1.03
DA B	FITC anti-(Lewis anti-DA) diluted 1:2	614	0	0
L T	FITC rabbit anti-rat Ig diluted 1:20	213	1	0.47
DA T	FITC rabbit anti-rat Ig diluted 1:20	133	1	0.75
L B	FITC rabbit anti-rat Ig diluted 1:20	168	165	98.21
DA B	FITC rabbit anti-rat Ig diluted 1:20	211	207	98.10

[a]T lymphocytes were prepared by using an anti-Ig column, B lymphocytes by using a rabbit anti-rat T cell antiserum (Binz and Wigzell, 1975b). Experiments were carried out under noncapping conditions.

roughly the same as that obtained in the mouse system. That these stained lymphocytes are indeed the very same that have the capacity to react against alloantigens could later be demonstrated, as shown in Section VI of this chapter.

Similar experiments were carried out using the fluorescence technique. A typical anti-DA idiotype-positive Lewis T lymphocyte is shown in Fig. 4 using rabbit anti-rat labeled with fluorescein isothiocyanate (FITC) indicator on top of anti-Lewis anti-DA antiidiotypic antibodies. Figure 5 shows idiotype-positive Lewis T lymphocytes of the same specificity after purification on anti-Ig columns as described in detail in Section VI. The staining in both cases (Figs. 4 and 5) was carried out under noncapping conditions.

Sandwich techniques cannot be applied to study the frequency of idiotype-positive B lymphocytes, since the cells carry conventional immunoglobulins on their surfaces. Direct labeling of the antiidiotypic antibodies with FITC or another marker is necessary. Antiidiotypic antibodies of specificity anti-(Lewis andi-DA) were directly labeled with FITC (Binz and Wigzell, 1975b). Lewis T lymphocytes were prepared with the standard anti-Ig columns (Binz and Wigzell, 1975b), and Lewis B lymphocytes with a heterologous rabbit anti-rat T-cell serum (Binz and Wigzell, 1975b). DA T and DA B lymphocytes were prepared in exactly the same way. Such cell preparations were then incubated with FITC labeled antiidiotypic antiserum. The results obtained are shown in Table XVII. They demonstrate that it is possible to stain idiotype-positive lymphocytes by direct FITC-labeled antiidiotypic antibodies. The results with regard to T lymphocytes are essentially the same as already obtained with autoradiographs, and the fluorescent staining observed is a typical membrane staining (see Figs. 3 and 4). These experiments were carried out under antibody excess, since the same antiidiotypic antiserum used in a dilution of 1:5 gave the same results. Again, about 6% of Lewis T lymphocytes were heavily labeled with FITC-labeled antiidiotypic antibodies. The specificity of the antiserum is demonstrated by the fact that DA and (Lewis X DA)F_1 purified T and B lymphocytes did not bind antiidiotypic antibodies to a significant extent. The frequency of idiotype-positive B lymphocytes is much lower compared with the frequency of idiotype-positive T lymphocytes. About 1% of Lewis B lymphocytes fixed antiidiotypic antibodies. This figure is quite high compared with some reports (Natvig et al., 1975), but not in comparison with others (K. Eichmann, personal communication). The fluorescence intensity of T and B cells as judged by the naked eye seemed to be about the same. To quantitate the fluorescence intensity on the single-cell level, however, quantitative cytofluorospectrophotometry was carried out (Binz and Wigzell, 1975d). The frequency distribution of idiotype-positive T lymphocytes was essentially the same as found before, while the cell numbers counted were too low to allow statements of idiotypic B cell frequencies. That the antigen-binding receptors on T lymphocytes are actually produced by the cells themselves and not acquired as cytophilic antibodies is indicated by several sets of data. Trypsin removal of the T-lymphocyte receptors with subsequent recovery *in vitro* had no influence on the high frequency of idiotype-positive T lymphocytes. In other experiments involving internal labeling with radiolabeled amino acids, actual synthesis of the receptors by the cells could be demonstrated (see Section VII). Finally, no constant-region markers of conventional immunoglobulins could be demonstrated on T lymphocytes.

In conclusion, we can say that it is possible to visualize idiotype-positive T and B lymphocytes by different methods such as autoradiography, fluorescence technique, and electron microscopy. Frequency studies showed that about 6% of normal Lewis T cells, and about 1% of the corresponding B lymphocytes, express anti-DA idiotypic determinants. Intensity studies on the single-cell level showed that T and B lymphocytes express similar "amounts" of idiotypic determinants. Whether this intensity is directly proportional to the actual number of antigen-binding T-cell receptors is, however, not clear.

VI. SPECIFIC ACCUMULATION AND PURIFICATION OF IDIOTYPE-POSITIVE T LYMPHOCYTES

To study the function and specific immunocompetence of the idiotype-positive, alloantigen-reactive T lymphocytes, it is important to have these cells in a highly enriched or even in a pure form. We describe here several methods that allow a specific accumulation of such T lymphocytes. It is possible to obtain them in a "pure" form to be subsequently analyzed by functional studies or direct visualization using fluorescein-labeled antiidiotypic antibodies. A positive correlation between the expression of idiotypic determinants and the capacity to react as GvH-reactive lymphocytes in semiallogeneic animals could be found.

A. Specific Accumulation of Idiotype-Positive Lymphocytes in Lymph Nodes Draining a Corresponding Skin Graft

It is known that in the course of an allograft rejection, there is an accumulation of effector lymphocytes and antibody-producing cells in the draining lymph nodes (Gowans and McGregor, 1965; Hildemann 1967). This knowledge served as the basis for the first series of experiments. An animal simultaneously carrying two allografts from genetically different donors will simultaneously enrich two populations of cells carrying different idiotypes in the draining lymph nodes of the corresponding allografts. It is known that antiidiotypic antibodies produced in F_1 animals directed against the variable part of alloantibodies of the variable part of T-cell receptors can be radiolabeled. Such labeled antibodies show

Table XVIII. Accumulation of Radiolabeled Antiidiotypic Antibodies in Lymph Nodes Draining a Corresponding Skin Graft[a]

Host	Radioactive antiidiotype injected	Mean activity (cpm/mg tissue) in 5 or 6 nodes draining grafts of:			Mean of differences ± S.D.
		Lewis	DA	BN	
Lewis	Anti-(Lewis anti-DA)	–	349.3	236.3	113 ± 38.12[b]
DA	Anti-(DA anti-Lewis)	473.3	–	244.5	228.8±112.75[b]
Lewis	Anti-(DA anti-Lewis)	–	212.0	217.8	–5.8± 35.45
DA	Anti-(Lewis anti-DA)	198.2	–	192.2	6.0± 26.55

[a]Seven days after skin allografts, hosts were injected intravenously with ^{125}I-radiolabeled antiidiotypic antibodies. Twenty-four hours later, the draining axillary lymph nodes were removed, injected, and counted in a gamma counter. For further details, see Binz and Lindenmann (1972b).
[b]Values differ significantly from 0 ($P < 1\%$).

specificity for the relevant parental lymphocytes (Binz and Lindenmann, 1972a).

Radiolabeled antiidiotypic antibodies of a given specificity systemically injected in excess should be accumulated in the lymph nodes draining the corresponding skin graft if lymphocytes carrying the corresponding idiotype are enriched at these nodes. Antiidiotypic antibodies of specificity anti-(Lewis anti-DA) and anti-(DA anti-Lewis) were iodinated with ^{125}I by standard procedures (Hunter and Greenwood, 1962; Binz and Lindenmann, 1972b). On day 0, rats of the Lewis and DA strains received two skin grafts each. DA skin was placed on the left side of a Lewis animal and BN skin on the right side. In the same way, Lewis skin was placed on the left side of a DA animal and BN skin on the right side. On day 7 after grafting, 0.5 ml of radiolabeled antiidiotypic antibodies was injected into the tail vein of each animal. Twenty-four hours later, the animals were killed, and the draining axillary lymph nodes were removed, weighed, and finally counted in a gamma counter for ^{125}I. The radioactivity was expressed as counts per minute per milligram of lymph node tissue. Table XVIII shows an experiment carried out under this protocol. In DA rats bearing Lewis and BN skin grafts and injected with radiolabeled anti-(DA anti-Lewis) and in Lewis rats bearing DA and BN skin grafts and injected with radioactive anti-(Lewis anti-DA) antibodies, a specific accumulation of radioactivity could be demonstrated in the lymph nodes draining the corresponding skin graft. On the other hand, if Lewis rats bearing DA and BN skin grafts and DA rats bearing Lewis and BN skin grafts were injected with anti-(DA anti-Lewis) or anti-(Lewis anti-DA), respectively, no differential accumulation in either lymph nodes could be demonstrated.

These data can be interpreted as follows: Idiotype-positive, antigen-binding lymphocytes accumulate in lymph nodes draining a corresponding skin graft. Antiidiotypic antibodies of corresponding specificity that have been radio-labeled are fixed by the relevant lymphocytes. Alternatively, the antiidiotypic antibodies were fixed by locally produced alloantibodies. However, in later experiments using fluorescent-labeled antiidiotypic antibodies (see below), we could demonstrate that idiotype-positive lymphocytes are in fact enriched in lymph nodes draining a corresponding skin graft.

B. Trapping of Idiotype-Positive T Lymphocytes in Popliteal Lymph Nodes Draining an Allograft

Immunocompetent lymphocytes have the capacity to recognize antigenic determinants. They are also able to circulate in the body, and it has been shown that specific reactive lymphocytes are able to travel toward injected antigen (Ford, 1975).

A similar system was chosen to try to accumulate specific alloantigen-reactive T lymphocytes. In experiments carried out using MLC as the test system it could be shown that alloantigen-reactive T lymphocytes accumulate in the draining popliteal lymph nodes when allogeneic spleen cells are previously injected into the corresponding footpad (Peck and Binz, unpublished results). In addition, it could be shown that the spleens of such animals are partially depleted of the corresponding alloantigen-reactive T lymphocytes. This partial depletion could still be demonstrated 1 month after injection of allogeneic cells if amputation of the corresponding leg lodging the popliteal lymph node was done 24 hr after the injection of the allogeneic cells.

In additional experiments, normal Lewis rats were injected with 1×10^7 DA spleen cells into the right footpad and 1×10^7 female Lewis cells into the left. Normal Lewis rats and (Lewis $\times$ DA)F_1 rats injected with saline only into the footpads were used as control animals. Twenty-four hours later, the animals were killed, and the spleens and popliteal lymph nodes were separately removed. Cell preparations of these organs were incubated with a fluorescein-labeled anti-(Lewis anti-DA) antiidiotypic antibody and finally analyzed for positive cells. Table XIX shows the results of such an experiment. Spleen and lymph node cells from control Lewis animals (injected with PBS only) or from (Lewis $\times$ DA)F_1 animals showed normal values (see also Section V). About 5–7% positive lymphocytes were found in lymph nodes or spleens from normal Lewis rats, and only background levels for (Lewis $\times$ DA)F_1 animals. On the other hand, spleen cells from the Lewis rats injected with DA spleen cells into the right footpad showed slightly decreased values in idiotype-positive lymphocytes (4% positive cells in the experimental animals compared with 5.6% in the control

Table XIX. Specific Accumulation of Idiotype-Positive T Lymphocytes
in Popliteal Lymph Nodes Draining a Corresponding Allograft[a]

| Hosts | Footpads injected with: | | Exp. No. | Idiotype-positive lymphocytes (mean %) from: | | |
	Left side	Right side		Spleen	Left L N	Right L N
(L×DA)F₁	PBS	PBS	1	0.5	0.4	0.4
Lewis	PBS	PBS	1+2	5.6	8.1	5.8
Lewis	Lewis spleen cells	DA spleen cells	1	4.1	6.4	11.1
			2	3.9	5.4	10.6

[a]1×10^7 spleen cells from either Lewis or DA rats were injected into the footpads of Lewis rats. As a control, PBS alone was injected. Popliteal lymph nodes and spleens were removed 24 hr later and analyzed for idiotype-positive lymphocytes using FITC-labeled anti-(L-anti DA).

animals). Lymph node cells from the experimental animals obtained from the popliteal lymph nodes draining the footpad injected with syngeneic Lewis cells showed normal values of about 6% positive lymphocytes. Lymphocytes from the popliteal lymph nodes draining the footpad that had received allogeneic DA spleen cells, however, showed a twofold increase of idiotype-positive lymphocytes.

C. Cytolytic Activity and Idiotypic Expression on Allograft-Infiltrating Cells

It is known that host cells infiltrating an allograft can finally cause the rejection of the graft. The characteristics of these, however, are still largely unknown. Recently, an experimental model that allows quantitative recovery of allograft-infiltrating cells has been described (Roberts and Häyry, 1976). A sponge matrix tissue is first infiltrated *in vivo* by fibroblasts of a given strain. Such infiltrated "sponges" are then grafted into allogeneic animals, where they are subsequently infiltrated by host cells. The sponges can easily be removed and the infiltrating aggressor cells recovered. The system has recently been used to study the allograft-infiltrating cells with regard to cytolytic activity and idiotype expression (Binz *et al.*, 1976).

Sponge matrix material was placed into the peritoneal cavities of DA, Lewis, or BN rats in order to be infiltrated with fibroblasts. Five days later, the sponges were removed and transplanted subcutaneously into the necks of Lewis rats. The

Table XX. Expression of Lewis Anti-DA Idiotypes Correlated with Cytolytic Activity Against DA Target Cells

Rat	Cells from	Total L anti-DA idiotype-positive cells (%)[a]	L anti-DA idiotype	Percentage distribution of latex-positive or phagocytic cells within the idiotype-positive or -negative cells[b]			Cytolytic anti-DA activity[c]
				Latex-negative	Latex-positive on cell surface	Latex-positive phagocytes	
Lewis carrying DA graft	Graft	42.8	Pos.	51.2	7.2	41.6	44.8
			Neg.	49.1	3.2	47.8	
	Draining lymph node	21.2	Pos.	72.0	13.0	13.0	22.5
			Neg.	96.0	2.0	1.0	
	Nondraining lymph node	5.2	Pos.	92.3	1.9	5.8	4.8
			Neg.	89.9	10.6	0.7	
	Spleen	9.2	Pos.	72.8	21.7	5.4	26.0
			Neg.	58.3	37.3	4.4	
Lewis carrying Lewis graft	Graft	2.0	Pos.	60.0	40.0	0.0	−0.9
			Neg.	50.7	3.0	46.2	
	Draining lymph node	5.8	Pos.	86.2	12.1	1.7	1.2
			Neg.	79.2	9.9	10.9	
	Nondraining lymph node	5.0	Pos.	86.0	14.0	0.0	ND
			Neg.	85.5	14.1	0.4	
	Spleen	4.9	Pos.	67.4	18.4	14.3	0.4
			Neg.	63.0	33.6	3.4	

		a					c
Normal Lewis rat	Graft	3.9	Pos.	43.6	18.0	38.5	5.3
			Neg.	49.1	4.5	46.4	
	Draining lymph node	7.5	Pos.	80.0	6.7	13.3	3.4
			Neg.	81.3	8.6	10.1	
	Nondraining lymph node	5.4	Pos.	90.8	7.4	1.8	2.2
			Neg.	87.4	11.3	1.3	
	Spleen	5.7	Pos.	73.7	17.5	8.8	1.3
			Neg.	61.3	33.6	5.1	
Normal DA rat	Lymph node	0.1	Pos.	0.0	0.0	100.0	ND
			Neg.	85.6	13.7	0.7	
	Spleen	0.2	Pos.	0.0	0.0	100.0	ND
			Neg.	63.8	31.4	4.8	

[a] Total number of idiotype-positive cells as measured by FITC-conjugated anti-(L anti-DA).

[b] Cells were first incubated for 30 min at 37°C with heat-aggregated human-IgG-coated latex particles. Cells were then incubated with the antiserum and analyzed for the presence/absence of surface immunofluorescence, for the presence/absence of latex particles attached to the cell surfaces (Fc-receptor-carrying cells), and for latex inside the cells (phagocytic cells).

[c] The killer assay was run overnight in microtiter plates with a killer/target cell ratio of 100:1 using ^{51}Cr-labeled PHA blasts as target cells.

rats were killed 1 week after grafting (peak killer activity in the graft), and the sponges and the draining and nondraining lymph nodes, as well as the spleens, were removed and cell suspensions were prepared. Different markers were used to further define the recovered cells. FITC-labeled anti-Lewis anti-DA antiidiotypic antibodies were used to demonstrate the presence of idiotypic markers on the DA-reactive Lewis lymphocytes. Human IgG-coated latex particles were used to demonstrate the phagocytic capacity of the cells or to demonstrate the presence of Fc receptors (latex particles bound on the surface of the cell). Finally, the cells were tested for their cytolytic activity *in vitro* against the relevant allogeneic target cells (PHA-induced blasts). Table XX summarizes part of these experiments. First, we could demonstrate that Lewis rats that received a DA allograft expressed normal idiotype frequency in nondraining lymph nodes (popliteal lymph nodes). A slight increase in frequency could be found in the spleen, but a pronounced increase in the draining lymph node and especially in the allograft sponge was noted. A positive correlation between idiotype expression and cytolytic activity toward DA alloantigens in the various suspensions could be demonstrated. Analysis as to surface or functional markers revealed that a high proportion of idiotype-positive cells invading the allograft expressed phagocytic activities or Fc receptors (see Table XX). We consider it quite likely that these cells are host macrophages being coated or armed with idiotypic molecules. Whether these molecules are of T- or B-cell origin is unknown. All that can be said is that the present sponge allograft systems allow the recovery of a highly enriched idiotype-positive cell suspension with strong, specific cytolytic activity.

D. Purification of Alloantigen-Reactive T Lymphocytes by the Use of Antiidiotypic Antibodies

To be able to study in detail the structure and function of immunocompetent T lymphocytes, enrichment figures still higher than the ones reported above would be necessary. Several methods exist to achieve a specific depletion or enrichment of antigen-specific B lymphocytes (Wigzell, 1971), but no convincing methods have been described achieving similar results for T lymphocytes with specific antigen-binding capacity. Cellular immunoabsorbents have been used for a selective depletion or enrichment of antigen-reactive T lymphocytes (Wigzell, 1971). In this instance, however, depletion experiments seem to be more successful than enrichment experiments (Golstein *et al.,* 1971; Wekerle *et al.,* 1972, Elliot *et al.,* 1975).

We describe here a procedure that allows the purification of alloantigen-reactive T lymphocytes on the order of 90% or more. Lewis T lymphocytes were prepared by the standard Degalan-Ig-anti-Ig columns (Binz *et al.,* 1974a). Some

Table XXI. Specific Purification and Depletion of Two Antigen-Reactive T-Cell Subpopulations by the Use of Two Different Antiidiotypic Antisera

Lewis T Lymphocytes 1^b
incubated with anti-(Lewis anti-BN)
⎯⎯⎯⎯⎯ Degalan-Ig-anti-Ig column

Cells eluted
from the column
3^b

Cells Passed the Column 2^b
Incubated with anti-(Lewis anti-DA)
⎯⎯⎯⎯⎯ Degalan-Ig-anti-Ig column

Cells eluted
from the column
5^b

Cells Passed the Column 4^b

Cells injected[a]	Hosts	Mean of lymph node weights ± S.E.[c] (mg)	Mean of lymph node weights ± S.E.[c] (mg)	Mean log ratio ± S.E.[d]
1	(L×BN)F$_1$	31.5±2.2	–	*0.64±0.07*
2	(L×BN)F$_1$	–	7.6±1.0	
1	(L×DA)F$_1$	37.2±7.6	–	−0.04±0.12
2	(L×DA)F$_1$	–	38.0±4.1	
1	(L×Au)F$_1$	13.2±1.9	–	−0.06±0.05
2	(L×Au)F$_1$	–	16.0±4.0	
1	(L×BN)F$_1$	18.8±2.3	–	*−0.61±0.08*
3	(L×BN)F$_1$	–	75.6±9.7	
1	(L×DA)F$_1$	22.0±4.9	–	*0.76±0.08*
3	(L×DA)F$_1$	–	3.5±0.5	
1	(L×Au)F$_1$	15.9∓0.8	–	*0.65±0.07*
3	(L×Au)F$_1$	–	3.6±0.5	
1	(L×BN)F$_1$	20.7±2.0	–	*0.63±0.12*
4	(L×BN)F$_1$	–	5.3±1.1	
1	(L×DA)F$_1$	27.9±2.8	–	*0.80±0.06*
4	(L×DA)F$_1$	–	4.5±0.6	
1	(L×Au)F$_1$	14.0±1.3	–	−0.07±0.01
4	(L×Au)F$_1$	. –	16.7±2.0	
1	(L×BN)F$_1$	22.0±2.5	–	*0.74±0.09*
5	(L×BN)F$_1$	–	4.0±0.5	
1	(L×DA)F$_1$	21.0±1.1	–	*−0.70±0.07*
5	(L×DA)F$_1$	–	105.1±9.4	
1	(L×Au)F$_1$	11.3±1.1	–	*0.55±0.09*
5	(L×Au)F$_1$	–	3.2±0.4	

[a]$3×10^6$ viable cells were injected into each footpad. Popliteal lymph nodes were removed 7 days later. Rats: Lewis (Ag-B^1), DA(Ag-B^4), BN(Ag-B^3), August (Au) (Ag-B^5). Reproduced from *Journal of Experimental Medicine*, **142**:1231 (1975).
[b]Cell numbers: (1) 600×10^6; (2) 521×10^6; (3) 64×10^6; (4) 396×10^6; (5) 44×10^6.
[c]Mean weights of 3–10 lymph nodes.
[d]Values in italics significantly different from 0.00.

of these cells were kept as control cells (see Table XXI). The other part of the cells was incubated with anti-(Lewis anti-BN) antiidiotypic antibodies and subsequently passed over a second small anti-Ig column. Part of the cells passing the column were used for the induction of GvH reactions, but another part was incubated with anti-(Lewis anti-DA) antiidiotypic antibodies and passed over a third anti-Ig column. Cells passing this column were also used to induce GvH reactions. Cells retained in the second and third anti-Ig columns were separately eluted from the Degalan beads by mechanical means and used for induction of GvH reactions.

The normal Lewis T lymphocytes (purified by passing spleen and lymph node cells through an anti-Ig column) were used as a control cell population for the induction of GvH reactions in (Lewis $\times$ DA)F_1, (Lewis $\times$ BN)F_1 and (Lewis $\times$ Au)F_1. Table XXI shows that Lewis T lymphocytes incubated with anti-(Lewis anti-BN) antiidiotypic antibodies and subsequently passed through a second anti-Ig column were completely depleted of BN-reactive lymphocytes. The reactivity toward DA and Au antigens were fully retained. Cells retained and eluted from the second anti-Ig column, however, showed *a highly increased activity against BN antigens* and *no reactivity toward DA or Au alloantigens.* Cells passing the second anti-Ig column, incubated with anti-(Lewis anti-DA)-antibodies and passed over a third anti-Ig column, were now not only depleted of BN-reactive lymphocytes (second column), but also of the T-cell subpopulation reactive against DA. On the other hand, the capacity to react against Au alloantigens was fully kept. Cells retained and eluted from the third anti-Ig column showed highly increased activity against DA alloantigens, but no reactivity against BN or Au. These data demonstrate that the T-cell subpopulation obtained by the present method was functionally pure, showing a highly enriched reactivity against the relevant alloantigens but with no significant reactivity against third-party antigens. This result would thus demonstrate that the percentage of double-reactive T lymphocytes in this system must be very low.

To further demonstrate the relationship between idiotypes and function of the T cells, experiments were carried out combining fluorescent staining and analysis of specific immune reactivity (Binz and Wigzell, 1975a). The percentage of idiotype-positive T lymphocytes in normal depleted or enriched cell populations as obtained via these procedures was plotted against the GvH reactivity. A striking positive correlation was found between the percentage of, for example, anti-DA (idiotype-positive) Lewis lymphocytes in a population and the GvH reactivity against DA alloantigens (Binz and Wigzell, 1975a). These experiments thus strongly suggested that the idiotype-positive T lymphocytes, as visualized by the fluorescence technique, are indeed the very same cells that express reactivity against the expected antigens.

VII. DEMONSTRATION AND CHARACTERISTICS OF NATURALLY OCCURRING, IDIOTYPIC, ANTIGEN-BINDING MOLECULES DERIVED FROM T AND B LYMPHOCYTES AND PRESENT IN NORMAL SERUM

Small B lymphocytes are known to be able to shed Ig molecules from their surfaces in detectable amounts (Andersson *et al.*, 1974). The presence of a comparatively high percentage of idiotype-positive T and a lower number of B lymphocytes in normal adult rats in the present antigenic systems (see Tables XVI and XVII) prompted a search for idiotypic molecules in the sera of normal rats. The principal technique used was the anti-T-cell idiotype radioimmuno-assay, using suboptimal concentrations of antiidiotypic antibodies in an attempt to inhibit the binding of these antibodies to the cells using normal serum as inhibitor (Binz and Wigzell, 1975b). The results of such experiments are shown in Table XXII, demonstrating that normal adult rats of, for example, the Lewis strain do indeed have in their sera idiotypic molecules of anti-DA specificity. Serum from (Lewis × DA)F_1 hybrids failed to inhibit, whereas immune Lewis-anti-DA serum as anticipated, was a significantly better inhibitor than Lewis

Table XXII. Capacity of Lewis Normal
and Lewis Anti-DA Immune Serum to Inhibit
Binding of (DA×L)F_1 Anti-Lewis
T Serum to Lewis T Cells

Cells[a]	In the presence of:	Mean cpm ± S.E. of duplicates[b]
Lewis T	L anti-DA 1:4	0.897±0.032
Lewis T	L anti-DA 1:16	1.030±0.083
Lewis T	L anti-DA 1:64	1.399±0.300
Lewis T	L anti-DA 1:128	2.251±0.498
Lewis T	L anti-DA 1:256	3.483±0.244
Lewis T	L normal serum 1:2	0.950±0.046
Lewis T	L normal serum 1:4	2.350±0.187
Lewis T	L normal serum 1:8	3.441±0.403
Lewis T	L normal serum 1:16	3.699±0.218
Lewis T	(DA×L)F_1 normal serum 1:2	2.606±0.768
Lewis T	(DA×L)F_1 normal serum 1:4	3.068±0.338

[a] $5×10^6$ T lymphocytes were added to each well containing a 1:20 dilution of a (Lewis × DA)F_1 anti-Lewis T cell serum (Binz and Wigzell, 1975b).
[b] ^{125}I-labeled protein A was added to each sample (Binz and Wigzell, 1975b).

normal serum. Complete inhibition of binding of anti-(Lewis-anti-DA) antibodies
to Lewis T cells could also be achieved, however, by using Lewis normal serum
at high concentration as inhibitor. Sera from several different colonies of Lewis
rats were tested with the same results, demonstrating the occurrence of idiotypic
molecules irrespective of whether or not they had been bred in colonies containing other strains of rats. Further proof of similarity between the "natural"
idiotype-positive molecules and conventional Lewis-anti-DA antibodies was provided for by the demonstration that such idiotypic material could be selectively
absorbed away using the proper alloantigen-containing cells. Thus, the idiotype-
positive molecules in normal rat serum do also express the expected specific
antigen-binding reactivity.

In some preliminary experiments, normal serum of Lewis origin was allowed
to pass through an anti-Lewis-anti-DA idiotype immunoabsorbent column to which
the idiotype-positive molecules were bound, eluted at low pH, neutralized,
labeled with ^{125}I, and fractionated over G-200 columns (Binz and Wigzell,
1975c). The various fractions were analyzed as to radioactivity as well as binding
capacity to (Lewis × DA)F_1 spleen cells using Lewis spleen cells as negative
controls. The elution profile of such purified normal serum molecules are shown
in Fig. 6, which shows peak activity at the IgG- and albumin-size peaks. As
indicated, the radiolabeled molecules expressed specific binding to the F_1 spleen
cells, thus demonstrating antigen-binding ability as well as idiotypic markers on

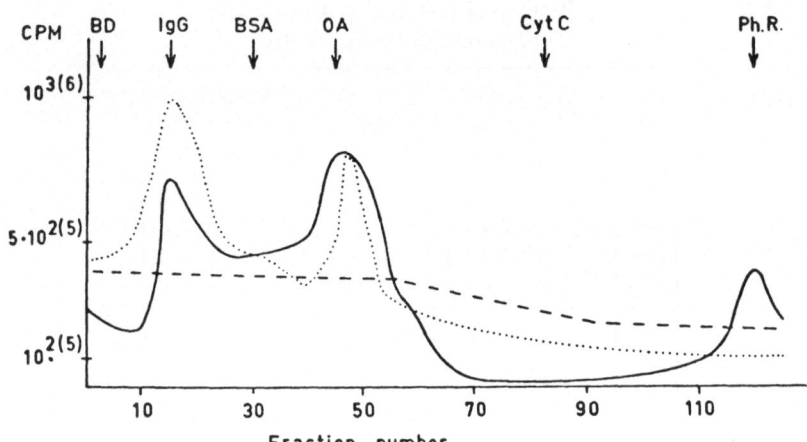

Fig. 6. Elution profile of Lewis normal serum filtered through an IgG anti-(Lewis
anti-DA) immunosorbent. The acid-eluted protein was labeled with ^{125}I and filtered
through a Sephadex G-200 column as indicated in the text. (BD) Blue dextran; (IgG)
normal rat IgG; (BSA) bovine serum albumin; (OA) ovalbumin; (Cyt C) cytochrome
C; (Ph.R.) phenol red. Fractions were tested for binding to Lewis (– – –) or (Lewis
×DA)F_1 (·····) spleen cells. (——) Total radioactivity, scale 5–6.

the respective molecules. When the procedures for isolating idiotypic material from normal rat serum were changed by using inhibitors of proteolysis, as well as by eliminating the 56°C treatment for 30 min, we noted that the low-molecular-weight peak is shifted into a peak of molecules of a size of about 70,000.

The factors found in the normal Lewis serum were thus subsequently analyzed in a more detailed form. Serum from normal adult Lewis rats (either sex) was collected and allowed to coagulate for 30 min at room temperature, after which phenylmethylsulfonfluoride was added to a final dilution of 1 mM to inhibit proteolysis. After an additional 1½ hr, the serum was centrifuged for 5 min at 4000g, and the serum was finally kept at −20°C until use. A quantity of 200 ml of normal serum was first passed over a 1.5×10 cm Sepharose 4 B column in order to absorb material that shows nonspecific binding to Sepharose. The serum was then passed over an F_1 anti-(Lewis anti-DA) antiidiotypic Sepharose immunoabsorbent (0.5 × 3 cm). The passed serum was collected on ice and passed again over the same column. The column was then washed at 4°C with PBS for 20 hr. The bound material was eluted in two steps. For the first step, 10 ml isotonic glycine−HCl buffer, pH 2.8, containing 2 M NaCl was used. The eluate was immediately neutralized with 0.4 N NaOH and kept on ice. For the second step, 10 ml 3 M $MgCl_2$ was used. The eluates were pooled and dialyzed against PBS containing 0.1% NP-40. Finally, the material was concentrated by negative pressure and kept at −70°C until use.

The isolated material was iodinated with ^{125}I by the chloramine T method (Hunter and Greenwood, 1962). To 20 μg isolated material (100 μl), 10 μl chloramin T (0.5 mg/ml PBS) was added, followed by 1 mCi iodine (Radiochemical Centre, Amersham, England). The mixture was allowed to react for 1 min at room temperature with constant shaking, after which 20 μl Na-metabisulfite (1 mg/ml PBS) was added. Free iodine was separated by passing the mixture over a Sephadex G-25 column. The iodinated material was kept at −70°C.

In exactly the same way, normal Lewis serum was also absorbed on a normal (Lewis × DA)F_1 Ig immunoabsorbent, and the eluted material was treated in the same way as described above. Since no specific protein was found in this preparation, we will refer below only to the material that was absorbed on the antiidiotypic immunoabsorbent. To prove that we were dealing with a molecule demonstrating both idiotypic specificity and antigen-binding capacity, the iodinated material was incubated with Lewis or DA spleen cells. The results in Table XXIII show that the isolated material has the capacity to recognize DA alloantigens. Material isolated over a normal F_1 Ig immunoabsorbent showed no specificity. The ability to recognize DA alloantigen by these isolated molecules is rapidly lost after iodination, normally within 24−48 hr.

Once the specificity of the isolated molecules was established, the material was analyzed on SDS polyacrylamide gels. Figure 7 shows a profile on a 10%

Table XXIII. Specificity of the Isolated
Normal Lewis Serum Factors

Normal Lewis serum absorbed and eluted from:	Incubated with spleen cells from[a]:	Mean cpm of triplicate wells±S.E.
Anti-(Lewis anti-DA)	Lewis	4,397±437
Anti-(Lewis anti-DA)	DA	12,568±851
Normal (L×DA)F$_1$ Ig	Lewis	4,803±769
Normal (L×DA)F$_1$ Ig	DA	4,531±385

[a]1×10^7 spleen cells were used per well, and about 250,000 cpm was added to each well. Incubation was carried out for 1 hr at 4°C.

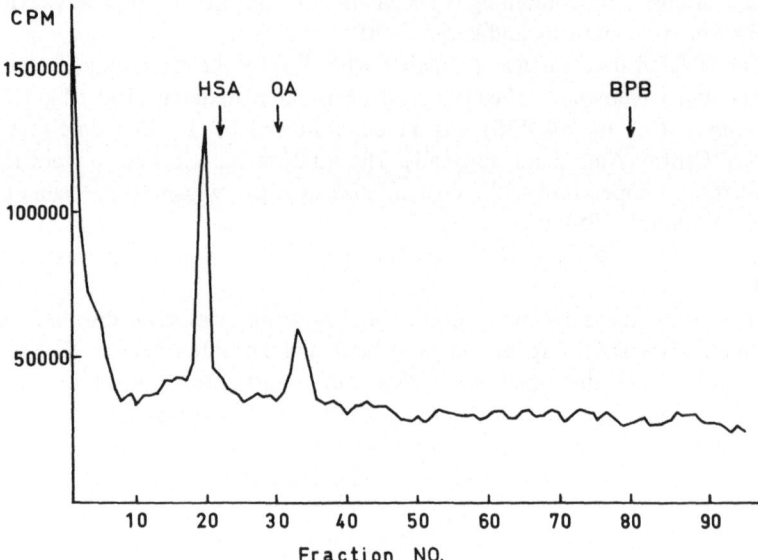

Fig. 7. ^{125}I-Labeled purified normal Lewis serum factor analyzed on a 10% (wt/vol) polyacrylamide gel containing 0.1% (wt/vol) sodium dodecyl sulfate. Following electrophoresis, the gel was sliced into 1-mm segments and radioactivity was determined. ^{125}I-Labeled human serum albumin (HSA) and ovalbumin (OA) were used as markers on parallel gels.

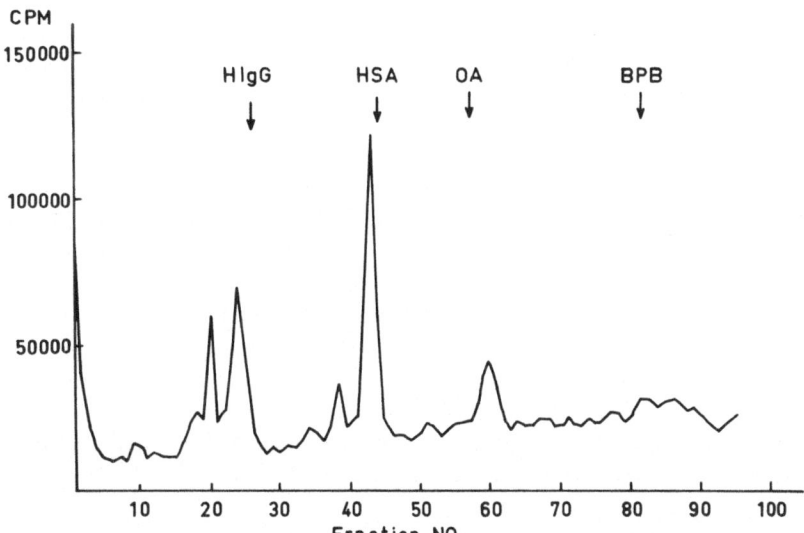

Fig. 8. ^{125}I-Labeled purified normal Lewis serum factor analyzed on a 5% (wt/vol) polyacrylamide gel. The conditions were otherwise the same as in Fig. 7. (HIgG) ^{125}I-Labeled human IgG run as a marker on a parallel gel.

gel. Two distinct peaks can be found, the first one corresponding to a molecular weight of about 70,000 and a second smaller one corresponding to about 35,000. Substantial amounts of radioactivity of larger-sized molecules did not enter the gel. In repeated experiments, the first peak was always found in the same position. The smaller peak, on the other hand, was found in positions corresponding to molecular weights between 30,000 and 40,000. In some experiments, the second peak was absent.

The same material was also analyzed on 5% SDS Gels. Figure 8 shows such an experiment. The dominant peak could again be detected in a position corresponding to about 70,000 daltons. Two distinct peaks could be found in the region where human IgG, used as a marker, appeared.

Thus far, we have been unable to identify these two peaks definitively. The larger one seems to correspond to 7S IgM and the second one to a dimer of molecules appearing in the 70,000-dalton peak. This was assessed by using reducing conditions. The first peak could be split into heavy and light chains of conventional nature, and the second one only into molecules corresponding to a molecular weight of about 70,000. Using supernatants from either a mixture of Lewis T and B cells or purified Lewis T lymphocytes and extracting shed receptors in a way similar to that described for the normal Lewis serum it could be shown that the peak appearing in the position corresponding to a molecular weight of about 70,000 is indeed formed by molecules derived from T lymphocytes. In addition, receptors from purified Lewis T lymphocytes can be internally labeled with ^{3}H-labeled amino acids. Supernatants from such lymphocytes absorbed on anti-(Lewis anti-DA) immunoabsorbents contain molecules that express idiotype specificity as well as alloantigen-binding capacity, as shown in Table XXIV.

It is thus quite likely that the low-molecular-weight molecules of approximately 35,000 daltons represent a degradation product from a larger molecule. When we found in the earlier experiments that the size of the low-molecular-weight peak (see Fig. 6) was probably in the size range of molecules being filtered out through the kidney,s we started to look for the presence of idiotypic material in the urine of normal adult rats. Urine was collected in metabolic cages, concentrated during dialysis against PBS, and tested for idiotypic material in the inhibition assay. Table XXV shows representative results proving the existence of such molecules in normal rat urine. Size determinations of these molecules showed that in the urine, virtually all idiotypic molecules were of the low-molecular-weight size (Binz and Wigzell, 1975c).

These results on T-cell receptors for antigen are still preliminary. However, the molecules seem to be distributed in three forms, one in the form of a molecule of about 150,000 daltons, composed of two chains with an approximate molecular weight of about 70,000. Whether these two chains are identical or not is unknown. The single chains of 70,000 size also found in normal serum can seemingly also be recovered as a fragment in the size range of 30,000–40,000 daltons. All these molecules can be shown to express both antigen-binding and idiotypic markers (Binz and Wigzell, 1975c, and this chapter), a finding of quite unorthodox nature as compared with conventional immuno-

Table XXIV. Isolation of Internally Labeled Alloantigen-Binding Molecules from Supernatants of Lewis Lymphocytes

Supernatant of[a]:	Incubated with spleen cells of[b]:	Mean ^{3}H cpm of duplicates ± S.E.
Lewis T + B cells	Lewis	1526± 223
Lewis T + B cells	(Lewis × DA)F$_1$	4591±1810
Lewis T + B cells	DA	9529± 893
Lewis T cells	Lewis	₋906± 284
Lewis T cells	(Lewis × DA)F$_1$	1898± 149
Lewis T cells	DA	3580±1012

[a]Supernatants were absorbed and eluted from anti-(Lewis anti-DA) immunoabsorbents.
[b]150,000 cpm, corresponding to 0.05 ml of isolated material, was incubated with 10^7 spleen cells.

Table XXV. Presence of "Natural" Factors with "L-Anti DA Idiotypes" in Normal Serum or Urine

Cells[a]	In the presence of:	Mean cpm ± S.E. of duplicates[b]
Lewis T	L normal serum	7.188±0.099
Lewis T	F_1[c] normal serum	14.206±0.805
Lewis T	DA normal serum	14.202±0.312
Lewis T	L urine	5.869±0.591
Lewis T	F_1[c] urine	12.551±1.232

[a] 1×10^7 T lymphocytes were added to each well containing a 1:20 dilution of a (Lewis × DA)F_1 anti-Lewis T serum (Binz and Wigzell, 1975c).
[b] ^{125}I-Labeled protein A was added to each sample.
[c] F_1: (L×DA)F_1.

globulin molecules. Attempts to dissociate the 70,000-dalton chain by reducing conditions using 6 M guanidine hydrochloride or 6 M urea have failed, strongly suggesting the true single-chain nature of this molecule.

As to other serologic markers, we have no evidence so far that the T-cell-derived molecules carry any conventional Ig markers. Three different rabbit—anti-rat Ig immunosorbent columns removed to completion only the naturally occurring B-cell-derived molecules without having any impact on the passing T-cell-derived molecules. Further attempts along this line will be carried out. Also, there is no evidence that the T-cell molecules have any serologic determinants coded for by the major histocompatibility complex genes, since three different DA-anti-Lewis alloantiserum immunosorbent columns all failed to remove these molecules. The same negative results were obtained when using a rabbit-anti-human B_2 microglobulin (showing detectable cross-reactivity with rat B_2 microglobulin) as immunoabsorbent. For further discussion of the characteristics of the T-cell molecules, see Section IX.

The present findings are important in two ways. First, they allow the investigator to readily isolate and analyze T-cell-receptor molecules with antigen-binding specificity using either internal or external isotope labeling procedures. Furthermore, the possibility of isolating from a nonimmune individual idiotypic receptors signifying the potential immune reactivity of that individual against certain major histocompatibility antigens allows an entirely new approach to induction of transplantation tolerance. Our experiments along these lines using purified idiotypic molecules from normal serum as immunogen in the strain of production, thereby causing autoantiidiotype antibody production and transplantation tolerance, will be discussed in detail in the following section.

VIII. SPECIFIC TRANSPLANTATION TOLERANCE RESULTING FROM AUTOIMMUNITY AGAINST NATURALLY OCCURRING IDIOTYPE-POSITIVE RECEPTOR MOLECULES

No evidence exists that genes the products of which create the antigen-binding sites of immunoglobulin molecules have been under any phylogenetic selective pressure so as to avoid creating sites with reactivity against self-components. Failure of an individual to react against self-components can thus frequently be ascribed to a successful induction of immune tolerance during ontogeny. There are several levels of tolerance that involve the different subsets of lymphocytes to varying extents. The concentration of the respective self-components in the body fluids is here a decisive factor. The antigen-binding sites of the autochthonous molecules can function as immunogens, resulting in production of antoantiidiotypic antibodies (Rodkey, 1974). In a few cases in which failure or difficulty to achieve such autoantiidiotype antibody synthesis has been reported, the failure or difficulty arose from the presence of idiotypes in normal serum in unusually high concentrations (Janeway, personal communication).

We know that in the present antigenic system, idiotypic anti-Ag-B-reactive receptor molecules are released in detectable form into the serum or urine of unimmunized rats (Binz and Wigzell, 1975c). The concentration of these naturally occurring idiotypic molecules is not high enough, however, to impede the successful induction of autoantiidiotypic antibodies (McKearn et al., 1974b). Autoimmune reactions are mostly considered to be bad or at most neutral for the individual. The present immunization procedures, however, can be shown to result in the specific induction of long-lasting tolerance with regard to the relevant transplantation antigen(s). In this section, details of such experiments will be presented, and the theoretical and practical implications of the present procedure in providing a new approach to transplantation tolerance via specific immunization will be discussed.

Rats can be immunized against their own alloantibodies. For instance, a Lewis rat immunized against BN cells will under repeated immunization frequently develop autoantiidiotypic antibodies reactive with some of its own alloantibodies with specificity for Ag-B antigens of BN type (McKearn et al., 1974a). The exact consequences of such simultaneous alloantibody and antiallo-antibody production as to transplantation immune reactivity have not been analyzed in detail. However, survival of kidney grafts containing BN alloantigens would seem optimal if transplanted at the peak of the autoantiidiotype production in these animals (McKearn, personal communication).

Our own approach to this problem has been primarily to try to use the individual's own "natural" idiotypic molecules with specificity for Ag-B antigens (Binz and Wigzell, 1975c) as immunogen in the host of production. We chose the present experimental attack for the following reasons: (1) To lead to complete transplantation tolerance, optimal induction of autoantiidiotypic antibody production should be directed against as many potential idiotype-positive, relevant specificities as possible. From this point of view, the normal serum factors would represent the very best, nonselected example of the individual's own immune potential with regard to reactivity toward the antigens. (2) A system that allows the use of normal serum or urine as a source for potential idiotypic immunogenic molecules in the host would, from the clinical point of view, have many obvious advantages.

Our system was therefore chosen as follows: Serum or urine from Lewis normal adult rats was collected, and the urine was dialyzed against phosphate-buffered saline at 4°C. Serum samples of 100–200 ml or urine samples of 300–500 ml were then filtered through columns containing 2 ml normal Sepharose beads (to remove anti-Sepharose-reactive material), followed by filtration through second columns coupled with antiidiotypic antibodies [(Lewis X DA)F_1 or (Lewis X BN)F_1 anti-Lewis T cell antibodies] (Binz and Wigzell, 1975c). The second columns were then washed extensively with saline until no detectable protein was coming out from the bottom of the column (less than 10 μg/ml protein). The bound, idiotype-positive molecules from serum or urine were then recovered using standard acid-elution procedures, neutralized, and concentrated using negative-pressure dialysis. The total recovered material from such a column was on the order of a few hundreds of micrograms of protein, but the exact "purity" of these materials as to idiotypic molecules has not been analyzed. The protein was then polymerized with an immunogenic carrier via glutaraldehyde, using different heterologous proteins as carriers. Subsequently, the polymerized complexes were emulsified in Freund's complete adjuvants and used for immunization in normal adult Lewis rats. Attempts to use DA or BN spleen cells as immunosorbents for the natural Lewis anti-DA or anti-BN molecules instead of the antiidiotype columns have so far provided an unsuccessful approach in the present system.

A. Evidence for Induction of Autoantiidiotypic Antibodies

Lewis rats immunized with Lewis-anti-DA or anti-BN molecules isolated from normal Lewis serum or urine will produce autoantiidiotypic antibodies with the expected specificity (Binz and Wigzell, unpublished results). Figure 9 shows some experiments denoting the production of such autoantiidiotypic antibodies after immunization with idiotypic molecules isolated from urine via antiidiotypic immunosorbents. It can be seen from Fig. 9 that the induction of autoantibodies is a swift process, with detectable IgG autoantiidiotypic antibodies (measured by protein A assay; Binz and Wigzell, 1975b) already at the first bleeding, day 14 after immunization. The results in Fig. 9 demonstrate only

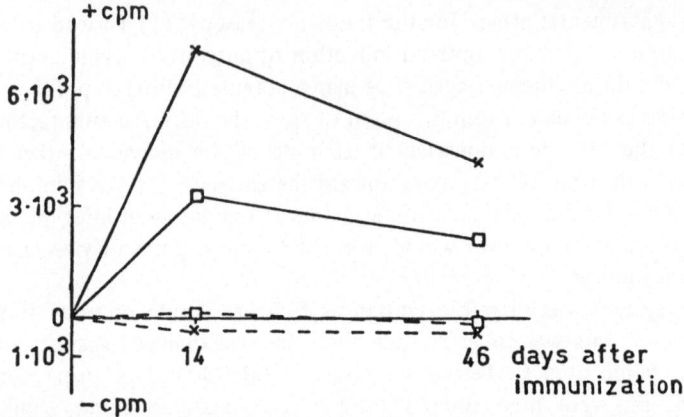

Fig. 9. Production of autoantiidiotypic antibodies. Idiotypic anti-DA or anti-BN molecules were isolated from Lewis normal urine by filtration over antiidiotype-specific immuno-absorbents [(L×DA)F$_1$ anti-Lewis T or (L×BN)F$_1$ anti-Lewis T cell idiotype Sepharose columns). The acid-eluted material was conjugated with human IgG molecules via glutaralde-hyde and used as immunogen in Lewis rats using Freund's complete adjuvants. Antisera were obtained at the days indicated and tested in [^{125}I]protein A assay. (X) Immunized with anti-BN receptors; (□) immunized with anti-DA receptors; (———) tested against Lewis T lymphocytes; (————) tested against the respective (L×DA)F$_1$ X or (L×BN)F$_1$ □ T cells. Subtraction of the background binding at day 0 gives the 0 level.

Table XXVI. Capacity of Autoantiidiotypic
Antibodies in the Presence of Complement
to Selectively Eliminate the Relevant
Mixed Leukocyte Culture Reactivity

Lewis lymphocytes	MLC against DA[a]	MLC against BN[a]
Treated with Lewis-anti (Lewis-anti DA) plus complement	28,303±2356	32,748±1818
Treated with Lewis normal serum plus complement	112,151±5622	34,811±3767

[a]Autoantiidiotypic sera obtained from individual Lewis rats 134 days after immunization with normal Lewis-anti-DA idiotypic factor. Individual antisera were assessed, and the group mean ± S.E. of thymidine uptake is given. Seven different autoantiidiotypic sera were tested.

Table XXVII. Absence of T Lymphocytes with "Anti-DA" Idiotypes
in Lewis Rats Autoimmunized Against Lewis-Anti DA Idiotypic Molecules

	Sera[b]			
Cells[a]	(L×DA)F$_1$ NS	(L×DA)F$_1$ anti-L T	(L×BN)F$_1$ NS	(L×BN)F$_1$ anti-L T
Lewis T from rats immunized with Lewis-anti DA idiotypes	2318± 60	2661±108	2556±52	4202± 80
Lewis T from normal rats	2567±207	5950±315	2554±57	5373±611

[a]The animals were killed on day 91 after immunization. The T cells were prepared over anti-Ig columns.
[b]Binding of antiidiotypic antibodies was determined by [^{125}I] protein A assay. Values are mean ± S.E. of ^{125}I-uptake. Cells from 5 individual immune rats were assessed separately.

the production of autoantibodies; they are not informative as to their true antiidiotypic nature. Evidence for this comes from the data shown in Table XXVI, from experiments in which sera containing supposed antiidiotypic antibodies were incubated in the presence of complement with Lewis normal T lymphocytes, and the cells were subsequently tested for reactivity in MLC. As shown, incubation with the antisera led to selective elimination of reactivity against the relevant alloantigens, while reactivity against third-party antigen was left intact. Thus, the supposed autoantiidiotypic antibodies were indeed such molecules and behaved exactly like "conventional" antiidiotypic antibodies in this system (Binz and Wigzell, 1975b).

The Lewis rats undergoing this autoimmunization procedure suffer no obvious harm. The presence of autoantiidiotypic antibodies, however, would be expected to lead to elimination of the respective idiotype-positive T and B lymphocytes, which in the present system would amount to a few percent of the total lymphocyte pool (Binz and Wigzell, 1975d). Lymphocytes of rats undergoing autoimmune reactions were thus used as targets in the antiidiotype radioimmunoassays studying the presence or absence of idiotypic receptors on lymphocytes. We could show (see Table XXVII) that these rats displayed selective reduction of the relevant idiotype-positive lymphocytes. Most likely, these cells were killed by the autoantiidiotypic antibodies *in vivo*.

B. Evidence That Autoantiidiotype Antibody Production Results in the Specific Elimination of Functional T Lymphocytes (Equivalent to a State of Specific Immune Tolerance)

The presence of autoantiidiotypic antibodies combined with the absence of the relevant idiotype-positive lymphocytes suggested that the autoimmunized rats should display specific absence of immune reactivity against the relevant

**Table XXVIII. Specific Loss of Mixed
Leukocyte Culture Reactivity in Lymphocytes
from Animals with Induced
Autoantiidiotype Immunity**

Days[a]	Cells[b]	MLC against DA[c]	MLC against BN[c]
14	Experimental	32,096± 2,561	39,825± 1,604
	Control	119,008± 6,117	42,503± 3,790
38	Experimental	20,458± 868	38,689± 1,096
	Control	133,898±18,035	42,984± 317
130	Experimental	17,142± 1,174	39,418± 1,546
	Control	156,190± 3,866	53,594±12,768

[a]Lewis rats immunized at day 0 with normal Lewis serum
anti-DA idiotypic factor, boosting at days 30 and 121.
[b]Spleen and lymph node cells from age-matched experimental (= immunized) or control Lewis rats.
[c]Mean cpm ± S.E. of tritiated thymidine uptake. The MLC
reactivity of each rat was determined in triplicate cultures.
The means of these triplicates were calculated and used to
calculate the mean ± S.E. as indicated.

**Table XXIX. Induction of Specific Skin
Graft Survival by the Induction of
Autoantiidiotype Immunity**

	Skin graft survival[b]	
Recipients	(L×BN)F$_1$	(Lewis × DA)F$_1$
Lewis normal	9–11	9–10
Lewis, immunized with Lewis-anti-DA molecules[a]	9–11	26.5±2.5

[a]Immunized with Lewis-anti-DA normal serum molecules
purified via anti-Lewis-anti-DA immunoabsorbents and subsequently polymerized with glutaraldehyde. Immunized
with Freund's complete adjuvant at day 0, boosted with
incomplete adjuvant at days 30 and 121. Skin grafted at day
144.
[b]Skin graft survival indicated either by range of survival of
grafts or by mean ± S.E.

alloantigens. Accordingly, lymphocytes from these animals were harvested from spleens and lymph nodes and assayed for the capacity to function in GvH or MLC assays. A summary of some representative MLC experiments is shown in Table XXVIII, from which it can be seen that Lewis-T-lymphocyte functions with regard to given Ag-B antigen(s) are selectively eliminated using the present autoimmunization procedure.

To further analyze the degree of specific immune suppression induced by the present procedures, we studied the survival of allogeneic skin grafts transplanted into the autoimmune Lewis rats. The results of such experiments are summarized in Table XXIX. A highly significant increased specific survival time of the relevant Ag-B incompatible skin grafts was observed, extending in some rats to more than 30 days without any further treatment. This increased survival time thus proves that a close to complete and specific elimination of immune reactivity against strong histocompatibility antigens can be induced using the present autoimmunization procedures. We will further discuss the implications of these thought-provoking findings in Section IX.

IX. GENERAL DISCUSSION

A problem frequently encountered in the studies of T-cell receptors for antigen has been the possibility of cytophilic Ig molecules being derived from B lymphocytes but adsorbed onto T cells. Whereas B lymphocytes express receptors for the Fc region of IgG molecules to a larger extent than T cells, there is by now little doubt that the latter cells are indeed able to bind low numbers of IgG molecules, especially if the molecules are in complexed form (Yoshida and Andersson, 1972). There are reports that within the T-cell pool, lymphoblasts and T lymphocytes of a certain subgroup are exceptionally able in binding such IgG complexes (Basten *et al.*, 1975). Lately, convincing evidence for the presence of a receptor for the Fc region of IgM on T lymphocytes has also been forthcoming (Moretta *et al.*, 1975). It is thus crucial for any system claiming to deal with "true" T-lymphocyte receptors for antigen to prove that these receptors are indeed manufactured by the cells themselves, or that they are essential for the cell to fulfill its specific immunopotential, or both. That both mammalian and avian B-deficient, agammaglobulinemic individuals can be shown capable of completely normal T-cell functions does exclude that cytophilic B-cell-derived Ig molecules on T cells are necessary structures for the T lymphocytes to react to the proper antigens.

In the present T-cell system, a series of experimental results supports the notion that we have indeed been studying antigen-binding, idiotypic receptors on the actual cells of production. Briefly, we have made the following findings:

Using anti-T cell idiotypic antisera, a low number of strongly positive T cells could be visualized among a majority of completely negative cells (Binz and Wigzell, 1975d). Polyvalent anti-Ig sera on the same T-lymphocyte suspensions failed to stain any cells except the occasional contaminating B cell. Thus, if the idiotypic molecules on the few positive T cells were derived from B cells, they would have to (1) be distributed in a nonrandom manner and (2) lack any conventional B-cell Ig serologic markers. Furthermore, these cells were derived from normal individuals, thus substantially reducing the problem of antigen–antibody complexes with sizable cytophilic activity. A second strong argument in favor of active T-cell synthesis of the idiotypic receptors stems from the functional inactivation or fractionation experiments, in which we could show decisively that idiotypic and expected immunoreactivity went in complete parallel as measured by GvH or MLC assays (Binz and Wigzell, 1975d). Finally, using highly purified T lymphocytes, we could remove their receptors via proteolytic treatment, allow them to recover *in vitro,* and demonstrate via internal labeling experiments that the cells produced and released such idiotype-positive, antigen-binding molecules with distinct physical features as compared with the Ig molecules released by B lymphocytes (Binz and Wigzell, unpublished results). We would thus conclude that the idiotype-positive, antigen-specific receptors found on or released by T lymphocytes in the present experimental system are active products of these very cells.

In this chapter, we have summarized the experimental results we have thus far obtained in the analysis of the idiotypic characteristics of the T-cell receptor for antigen. In place of entities that were considered "elusive" because of the failure to demonstrate them via use of conventional antiimmunoglobulin reagents (Crone *et al.,* 1972), we can now demonstrate these structures in a palpable form. Yet several uncertainties still remain. Beginning with the antigen-binding area of the T-cell receptor in comparison with a conventional immuno-globulin, similarities as well as dissimilarities would seem to exist. Using anti-idiotypic antibodies produced against idiotypic T receptors, we could demon-strate (see Tables I, II, and IV) that they would also react with conventional IgG antibodies with the same antigen-binding specificity as the T receptors. Using highly purified IgG antibodies as immunoabsorbent, we could show that this reaction was complete, since the IgG immunoabsorbent could remove all the anti-T idiotype-reactive antibodies. From this finding, one can conclude either that all T-cell idiotypes are also to be found on B-cell immunoglobulins or, alternatively, that the IgG immunsorbent perhaps did contain some T-cell receptors purifying in parallel with IgG molecules. We have no evidence for the latter (Binz and Wigzell, 1975b), and would thus favor the former alternative. Also, purified B lymphocytes could be shown to remove all anti-T-cell-reactive antibodies as well, thus further weakening the reasoning for the possibility that T-cell products contaminate the IgG preparations. On the other hand, earlier (Binz *et al.,* 1974a,b) as well as more recent data (see Table III) indicate or show that antiidiotypic antisera raised against conventional antibodies frequently contain two groups of antiidiotypic antibodies. One group shows complete cross-reactivity between B and T idiotypes, but the second population of antibodies demonstrates exclusive reactivity against B-cell receptors of immunoglobulin idiotypes.

Taken together, then, our data would suggest that whereas all idiotypic determinants found on T-cell receptors are also found on the corresponding B-lymphocyte products, the opposite is not true. This would suggest that the two lymphocyte groups are using some common variable genes in the creation of their respective antigen-binding receptors, but that the B-cell receptors also contain additional idiotypic determinants. It has long been known that idiotypic determinants on conventional immunoglobulin molecules are to a very large extent created via combination between heavy- and light-chain variable regions (Huser et al., 1975). It is thus possible that the T lymphocyte may fail to use all V gene pools available for the B lymphocyte, either lacking a part of a given V-gene cluster or one or more V-gene clusters altogether. In this context, it may also be relevant to recall that we have thus far been unable to find evidence for two variable regions of a two-chain type in the antigen-binding molecules released from T lymphocytes (Binz and Wigzell, unpublished results).

Exact localization as to which V genes are shared between T and B lymphocytes in their generation of antigen-binding receptors is still lacking. In the present system, two experiments have been performed using heavy and light chains from idiotype-positive alloantibodies as inhibitors of the anti-T idiotype reaction (Binz and Wigzell, unpublished results). In both experiments, considerable inhibitory activity could be shown to reside in the heavy-chain preparation, suggesting that T-cell receptors contain heavy-chain V-gene products. Although these results should be regarded with skepticism because of the very small body of experimental data, they are in accordance with the suggested evidence that T-cell-receptor-derived material in released form, although it is of single-chain type, can still express both idiotypic and antigen-binding characteristics (Binz and Wigzell, 1975c). In another system studying T-cell receptors via use of antiidiotypic antibodies (Eichmann and Rajewsky, 1975), preliminary data that provide similar support for a linkage between T-cell idiotypes and heavy-chain allotype have been presented. Heavy-chain immunoglobulin V genes participating in the T-cell receptor for antigen would thus seem to be both logical and supported by the meager existing data on this issue.

Our own data on the actual biochemistry of the T-cell receptor(s) for antigen should be considered preliminary. As already shown (see Figs. 6–8), we have been able to isolate from T lymphocytes in shed form three kinds of molecules, all expressing idiotypic as well as antigen-binding activity. A simple model to encompass these findings would be a polypeptide chain of around 70,000 daltons, which can also be found in a dimeric form (we have no evidence of identity of the two chains in the dimer) and can also be recovered as a degradation product in the molecular-weight range of 30,000—40,000. We have been unable thus far to demonstrate the presence of conventional immuno-globulin markers of constant-region types on these molecules. Also, alloantigenic markers signifying that the chain is produced by *Ag-b*-locus-linked genes have not been detected. Finally, we have no evidence that a second smaller chain exists in these molecules, at least in the form recovered by our isolation procedures. It is unclear how these findings are to be adjusted to fit the findings of other workers reporting on molecules, antigen-binding in a specific manner, and with alloantigenic markers of *H-2* linked type (Munro and Taussig, 1975; Takemori and Tada, 1975). Three alternative explanations do exist: (1) The antigen-binding receptors from T lymphocytes may initially be composed of two different chains, perhaps present in a dimeric form such as a conventional IgG molecules with the light-chain analogue bearing Ia-like antigenic markers. Our isolation procedures may allow a dissociation between the two chains, and since the Ia-determined chain would contain no idiotypic markers, we would then fail to detect it. (2) A more trivial explanation would be that our molecules are indeed coded for by *Ag-B*-linked genes in a manner analogous to the Ia genes in the mouse, but the antisera we have tried thus far may have failed to contain antibodies against the relevant antigenic determinants. It is already clear from the work in the mouse systems that the antigen-binding factor(s) from T lymphocytes will express only some, not all, of the conventional Ia-specificities (Munro and Taussig, 1975; Takemori and Tada, 1975). (3) Finally, although the explanation is unattractive, it is still not excluded that the T lymphocytes may use two distinct systems for the cognition and recognition of foreign structures.

Diversity of recognition of antigenic determinants seems to be of compara-tive extent for B and T lymphocytes. It is well known that a major reason for the heterogeneity of B-cell receptors (immunoglobulins) is the molecular buildup of the antigen-binding area of the molecules. Here, two variable polypeptide regions, each created by a separate gene, collaborate, thus allowing an exponen-tial buildup of potential combinations using relatively few genes. *If* the T-cell receptor does indeed depend for its antigen-binding area only on a single variable polypeptide chain (though it should be noted that the single chain expresses significant antigen-binding ability), problems do arise in creating enough antigen-binding areas for the T lymphocytes. It is unknown, however, whether a T lymphocyte is expressing allelic exclusion, and it is thus possible that the dimeric molecules isolated may be constructed by chains with nonidentical V regions. Also, the size of the chain may allow the housing of more than one V-region stretch on each chain. One might also return to the possibility that the receptor on the cellular level may contain a second chain of Ia-type, possibly of a comparatively constant type but existing in a few alternative forms (like the λ chains of the mouse; Hood *et al.,* 1974), thereby adding to the number of alternative antigen-binding regions of the T-cell receptors.

Another striking feature in the present system is the high frequency with which idiotypic T lymphocytes are present in the normal, unimmunized animal. Our figures on the numbers of idiotype-positive T lymphocytes denoting reactivity across the major histocompatibility barrier of the species (Binz et al., 1975b) are in striking agreement with the results of other, earlier workers studying the frequencies of cells participating in GvH or MLC reactions across similar barriers (Ford et al., 1975; Howard and Wilson, 1974; Nisbet et al., 1969; Wilson et al., 1968). Using the affinity chromatography approach, we could enrich and deplete for these idiotypic T cells and demonstrate that they are indeed responsible for such reactions (Binz and Wigzell, 1975a). The most obvious question arising from these findings is how to explain the high frequency of idiotypic T cells (the percentage of B lymphocytes with the same idiotypes is significantly lower). This would seem quite simple from one point of view, since the idiotypes on the T-cell receptor are still expressed at the single-chain level. Conventional idiotypes are generated by a combination of variable regions of heavy and light chains, with only minor idiotypic activities being left after dissociation into single chains (Huser et al., 1975). The gene frequency of a heavy-chain V gene times the gene frequency for the light-chain V gene would thus tend to generate a very low frequency of cells positive with this "composite" idiotype. However, when the antisera induced against the idiotypes created by a single chain (in the present system, according to this reasoning, this would correspond to our anti-T cell idiotypic antisera, whereas the antisera against the alloantibodies would contain mostly antibodies directed against "composite" idiotypes), cells expressing such single-chain-determined idiotypes would then be expected to occur at a frequency similar to the actual gene frequency of the particular V gene involved. In this case, that B lymphocytes would not express the same frequencies of idiotypic cells could then be explained on the basis of masking of variable regions of the relevant idiotypic chain by the variable regions of the second chain. That such masking can occur in conventional immunoglobulin molecules is well known (Epstein, 1965). Reasoning such as the foregoing could thus well explain the high frequencies of idiotypic T cells and also the lower frequency of B as compared with idiotypic T lymphocytes in the present system. The high frequency of T lymphocytes carrying a given idiotypic receptor (assuming now that our idiotypic groups do contain only a few distinct idiotypic determinants; Binz et al., 1975b) do, however, again bring up the complications as to diversity. Data already exist showing that T lymphocytes enriched in vitro for MLC reactivity against a given Ag-B locus in the rat demonstrate a reduced reactivity toward third-party Ag-B antigens, while retaining normal helper-T-cell activity against an unrelated antigen (Heber-Katz and Wilson, 1976). This may suggest, then, that the present idiotypic determinants are present on subgroups of T-cell-receptor molecules, which in addition may contain intragroup variations allowing for heterogenity of reactivity against "conventional" antigens. Such reasoning would be in line with the concept that major histocompatibility locus antigens constitute unique antigens against which the initial immune recognition system is tuned to react and in which sophisticated heterogeneity as for "conventional" epitopes has been added only late in phylogeny. We have no results as yet that can shed additional light on such reasoning.

In conclusion, one would now eventually have to regard the T-cell receptor for antigen as being eluseive (Crone *et al.*, 1972). A molecule is emerging that is present on the relevant immunocompetent T lymphocytes in high numbers and allows itself to be labeled by internal or external means. An obvious relationship between the T- and B-cell molecules with specificity for antigen is revealed by the analysis with antiidiotypic antibodies. More exact arguments as to identity or complete cross-reactivity at the level of the variable regions must await genetic and further biochemical analysis. A lack of self-tolerance to the idiotypic T-cell receptors has been demonstrated, allowing the induction of specific tolerance toward transplantation antigens via autoimmunization procedures using the individual's own, naturally occurring receptors. This latter approach may have far-reaching consequences in the regulation of transplantation immunity, autoimmune diseases, and allergic disorders.

ACKNOWLEDGMENTS

We are very grateful to Dr. Thomas Bächi, Department of Medical Microbiology, University of Zürich, who performed all the work on the electron-microscopic studies on the antiidiotype-coated lymphocytes. This work was supported by grants to H. Binz from the Swiss National Foundation for Scientific Research and the European Molecular Biology Organization, and by grants to H. Wigzell from the Swedish Cancer Society and NIH contract NOI-CB-335859.

X. REFERENCES

Abney, E.R., and Parkhouse, R.M., 1974, Candidate for immunglobulin D present on murine B lymphocytes, *Nature (London)* **252**:600.

Alm, G. V., and Peterson, R.D.A., 1970, Effect of thymectomy and bursectomy on the *in vitro* response of chicken spleen cells to PHA, sheep erythrocytes (SRBC) and allogeneic cells, *Fed. Proc. Fed. Amer. Soc. Exp. Biol.* **29**:430.

Andersson, J., Lafleur, L., and Melchers, F., 1974, IgM in bone marrow-derived lymphocytes. Synthesis, surface deposition, turnover and carbohydrate composition in unstimulated mouse B cells, *Eur. J. Immunol.* **4**:170.

Andersson, L.C., Nordling, S., and Häyry, P., 1973 Proliferation of B and T cells in mixed lymphocyte cultures, *J. Exp. Med.* **138**:324.

Bach, F.H., Widmer, M.B., Bach, M.L., and Klein, J., 1972, Serologically defined and lymphocyte defined components of the major histocompatibility complex in the mouse, *J. Exp. Med.* 136:1430.

Barchilon, J., and Gershon, R.K., 1970, Synergism between thymocytes and bone marrow cells in a graft-versus-host reaction, *Nature (London)* 227:71.

Basten, A., Miller, J.F.A.P., Warner, N.L., Abraham, R., Chia, E., and Gamble, J., 1975, A subpopulation of T cells bearing Fc receptors, *J. Immunol.* 115:1159.

Benacerraf, B., and McDevitt, H.O., 1972, Histocompatibility-linked immune response genes, *Science* 175:273.

Billingham, R.E., and Silvers, W.K. (eds.), 1961, *Transplantation of Tissues and Cells,* The Wistar Institute Press, Philadelphia.

Binz, H., 1975, Local graft-versus-host reaction in mice specifically inhibited by anti-receptor antibodies, *Scand. J. Immunol.* 4:79.

Binz, H., and Askonas, B.A., 1975, Inhibition of mixed leucocyte culture by anti-idiotypic antibodies, *Eur. J. Immunol.* 5:618.

Binz, H., and Lindenmann, J., 1972a, Cellular receptors: Binding of radioactively labelled anti-alloantiserum, *J. Exp. Med.* 136:872.

Binz, H., and Lindenmann, J., 1972b, Antibodies against recognition structures: Preferential accumulation in lymph nodes draining a corresponding skin graft, *Scand. J. Immunol.* 1:339.

Binz, H., and Lindenmann, J., 1974, Allotypes of anti-alloantibodies, *Cell. Immunol.* 10:260.

Binz, H., and Wigzell, H., 1975a, Shared idiotypic determinants on B and T lymphocytes reactive against the same antigenic determinants. III. Physical fractionation of specific immunocompetent T lymphocytes by affinity chromatography using anti-idiotypic antibodies, *J. Exp. Med.* 142:1231.

Binz, H., and Wigzell, H., 1975b, Shared idiotypic determinants on B and T lymphocytes reactive against the same antigenic determinants. I. Demonstration of similar or identical idiotypes on IgG molecules and T cell receptors with specificity for the same alloantigens, *J. Exp. Med.* 142:197.

Binz, H., and Wigzell, H., 1975c, Shared idiotypic determinants on B and T lymphocytes reactive against the same antigenic determinants. IV. Isolation of two groups of naturally occurring idiotypic molecules with specific antigen binding activity in the serum and urine of normal rats, *Scand. J. Immunol.* 4:591.

Binz, H., and Wigzell, H., 1975d, Shared idiotypic determinants on B and T lymphocytes reactive against the same antigenic determinants. II. Determination of frequency and characteristics of idiotypic T and B lymphocytes in normal rats using direct visualization, *J. Exp. Med.* 142:1218.

Binz, H., Lindenmann, J., and Wigzell, H., 1973, Inhibition of local graft-versus-host reaction by anti-alloantibodies, *Nature (London)* 246:146.

Binz, H., Lindenmann, J., and Wigzell, H., 1974a, Cell bound receptors for alloantigens on normal lymphocytes. I. Characterization of receptor-carrying cells by the use of antibodies to alloantibodies, *J. Exp. Med.* 139:877.

Binz, H., Lindenmann, J., and Wigzell, H., 1974b, Cell bound receptors for alloantigens on normal lymphocytes. II. Antialloantiserum contains specific factors reacting with relevant immunocompetent T lymphocytes, *J. Exp. Med.* 140:731.

Binz, H., Bächi, T., Wigzell, H., Ramseier, H., and Lindenmann, J., 1975a, Idiotype positive T cells visualized by autoradiography and electron microscopy, *Proc. Natl. Acad. Sci. U.S.A.* 72:3210.

Binz, H., Kimura, A., and Wigzell, H., 1975b, Idiotype-positive T lymphocytes, *Scand. J. Immunol.* 4:413.

Binz, H., Wigzell, H., and Häyry, P., 1976, Correlation between specific cytolysis and expression of idiotypic receptors of allograft-infiltrating cells, *Nature (London)* 259:401.

Cantor, H., 1972, The effect of anti-theta antiserum upon graft-versus-host activity of spleen and lymph node cells, *Cell. Immunol.* 3:461.

Click, R.E., Benck, L., and Alto, B.S., 1972, Immune responses *in vitro*. I. Culture conditions for antibody synthesis, *Cell. Immunol.* 3:264.

Crone, M.M., Koch, C., and Simonsen, M., 1972, The elusive T cell receptor, *Transplant Rev.* 10:36.

Dorval, G., Welsh, K.I., and Wigzell, H., 1974, Labelled staphylococcus protein A as an immunological probe in the analysis of cell surface markers, *Scand. J. Immunol.* 3:405.

Eichmann, K., and Rajewsky, K., 1975, Induction of T and B cell immunity by anti-idiotypic antibody, *Eur. J. Immunol.* 5:661.

Elliot, B.E., Haskill, J.S., and Axelrad, M.A., 1975, Rosette-forming ability of thymus-derived lymphocytes in humoral and cell mediated immunity. Delayed hypersensitivity and *in vitro* cytotoxicity, *J. Exp. Med.* 141:584.

Elves, M.V., 1973, The impairment of graft-versus-host reactions by immunization of F_1 hybrids with low doses of parental cells, *Transplantation* 16:403.

Epstein, W.V., 1965, Specificity of macroglobulin antibody synthesized by the normal human fetus, *Science* 148:1591.

Feldmann, M., 1974, T cell suppression *in vitro*. II. Nature of the suppressive specific factor, *Eur. J. Immunol.* 4:667.

Festing, M., and Staats, J., 1973, Standardized nomenclature for inbred strains of rats, *Transplantation* 16:221.

Ford, W.L., 1975, Lymphocyte migration and immune responses, *Prog. Allergy* 19:1.

Ford, W.L., Burr, W., and Simonsen, M.M., 1970, A lymph node weight assay for the graft-versus-host activity of rat lymphoid cells, *Transplantation* 10:258.

Ford, W.L., Simmonds, S.I., and Atkins, R.C., 1975, Early events in a systematic graft-versus-host reaction. II. Autoradiographic estimation of the frequency of donor lymphocytes which respond to each Ag-B determined antigenic complex, *J. Exp. Med.* 141:681.

Forsgren, A., and Sjöqvist, J., 1966, "Protein A" from *Staphylococcus aureus*. I. Pseudo-immune reaction with human gamma globulin, *J. Immunol.* 97:822.

Fröland, S.S., and Natvig, J., 1971, Effect of poly-specific rabbit anti-immunglobulin antisera on the response of human lymphocytes in mixed lymphocyte cultures, *Int. Arch. Allergy Appl. Immunol.* 41:248.

Golstein, P., Svedmyr, E.A.J., and Wigzell, H., 1971, Cells mediating specific *in vitro* cytotoxicity. I. Detection of receptor-bearing lymphocytes, *J. Exp. Med.* 134:1395.

Gowans, J.L., and McGregor, D.D., 1965, The immunological activities of lymphocytes, *Prog. Allergy* 9:1.

Grey, H.M., Kubo, R.T., and Cerottini, J.C., 1972, Thymus derived (T) cell immunglobulins. Presence of a receptor site for IgG and absence of large amounts of "buried" Ig determinants on T cells, *J. Exp. Med.* 136:1323.

Hämmerling, U., and Rajewsky, K., 1971, Evidence for surface associated immunoglobulin on T and B lymphocytes, *Eur. J. Immunol.* 1:447.

Heber-Katz, E., and Wilson, D.B., 1976, Sheep red blood cell-specific helper activity in rat thoracic duct lymphocyte populations positively selected for reactivity to specific strong histocompatibility alloantigens, *J. Exp. Med.* 143:701.

Hildemann, W.H., 1967, Early antibody production in relation to skin allograft reactions in mice, *Transplantation* 5:1001.

Hood, L., Barstad, P., Lok, E., and Nottenburg, C., 1974, in: *The Immune System: Genes, Receptors, Signals,* p. 119 (Sercarz, Williamson, and Fox, eds.), Academic Press, New York and London.

Hopper, J.E., and Nisonoff, A., 1971, Individual antigenic specificity of immunoglobulins, *Adv. Immunol.* **13**:58.

Howard, J.C., and Wilson, D.B., 1974, Specific positive selection of lymphocytes reactive to strong histocompatibility antigens, *J. Exp. Med.* **140**:660.

Hunter, W.M., and Greenwood, F.C., 1962, Preparation of iodine-131 labelled human growth hormone of high specific activity, *Nature (London)* **194**:195.

Huser, H., Haimovich, J., and Jaton, J.C., 1975, Antigen-binding and idiotypic properties of reconstituted IgG derived from homogeneous rabbit anti-pneumococcal antibodies, *Eur. J. Immunol.* **5**:206.

Joller, P.W., 1972, Graft-versus-host reactivity of lymphoid cells inhibited by anti-recognition structure serum, *Nature (London) New Biol.* **240**:214.

Katz, D.H., and Benacerraf, B., 1975, The function and interrelationship of T-cell receptors, Ir genes and other histocompatibility gene products, *Transplant Rev.* **22**:175.

Katz, D., and Osborne, D.P., 1972, The allogeneic effect in inbred mice. II. Establishment of the cellular interactions required for enhancement of antibody production by the graft-versus-host reaction, *J. Exp. Med.* **136**:455.

Klein, J., and Park, J.M., 1973, Graft-versus-host reaction across different regions of the *H-2* complex of the mouse, *J. Exp. Med.* **137**:1213.

Lisowska-Bernstein, B., Rinuy, A., and Vasalli, P., 1973, Absence of IgM in enzymatically or biosynthetically labelled thymus derived lymphocytes, *Proc. Natl. Acad. Sci. U.S.A.* **70**:2879.

Marchalonis, J.J., Atwell, J.L., and Cone, R.E., 1972a, Isolation of surface immunglobulin from lymphocytes from human and murine thymus, *Nature (London) New Biol.* **235**:240.

Marchalonis, J.J., Cone, R.E., and Atwell, J.L., 1972b, Isolation and partial characterization of lymphocyte surface immunglobulin, *J. Exp. Med.* **135**:956.

McKearn, T.J., 1974, Antireceptor antiserum causes specific inhibition of reactions to rat histocompatibility antigens, *Science* **183**:94.

McKearn, T.J., Stuart, F.P., and Fitch, F.W., 1974a, Anti-idiotypic antibodies in rat transplantation immunity. I. Production of antiidiotypic antibodies in animals repeatedly immunized with alloantigens, *J. Immunol.* **113**:1876.

McKearn, T.J., Hamada, Y., Stuart, F.P. and Fitch, F.W., 1974b, Antirecptor antibody and resistance to graft-versus-host disease, *Nature (London)* **251**:648.

Mond, J.J., Luzzati, A.L., and Thorbecke, G.J., 1972, Surface antigens of immunocompetent cells. IV. Effect of anti-G 5 allotype on immunologic response of homozygous b 5 rabbit cells *in vitro, J. Immunol.* **108**:466.

Moretta, L., Ferrarini, M., Durante, M.L., and Mingari, M.C., 1975, Expression of a receptor for IgM on human T cells *in vitro, Eur. J. Immunol.* **5**:565.

Munro, A.J., and Taussig, M., 1975, Two genes in the major histocompatibility complex control immune response, *Nature (London)* **256**:103.

Natvig, J., Salason, F., Fröland, S., and Stavhem, P., 1975, Same idiotype of membrane bound IgD and IgM on single cells, in: *International Symposium on Membrane Receptors of Lymphocytes,* p. 13 (M. Seligman, ed.), North-Holland Publishing Co., Amsterdam.

Nisbet, H.W., Simonsen, M., and Zaleski, M., 1969, The frequency of antigen-sensitive cells in tissue transplantation, *J. Exp. Med.* **129**:459.

Peck, A.B., Alter, B.I., and Lindahl, K.F., 1976, Specificity in T cell mediated lympholysis:

Identical genetic control of the proliferative and effector phases of allogeneic and xenogeneic reactions, *Transplant Rev.* **29**:189.

Raff, M., Feldmann, M., and de Petris, S., 1973, Monospecificity of bone-marrow derived lymphocytes, *J. Exp. Med.* **137**:1024.

Rajewsky, K., and Mohr, R., 1974, Specificity and heterogeneity of helper T cells in the response to serum albumin in mice, *Eur. J. Immunol.* **4**:111.

Ramseier, H., 1973, Antibodies to receptors recognizing histocompatibility antigens, *Curr. Top. Microbiol. Immunol.* **60**:31.

Ramseier, H., 1974a, Spontaneous release of T cell receptors for alloantigens. I. Recognition of alloantigens and receptor release dynamics, *J. Exp. Med.* **140**:603.

Ramseier, H., 1974b, Antibodies to T cell receptors and to histocompatibility antigens, *Cell. Immunol.* **8**:177.

Ramseier, H., 1975, Spontaneous release of T cell receptors for alloantigens. II. Induction of antibodies to T cell receptors, *Eur. J. Immunol.* **5**:23.

Ramseier, H., 1976, T-lymphocyte receptors for alloantigens, *Immunol. Commun.* **5**:303.

Ramseier, H., and Lindenmann, J., 1969, F₁ hybrid animals: Reactivity against recognition structures of parental strain cells, *Pathol. Microbiol.* **34**:379.

Ramseier, H., and Lindenmann, J., 1972a, Aliotypic antibodies, *Transplant Rev.* **10**:57.

Ramseier, H., and Lindenmann, J., 1972b, Similarity of cellular recognition structures for histocompatibility antigens and of combining sites of corresponding alloantibodies, *Eur. J. Immunol.* **2**:109.

Roberts, P.I., and Häyry, P., 1976, Sponge matrix allograft: A model for analysis of killer cells infiltrating mouse allografts, *Transplantation* **21**:437.

Rodkey, L.S., 1974, Studies of idiotypic antibodies. Production and characterization of auto-anti-idiotypic antisera, *J. Exp. Med.* **139**:713.

Shevach, E.M., Green, I., and Paul, W.E., 1974, Alloantiserum-induced inhibition of immune response gene product function. II. Genetic analysis of target antigens, *J. Exp. Med.* **139**:679.

Takemori, T., and Tada, T., 1975, Properties of antigen-specific suppressive T cell factor in the regulation of antibody response of the mouse. I. *In vivo* activity and immunochemical characterization, *J. Exp. Med.* **142**:1241.

Vitetta, E.S., Bianco, C., Nussenzweig, V., and Hur, J.W., 1972, Cell surface immunglobulin. IV. Distribution among thymocytes, bone-marrow cells and their derived populations, *J. Exp. Med.* **136**:81.

Wekerle, H., Lonai, P., and Feldmann, M., 1972, Fractionation of antigen reactive cells on a cellular immunabsorbent. Factors determining recognition of antigen by T lymphocytes, *Proc. Natl. Acad. Sci. U.S.A.* **69**:1620.

Wells, J.V., Wang, A.-C., Thornsvard, C.T., Schanfield, M.S., Bleumers, J.F., and Fudenberg, H.H., 1973, Detection of idiotypic determinants on human monoclonal proteins with specific rabbit antisera and hemagglutination–inhibition, *J. Immunol.* **111**:841.

Wigzell, H., 1971, Cellular immunabsorbents, *Prog. Immunol.* **1**:1105.

Wigzell, H., 1973, On the relationship between cellular and humoral antibodies, *Contemporary Topics in Immunobiology,* Vol. 3, pp. 77–96 (M.D. Cooper and N.L. Warner, eds.), Plenum, New York.

Wigzell, H., and Andersson, B., 1969, Cell separation on antigen coated columns. Elimination of high rate antibody forming cells and immunological memory cells, *J. Exp. Med.* **129**:23.

Wilson, D.B., Silvers, W.K., and Nowell, P.C., 1967, Quantitative studies on the mixed lymphocyte culture interaction in rats. II. Relationship of the proliferative response to the immunological status of the donors, *J. Exp. Med.* **126**:655.

Wilson, D.B., Blyth, I.L., and Nowell, P.C., 1968, Quantitative studies on the mixed lymphocyte interaction in rats. Kinetics of the response, *J. Exp. Med.* **128**:1157.

Wu, T., and Kabat, E., 1970, Analysis of the sequence of the variable regions of Bence Jones proteins and myeloma light chains and their implications for antibody complementarity, *J. Exp. Med.* **132**:211.

Yoshida, T.O., and Andersson, B., 1972, Evidence for a receptor recognizing antigen-complexed immunoglobulin on the surface of activated mouse thymus lymphocytes, *Scand. J. Immunol.* **1**:401.

Chapter 5

Major Transplantation Antigens, Viruses, and Specificity of Surveillance T Cells

Rolf M. Zinkernagel

Department of Immunopathology
Scripps Clinic and Research Foundation
La Jolla, California

and

Peter C. Doherty

The Wistar Institute
Philadelphia, Pennsylvania

I. INTRODUCTION

The altered-self hypothesis is an attempt to explain why thymus-derived lymphocytes (T cells) apparently lyse only virus-infected target cells with which they share major transplantation antigens (Zinkernagel and Doherty, 1974a–c; Doherty and Zinkernagel, 1974, 1975a). Specific T-cell-mediated lysis of cells infected with lymphocytic choriomeningitis virus (LCMV), ectromelia virus (mouse pox), or vaccinia- or paramyxovirus (Sendai) requires homology of the K or D regions but not the I region of the major murine histocompatibility (H-2) gene complex (Doherty *et al.*, 1976a; Zinkernagel and Doherty, 1975; Blanden *et al.*, 1975a; Doherty and Zinkernagel, 1976; Koszinowski and Thomssen, 1975; Zinkernagel, 1976a). H-2K and H-2D code for major histocompatibility (H) or transplantation antigens that are expressed independently on the cell surface and that are responsible for rapid allogeneic graft rejection (reviewed in Schreffler and David, 1975, and Klein, 1975).

Table I. Requirement for H-2 Compatibility of T Cells and Cells with Which They Interact in Cell-Mediated Immunity

T-cell function	Model[a]	Target cell[b]	Favorite interpretation	References
In Vitro				
T helper	2° response	B,M?	Physiological interaction	Katz et al. (1973, 1975)
	1° response	M,B	Altered Ia?	Erb and Feldman (1975)
Cytotoxicity	LCMV	Virus-infected	Altered H-$2K$ or D	Zinkernagel and Doherty (1974b, 1975)
	Ectromelia	Target cell	Altered H-$2K$ or D	Blanden et al. (1975a)
	Vaccinia			Koszinowski and Thomssen (1975) Zinkernagel (1976a)
				Herbermann et al. (1973)
	MSV		?	Doherty and Zinkernagel (1976)
	Sendai			Shearer (1974)
	TNP	TNP-target	Altered H-2	Wainberg et al. (1974)
	Rous sarcoma	Virus-target		Bevan (1975a,b)
	Minor H-antigens		H-2 modifier	Gordon et al. (1975)
	Male Y antigen		Altered H-2	
Proliferation	Guinea pig	M	?	Rosenthal and Shevach (1973, 1976)
	1° response			
	2° response			
In Vivo				
Helper	Nude mice	?	?	Kindred and Shreffler (1972)
	F$_1$	?	Physiological interaction	Katz et al. (1973, 1975)
Macrophage activation	Listeriosis	M?	?	Zinkernagel (1974)
Immunopathology	Acute fatal LCM	?	Altered H-$2K$ or D	Doherty et al. (1976a)
Antiviral effect	Ectromelia	?	Altered H-$2K$ or D	Blanden et al. (1975a)
	LCMV			Zinkernagel and Welsh (1976)
Delayed-type hypersensitivity	Fowl γ-globulin	?	I region?	J.F.A.P. Miller et al. (1975)
	LCMV	?	K or D region	Zinkernagel (unpublished results)

[a] LCMV: lymphocytic choriomeningitis virus; MSV: murine sarcoma virus; 1°: primary, 2°: secondary immune response; F$_1$: hybrid mouse.
[b] B: bone-marrow-derived or bursa-equivalent lymphocyte; M: macrophage.

It seems that virus-immune T cells are sensitized to "altered-self" cell-surface antigens specified at, or near, *H-2K* or *H-2D*. Thus, at least from an immunologic point of view, alloantigens and altered-self may be similar antigens, which are singled out on the cell surface and attacked by T cells because they differ from the "normal" self-marker (Zinkernagel and Doherty, 1974c; Doherty and Zinkernagel, 1975d). Similar conclusions have been reached for the specificity of T cells cytotoxic for trinitrophenyl (TNP)-modified lymphocytes (Shearer, 1974; Shearer *et al.,* 1975; Forman, 1975), minor H antigens (Bevan, 1975a,b), or the male Y antigen (Gordon *et al.,* 1975).

The altered-self concept, which stresses the role of *H-2* antigens in defining the immunologic specificity of T cells, is by no means the only hypothesis that could fit the available experimental data (Doherty *et al.,* 1976a; Zinkernagel, 1976a). A dual recognition model similar to the one originally proposed by Katz and Benacerraf to explain the *H-2* restriction of T—B cell cooperation (Katz *et al.,* 1973; Katz and Benacerraf, 1975) may be correct. In contrast to the single recognition model of altered self this dual recognition model emphasizes that *H-2* markers are unidirectionally recognized separately from viral antigens by a second T-cell receptor. Whatever the explanation for the *H-2* association of immune phenomena (Table I), they are too diverse and clear-cut to be simply experimental artifacts, and they probably reveal fundamental biological mechanisms, the functional integrity of which may be central for general and immunologic homeostasis of multicellular organisms.

We do not attempt to present a comprehensive and completely updated review of this expanding and rapidly changing domain of cellular immunology (Table I). This account is a summary of our own struggle with one example of *H-2*-associated experimental phenomenology.

Our work could only evolve based on the previous and concurrent work of many others. We are especially grateful to the mouse geneticists who provided us generously with genetically defined strains (Gorer, 1937; Snell, 1974; Stimpfling, 1971; Bailey *et al.,* 1971; Shreffler and David, 1975; Klein, 1975) and to the immunologists who recently presensitized us to the importance of the *H-2* gene complex (Kindred and Schreffler, 1972; Benacerraf and McDevitt, 1972; Katz *et al.,* 1973; among many others). In this chapter, we examine the *H-2* compatibility requirement for virus-specific T-cell effector functions *in vitro* and *in vivo,* explain the derivation of the altered-self concept, and compare it with the dual recognition model. Furthermore, possible implications for a more general concept of immunologic surveillance and a possible biological role for major transplantation antigens are considered and discussed.

II. VIRUS-SPECIFIC CYTOTOXIC T CELLS *IN VITRO*

A. Experimental Model and Cellular Parameters

Cell-mediated immunity to LCMV infections in mice has been tested repeatedly *in vitro* by measuring ^{51}Cr release (Fig. 1) (Brunner *et al.*, 1968; Oldstone *et al.*, 1969; Oldstone and Dixon, 1970; Marker and Volkert, 1973; Cole *et al.*, 1973; Gardner *et al.*, 1974a,b; Zinkernagel and Doherty, 1974a; Doherty *et al.*, 1974). LCMV-immune lymphocytes lyse target cells infected with the same virus, but not normal uninfected target cells or targets infected

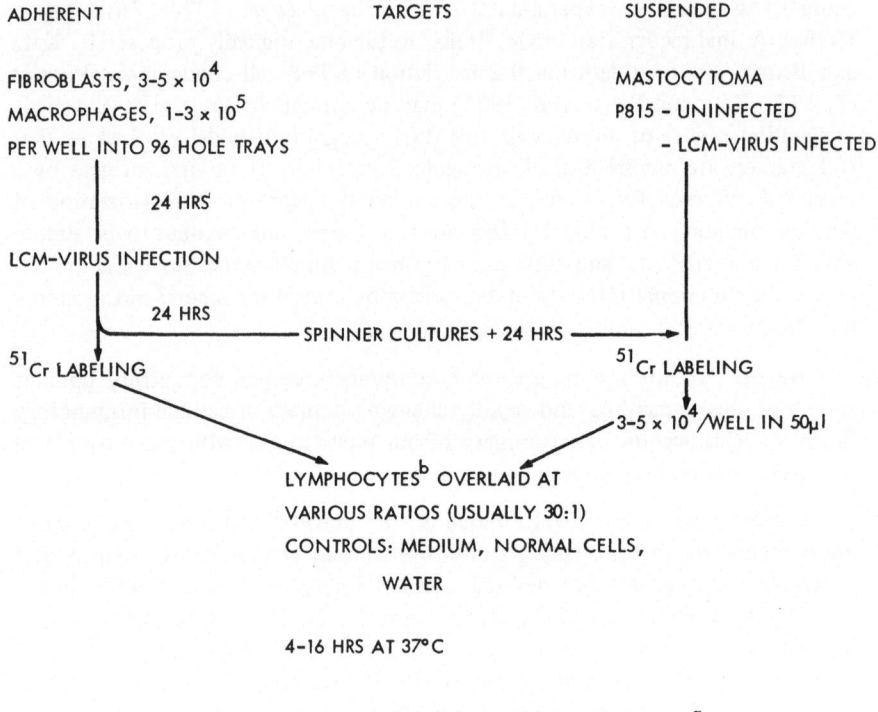

$$\% \text{ SPECIFIC }^{51}\text{Cr RELEASE} = \frac{\% \text{ RELEASE (IMMUNE ON LCM)} - \% \text{ (CONTROL}^a)}{\% \text{ (H}_2\text{O RELEASE)} - \% \text{ (CONTROL)}} \times 100$$

[a]   % Control: Higher value % release of immune cells on normal targets, or normal cells on virus-infected targets.

[b]   Immune lymphocytes were spleen cells harvested 7 d after intravenous injection of 10^3 i.c. LD_{50} of WE3 LCM-virus.

Fig. 1. ^{51}Cr-release assay for virus-specific cytotoxic T cells.

with pox or paramyxoviruses (Doherty and Zinkernagel, 1976; Doherty *et al.*, 1976a). The effector cell is a T cell by several criteria (Doherty *et al.*, 1974; Zinkernagel and Doherty, 1973; Gardner *et al.*, 1974a,b), and with parameters that are virtually identical to those of alloantigen-reactive cytotoxic T cells (Table II).

B. Apparent Requirement for *H-2* Compatibility for Virus-Specific Cytolytic Interactions *in Vitro*

Oldstone *et al.* (1973) described variation in susceptibility to infection with LCMV in congenic mice, which differ only at *H-2*; *H-2^q* mice were more susceptible than *H-2^k* mice. This difference may reflect a regulatory influence by *Ir* genes (Oldstone *et al.*, 1973). However, in more recent experiments with the same strains of mice used in the original study (Oldstone *et al.*, 1973), overall susceptibility, as determined by the 50% lethal dose (LD_{50}) of LCMV injected intracerebrally (i.c.), did not differ substantially, but the kinetics of dying was accelerated in *H-2^q* mice (Oldstone, 1976). Thus, a clear-cut example for a role of immune response (Ir) genes in a viral infection is still missing. Nevertheless, it was this report that led us to investigate a possible link between susceptibility to infection and capacity to generate cytotoxic T cells.

Based on the prediction that the cell-mediated immune response may be more acute and of greater magnitude in the more susceptible mouse strains, a wide variety of mouse strains were infected intracerebrally with the WE3 strain of LCMV, and the animals' lymphoid cells were assayed for cytotoxic activity against LCMV-infected L cells (mouse fibroblasts). The totally unexpected finding was that lytic interactions occurred only when virus-immune T cells and infected target cells were compatible at the *H-2* gene complex (Zinkernagel and Doherty, 1974b; Doherty and Zinkernagel, 1975b). Immune lymphocytes from F_1 or *H-2* genetic recombinant mice were capable of lysing both parental targets and vice versa (Fig. 2). Lymphocytes from *H-2*-incompatible donors did not cause any specific lysis, although these mouse strains died of acute LCM to a comparable extent. Xenogeneic targets also were not lysed (Zinkernagel, 1975; Table III).

The use of *H-2* congenic mouse strains rigorously proved that compatibility at *H-2* alone was crucial for virus-specific cytolysis (Doherty and Zinkernagel, 1975b; Gardner *et al.*, 1975); non-*H-2* genetic background (like the *M*-locus; Festenstein, 1973) was irrelevant. Also, up to 12 shared public specificities were not sufficient for lysis to occur (Table IV).

One of the striking initial findings, which in retrospect is more easily understood, was that ectromelia virus-specific cytolysis could be blocked much more readily with anti-*H-2* sera than with hyperimmune antivirus antisera (Gardner *et al.*, 1974a; Koszinowski and Ertl, 1975; Zinkernagel, 1975). More

Table II. Characteristics of Cytotoxic T Cells

Parameter	Anti-alloantigen	References	Anti-LCMV
Identity of Effector Cell			
AKR-anti-Θ C3H + C' sensitive	+	Cerottini et al. (1970b)	+
Rabbit anti-mouse-Ig + C' sensitive	−	Mauel et al. (1970)	−
Macrophage involvement	−	Brunner et al. (1970)	−
Lymphocyte-dependent, antibody-mediated	−	Brunner et al. (1968)	−
Lymphotoxin involvement	−	Häyry et al. (1972)	−
		Cerottini and Bruner (1974)	
Cortisone resistance	+	Mauel et al. (1970 in vitro)	+(in vivo)
850 rad resistance in vitro	+	Cerottini and Brunner (1974)	+
Blast cells present, or cell size > 9µm	+	Häyry et al. (1972)	+
Specificity			
H-2 specific	+	Brunner et al. (1970)	+
Distinct specificities related to H-2K or H-2D	+	Nabholz et al. (1974)	+
Efficiency difference, specific–nonspecific target	> 300	MacDonald et al. (1973)	> 100
		Lafferty et al. (1974)	
Cold target competitive inhibition	+	Cerottini and Brunner (1974)	+
Anti-H-2 serum blocks target	+	Brunner et al. (1968)	+
Blocking with antivirus serum			−

Generation *In Vivo*			
First detectable day after immunization (P815)	3(−7)	5	Cerottini and Brunner (1974)
In vivo peak activity days after immunization (P815)	4−5(−11)	5−9	Cerottini and Brunner (1974)
Peak activity: sensitized lymphocytes to lyse one target (P815) per hour	10−30	10−30	Henney (1974)
Loss of activity by day after immunization	7−8 (>20)	9∓15	Cerottini and Brunner (1974)
In Vitro Parameters			
Contact requirement	+	+	Rosenau and Moon (1966)
			Brunner *et al.* (1970)
Geometric limitations	20:1	20:1	Henney (1971)
Linear ^{51}Cr release with time	+	+	Brunner *et al.* (1968)
"One-hit" mechanism for target lysis	+	+	R. G. Miller and Dunkley (1974)
Kill probably more than 1	+	+	Brunner *et al.* (1970)
			R. G. Miller and Dunkley (1974)
Temperature-sensitive	+	+	Brunner *et al.* (1968)
Target cells: P815	+	+	
Macrophages	+	+	
Fibroblasts	+	+	Häyry *et al.* (1972)

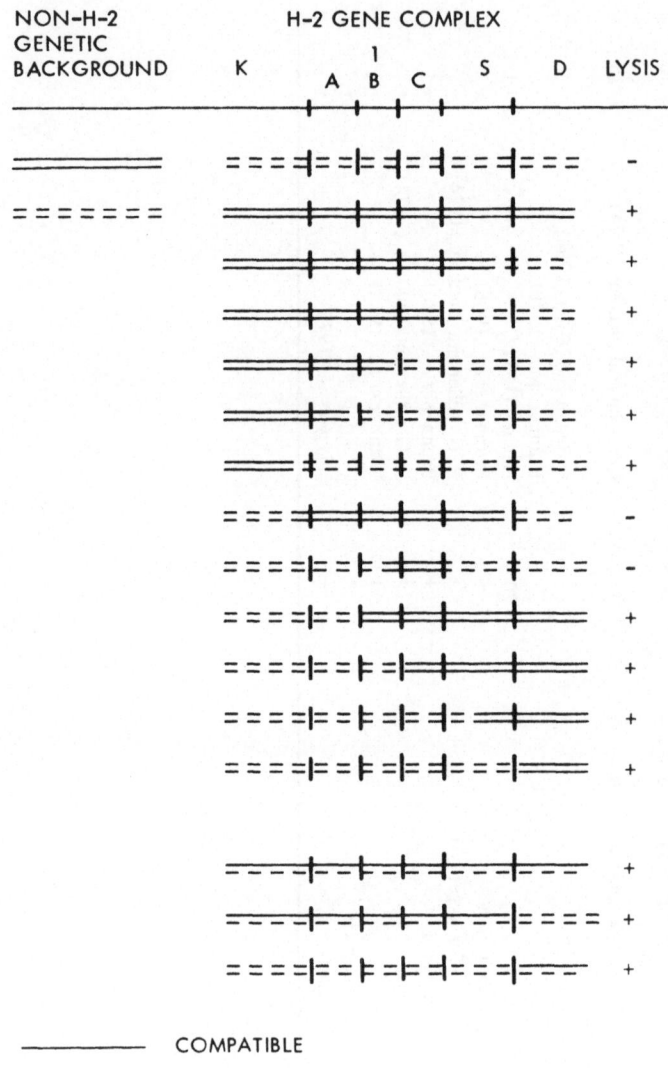

COMPATIBLE

INCOMPATIBLE

Fig. 2. Summary of the tested *H-2* compatibility combinations for LCMV-specific cytotoxicity. From Zinkernagel and Doherty (1974b), Doherty and Zinkernagel (1975b), Blanden *et al.* (1975a), and Zinkernagel *et al.* (1976).

**Table III. LCMV-Immune Mouse Lymphoid Cells Assayed on
Various Xenogeneic LCMV-Infected Target Cells**

Target cell[a]	Origin	Immunofluorescent anti-LCMV staining	Specific ^{51}Cr release[b]
Vero	Monkey	+++	−
HeLa	Human	+++	−
BHK-21	Hamster	+++	−
L cell	Mouse (H-2^k)	++	+++

[a]Infected with a high multiplicity of LCMV for 24 hr before assay.
[b]Overlaid at 30:1 and assayed for 14 hr at 37°C.

detailed studies by Germain *et al.* (1975) and subsequently by Schrader *et al.*
(1975) revealed that for blocking anti-*H-2* sera had to be directed against the *H-2*
specificity of the target cell only and that antiviral antibodies blocked in a tumor
virus model. The controversy over the fact that antiviral antibodies do block
lysis in the vaccinia model, but do not in the ectromelia model, and that sera
sampled 7–9 days after infection block only weakly in the LCMV model is
unresolved as yet. Comparable restrictions of T-cell-mediated virus-immune
cytotoxicity have been found *in vitro* for ectromelia (Gardner *et al.*, 1975),
vaccinia (Koszinowski and Thomssen, 1975), Sendai (Doherty and Zinkernagel,
1976), Friend-virus (Blank *et al.,* 1976), and probably murine sarcoma viruses

**Table IV. Public *H-2* Specificities Shared Between Immune Spleen Cells and
Infected Target Cells Without Significant Expression of Cytotoxicity[a]**

Immune spleen cell donors	Infected target cell	Shared *H-2* public specificities[b]
H-2^d	H-2^k	3, 8, 47, 49
H-2^b	H-2^k	5
H-$2^{d/b}$	H-2^k	3, 5, 8, 47, 49
H-2^s	H-2^k	1, 3, 5, 45, 49
H-2^q	H-2^k	1, 3, 5, 11, 45, 49, 52
H-2^b	H-2^d	6, 14, 27, 28, 29, 35, 36, 46
H-$2^{k/b}$	H-2^d	3, 6, 8, 14, 27, 28, 29, 35, 36, 46, 47, 49
H-2^s	H-2^d	3, 6, 28, 36, 42, 49
H-2^q	H-2^d	3, 6, 13, 27, 28, 29, 34, 49

[a]Summarized from Zinkernagel and Doherty (1974a), Doherty and Zinkernagel (1975b),
and unpublished data.
[b]From Klein (1975).

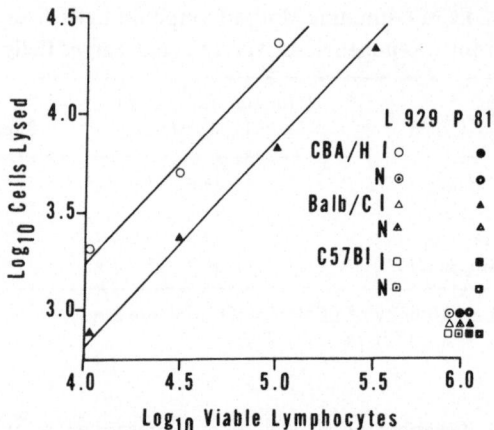

Fig. 3. Dose effect on the lytic activity of LCMV-immune lymphocytes against *H-2*-compatible (o, ▲) or -incompatible virus-infected targets (all other combinations). (I) Immune, (N) normal lymphocytes on infected targets.

(MSV) (Herbermann *et al.*, 1973; Plata, Cerottini, and Brunner, personal communication).

Activity against *H-2*-compatible LCMV-infected targets is more than 100 times greater than against incompatible ones (Doherty and Zinkernagel, 1975b; Fig. 3). This apparent restriction of cytotoxic T-cell activity over the entire period of a measurable primary immune response by the *H-2* gene complex is thus a biological "all-or-none" phenomenon that makes the difference more qualitative than quantitative.

C. Association of Specificity with Structures Coded in *K* or *D* of *H-2*

In the *H-2* gene complex, several regions and subregions have been defined with the help of crossover events within *H-2* (reviewed in Schreffler and David, 1975, and Klein, 1975). Virus-immune spleen cells from *H-2* recombinant mice, having part of the *H-2* gene complex in common with original *H-2* type targets, or vice versa, were assayed in several combinations (Fig. 2; Blanden *et al.*, 1975a; Zinkernagel *et al.*, 1976). Compatibility at *H-2K* or *H-2D* alone was sufficient for cytolysis. Compatibility at only one of the possible four *K* and *D* regions in heterozygous mice was the minimal requirement for lysis (Fig. 2; Zinkernagel *et al.*, 1975). Furthermore, at the effector level, *I*-region compatibility alone was not sufficient for lytic interactions, nor did *I*-region compatibility improve cytolysis for *K*- and *D*-compatible interactions. This contrasts sharply with T helper cells, for which *I* but not *K* or *D* compatibility alone allows collaboration with B cells (Katz *et al.*, 1975; Erb and Feldman, 1975).

The failure of *I*-region compatibility to enable lytic interaction most likely does not reflect absence of the relevant *I*-region-coded structures, e.g., *Ia* antigens, on the surfaces of target cells. Macrophages, which were used for these studies, are known to express *Ia* antigens (Delovitch and McDevitt, 1975; Unanue *et al.*, 1974; Hämmerling *et al.*, 1975), but were not lysed by virus-specific cytotoxic T cells, which were compatible only for *H-2I*. Nevertheless, the total failure of only *I*-region-compatible LCMV-immune spleen cells to adoptively transfer any antiviral protection, as will be discussed in a later section, may more convincingly indicate that at the effector level, *I*-region-coded structures are not of crucial importance in these models.

This exclusive association of virus-specific cytotoxicity with *H-2K* or *D* can be used for *H-2* typing of outbred or wild mice and more generally in other species. Mice from outbred mouse strains, which revealed positive mixed lymphocyte reactions *in vitro* when reciprocally tested, behaved like inbred mice when assayed for LCMV-immune cytotoxic lymphocytes. Reactivity was restricted between them, but not within them, reflecting a restricted repertoire of different *H-2K* or *H-2D* regions within one particular outbred strain of mice (Zinkernagel *et al.*, 1975).

D. Roles of the *H-2I* Region and Non-*H-2* Genes in Regulating Cytotoxic Immune Responses to Lymphocytic Choriomeningitis Virus

Although *I*-region compatibility is not required at the effector level for cytolytic interaction, it could well be of importance for triggering virus-specific cytotoxic T-cell responses. Six *H-2* recombinant mouse strains, all of which possessed the D^d region but had different *I*-region specificities, did not differ greatly in their capacities to generate LCMV-specific cytotoxic activity associated with D^d. The I^d specificity of the *I* region did not confer the capacity to generate greater cytotoxic activity than non-I^d specificities (Zinkernagel *et al.*, 1976). Because this result was basically negative, however, it is not conclusive. It may reflect either wide "cross-reactivity" of the relevant *I*-coded structures in the examples studied or that minor effects were missed. A role for *I* genes might still be found if many more strain combinations are tested.

When a wide variety of *H-2* recombinant mouse strains was assayed for LCMV-specific cytotoxicity, D2.GD ($H-2K^d|D^b$) mice failed to generate high activity. Further analysis revealed that DBA/2 ($H-2^d$) mice, from which the D2.GD mice are derived, were also low responders when infected intravenously (i.v.) with the standard 10^3 i.c. LD_{50} of viscerotropic WE LCMV as assessed by *in vitro* cytotoxicity. Yet, with an infectious dose 100 times lower, some LCMV-specific activity was measurable by day 7. This virus–dose dependent low responsiveness is recessive, since C3H×DBA/2 F_1 mice are highly responsive when injected with the entire range of the same virus doses (Zinkernagel *et al.*, 1976). BALB/c or B10.D2 (both *H-2^d*) mice generate LCMV-specific cytotoxicity at low and high virus doses. The factor(s) regulating this low responsiveness in DBA/2 mice is thus coded for by non-*H-2* genes. These genes have not been defined further as yet, but may well reflect factors that control the initial spread and multiplication of infectious agents. Thus, easier and wider spread of virus in an organism could cause high-dose immune paralysis (Hotchin, 1971; Doherty and Zinkernagel, 1974) and/or might recruit effector cells to organs other than those normally examined during immunologic testing (i.e., spleen), enabling them to escape *in vitro* detection (Zinkernagel *et al.*, 1976). Characteristics such as the antigen-dose-dependent role of the *I* region and the high–low response phenomena with viruses mark an important difference between soluble, chemically defined inert antigens and infectious agents in an intact animal. This difference is probably one of the keys to explaining the differential association of soluble antigens with *I*-region-coded structures and that of viruses with *K*- or *D*-coded cell-surface components.

E. Specificity of Cytotoxic T Cells from *H-2K* Mutant Mice

H-2 mutant mice differ from the original strain only by one very small part of the genome, probably the size of one cistron (Klein, 1975, 1976; Shreffler and David, 1975; Bailey *et al.*, 1971). Most of these mutants described so far carry a mutation in the *K* region of *H-2*.

Two mutants Hz1 (C57BL/6, *H-2K^{ba}*) and Hz170 (C57BL/6, *H-2k^{bf}*), and the original C57BL/6 have been shown to reject mutual skin grafts *in vivo*, to cause positive mixed lymphocyte cultures, and to generate cytotoxic T cells when mutually cultured *in vitro*, although they do not differ serologically (Bailey *et al.*, 1971; Widmer *et al.*, 1973; Klein, 1975). Spleen cells from LCMV- or vaccinia-virus-infected Hz1 or Hz170 mice could not lyse infected wild type *H-2K^b* targets of B10.A(5r) origin or vice versa (Zinkernagel, 1976a; Doherty *et al.*, 1976a). With cold target competition experiments, it could be demonstrated that this failure did not reflect a simple deletion of the *H-2K* structure, since these mutant mice generated cytotoxic T cells specifically associated with *H-2K^{ba}* or *H-2K^{bf}*. Similar results were obtained for ectromelia virus infection in Hz1 mice. Yet spleen cells from another mutant, C57BL/6 *H-2^{bh}*, cross-reacted extensively with the infected wild-type target, indicating that the mutation affected the relevant self-marker not at all or only slightly (reviewed in Doherty *et al.*, 1976a).

III. RESTRICTION OF VIRUS-SPECIFIC EFFECTOR-T-CELL FUNCTIONS *IN VIVO* BY *H-2K* OR *H-2D*

The protective or destructive roles of T cells in virus infections have been summarized in various reviews during recent years (Hotchin, 1971; Allison, 1974; Blanden, 1974; Doherty and Zinkernagel, 1974; Cole and Nathanson, 1975; Blanden *et al.*, 1975c; and many others). Virus-specific cytotoxicity is the most easily *in vitro* demonstrable T-cell function generated during LCMV infection. To what extent these cytotoxic T cells are actually involved in various immune

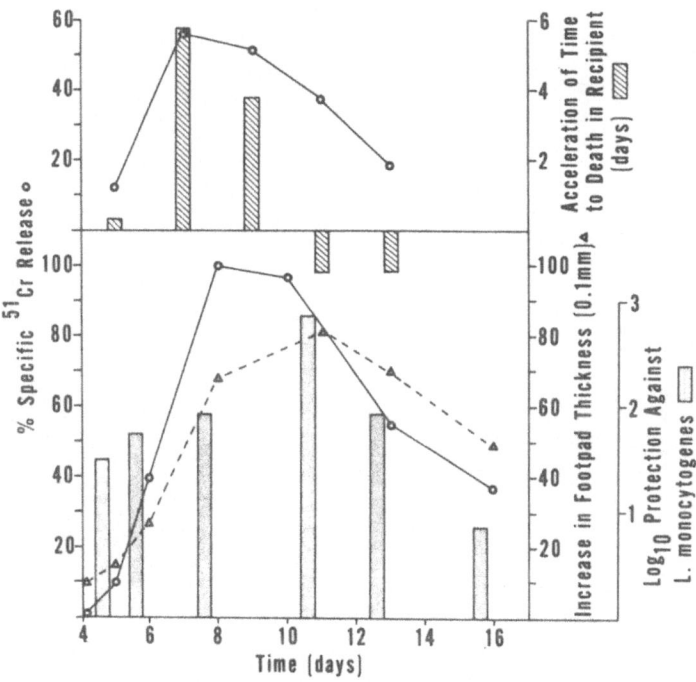

Fig. 4. *Top panel:* Kinetics of generation of cytotoxic T cells (o————o) during a primary immune response to a LCMV infection (1000 i.c. LD_{50} i.v. on day 0) in CBA/H mice, compared with the capacity of these cells to adoptively induce acute LCM in LCMV i.c. infected, immunosuppressed recipients (▨) Modified from Doherty and Zinkernagel (1975a). *Bottom panel:* Comparison of cytotoxic activity (o————o), magnitude of 24-hr DTH response (△—————△), and extent of macrophage activation as measured by their nonspecifically increased bactericidal capacity against *Listeria monocytogenes*, in CBA/H mice injected with 10^3 i.c. LD_{50} i.v. on day 0 (Zinkernagel, unpublished results). Protection against *L. monocytogenes* during 24 hr was assessed as described by Mackaness (1969).

Table V. Parameters of LCMV-Immune T Cells

Parameter	In vitro	In vivo		
	Cytotoxicity by ^{51}Cr-release assay	Adoptive induction of acute LCM or inflammation in CSF	Adoptive transfer of antiviral protection	Adoptive transfer of DTH
Specificity vs. normal or other viruses	+	+	+	+
Anti-Θ + C' sensitive	+	+	+	+
Anti-mouse Ig + C' insensitive	+	+	+	+
Peak activity (days after infection)	7–9	7–9	6–9	7–11
H-2 compatibility required at: K or D	+	+	+	+
I	–	–	–	–
Cross-reactivity between wild type H-$2K^b$ and H-2 mutants H-$2K^{ba}$ or H-$2K^{bf}$	–	–	–	–
References	Marker and Volkert (1973) Cole et al. (1973) Zinkernagel and Doherty (1973) Doherty et al. (1974) Blanden et al. (1975a)	Cole et al. (1972) Gilden et al. (1972) Doherty and Zinkernagel (1975a) Doherty et al. (1976b)	Blanden et al. (1975b) Zinkernagel and Welsh (1976)	Zinkernagel (1976d)

phenomena *in vivo* is poorly understood. Circumstantial evidence pointing to their biological function derives from the fact that cytotoxic T cells of great specific activity can be isolated from the cerebrospinal fluid of clinically affected mice (Zinkernagel and Doherty, 1973). Furthermore, as can be seen from Fig. 4, kinetics parallel remarkably for (1) cytotoxic activity *in vitro*, (2) onset of fatal LCM resulting from adoptive transfers of LCMV immune T cells, (3) delayed-type hypersensitivity (DTH) in animals challenged by injection of virus into footpads, (4) induction of macrophage activation as measured by their bactericidal activity against *Listeria monocytogenes* (Zinkernagel, unpublished results), and (5) antiviral protection as measured in an adoptive transfer system. Also, the cellular parameters are virtually identical (Table V).

LCMV-immune T cells were thus assessed *in vivo* with respect to their association with the various *H-2* regions. The three different adoptive transfer models represent the diverse immunologic phenomena observed in LCMV infections:

1. Adoptive transfer of acute LCM to assay for capacity of T cells to induce fatal immunopathology.
2. Adoptive transfer of antiviral protection to assess the potential of T cells to decrease viral growth or spreading or both.
3. Adoptive transfer of DTH as measured by induction of footpad swelling, a complex T-cell-mediated immunologic mechanism leading to predominantly mononuclear inflammation.

A. Adoptive Induction of Acute Lymphocytic Choriomeningitis

The evidence supporting the idea that T cells are essential for induction of acute LCM has been summarized extensively (Hotchin, 1971; Lehmann-Grube, 1971; Doherty and Zinkernagel, 1974; Cole and Nathanson, 1975). Acute LCM is a laboratory artefact initiated by intracerebral injection of LCMV and is usually a fatal neurological disease (Fig. 5). The disease can be adoptively transferred only when donors of LCMV-immune cells and recipients are *H-2* compatible (Doherty and Zinkernagel, 1975a). Furthermore, adoptive induction of inflammation in cerebrospinal fluid (CSF) is dependent on T cells and recipients sharing the *K* or *D* but not the *I* region of *H-2* (Doherty *et al.*, 1976b). Also, cells from Hz1 ($H\text{-}2K^{ba}D^b$) mutant mice did not transfer inflammatory processes to wild-type $H\text{-}2K^b$ recipients, but did so to $H\text{-}2D^b$-compatible mice.

B. Antiviral Protection by LCMV-Immune T Cells

The capacity of adoptively transferred immune T cells to protect the recipients from infection by subsequent exposure to *Listeria monocytogenes*

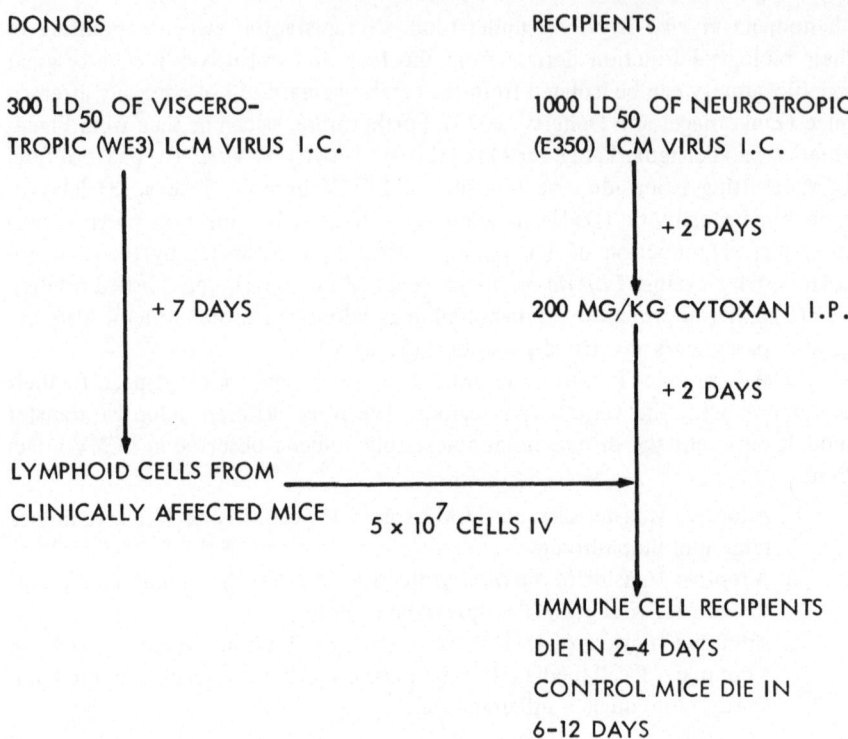

DONORS   RECIPIENTS

300 LD$_{50}$ OF VISCERO-   1000 LD$_{50}$ OF NEUROTROPIC
TROPIC (WE3) LCM VIRUS I.C.   (E350) LCM VIRUS I.C.

                                                              + 2 DAYS

              + 7 DAYS   200 MG/KG CYTOXAN I.P.

                                                              + 2 DAYS

LYMPHOID CELLS FROM
CLINICALLY AFFECTED MICE   5 x 10^7 CELLS IV

                                              IMMUNE CELL RECIPIENTS
                                              DIE IN 2-4 DAYS
                                              CONTROL MICE DIE IN
                                              6-12 DAYS

Fig 5. Experimental protocol for the adoptive transfer of acute LCM. Modified from Doherty and Zinkernagel (1975a).

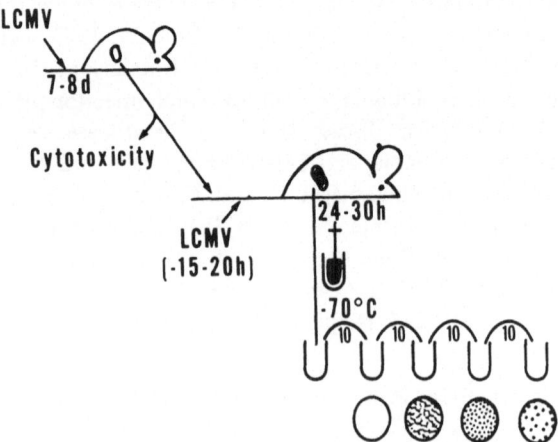

Fig. 6. Protocol for the adoptive transfer of anti-LCMV protection. (From Zinkernagel and Welsh, 1976.)

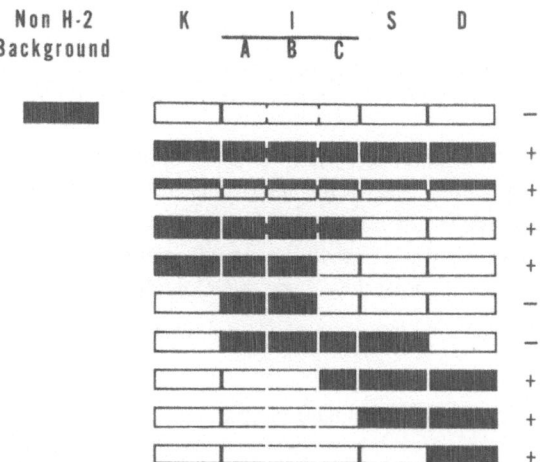

Fig. 7. Summary of the genetic requirement for the adoptive transfer of anti-LCMV protection. Modified from Zinkernagel and Welsh (1976).

bacteria or to ectromelia virus was clearly shown to be restricted by the *H-2* gene complex (Zinkernagel, 1974; Blanden *et al.*, 1975b). The classic transfer models described by Mackaness (1969) and Blanden (1971) to measure the capacity of LCMV-immune T cells (Mims and Blanden, 1972; Zinkernagel and Welsh, 1976) to control LCMV growth in infected recipients were used to map the genetic requirements (Fig. 6 and 7). Virus titers were greatly reduced only in recipients compatible at *H-2K* or *D* with the transferred T cells. *I*-region compatibility

Table VI. Adoptive Transfer of Anti-LCMV Protection in *H-2* Mutant Mice[a]

	Log_{10} PFU of LCMV per spleen of recipient mice[b]	
LCMV-immune donor	B10.A(5r) *b bbd d d*	C57BL/10 *b bbb b b*
B6 *H-2^bf* (Hz170) $K \begin{matrix} 1 \\ A \, B \, C \end{matrix} S D$ *bf b b b b b*	6.60±0.19	3.42±0.51
Control (no cells)	6.48±0.20	6.68±0.09

[a]For the experimental protocol, see Fig. 7. From Zinkernagel and Welsh (1976).
[b]Recipients were challenged with 10^3 PFU WE LCMV.

alone neither conferred protection nor improved the activity of T cells compatible at K or D. Also, immune spleen cells from $H\text{-}2K^{bf}D^b$ mutant mice did not protect wild-type $H\text{-}2K^b$ mice, but did protect $H\text{-}2D^b$-compatible recipients (Table VI).

How T cells, especially cytotoxic T cells, endow antiviral protection is unclear. Possibly they act directly by destroying infected cells before infectious virus is assembled or by releasing soluble mediators that activate macrophages nonspecifically. This pathway and other possible pathways of action will not be discussed further here, since they have been dealt with in a recent review (Blanden *et al.,* 1975c).

C. Adoptive Transfer of LCMV-Specific DTH

DTH (reviewed in Crowle, 1975) to LCMV is a T-cell-mediated phenomenon as judged by the following criteria. By using the experimental protocol summarized in Fig. 8 for eliciting DTH, effector cells were shown to be sensitive to AKR anti-Thy-1.2 + C', but were unharmed by rabbit anti-mouse Fab + C' treatment. Also, primary footpad swelling caused by local LCMV injection did not occur in T-cell-depleted mice (Zinkernagel, 1976d).

Evaluation of the genetic requirements for eliciting DTH in this model revealed again that T cells and recipients had to share K or D but not the I region of $H\text{-}2$. $H\text{-}2K^b$ wild-type LCMV-immune cells elicited positive DTH in $H\text{-}2K^b$ wild-type but not in $H\text{-}2K^{ba}$ mutant mice, further emphasizing that compatibility of T cells and recipients of IA^b and IB^b is not sufficient for initiating DTH (Table VII and Fig. 9).

This result is in good agreement with the results from the other two transfer models. J. F. A. P. Miller *et al.* (1975) rcently showed, however, that adoptive

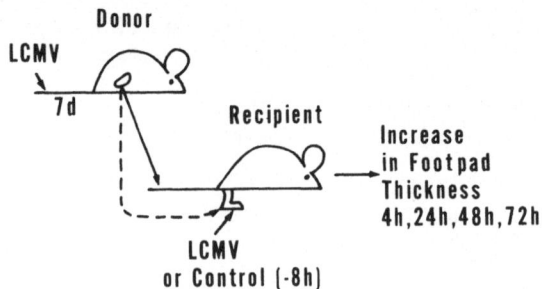

Fig. 8. Protocol for the adoptive transfer of LCMV-specific DTH. (From Zinkernagel, 1976d.)

Table VII. Adoptive Transfer of
LCMV-Specific DTH[a]

LCMV-immune donor[b]	Recipient	Mean increase in footpad thickness (%) at time after transfer (hr)		
		6	24	48
B10.A(3r)	B6.*H-2^{ba}*(Hz1)	4±3	4±2	4±2
	C57BL/6	2±2	25±2	53±3

[a]For the experimental protocol, see Fig. 8. From Zinkernagel (1976d).
[b]10^8 immune spleen cells were transferred intravenously.

transfer of fowl γ-globulin-specific DTH was restricted to *H-2I*-compatible strain combinations. Compatibility at either *K* or *D* was not sufficient. This discrepancy may well reflect the fundamentally different nature of the antigens used. Chemically defined soluble and inert antigens may quite generally associate with structures coded in *I*, and multiplying, infectious (i.e., actively penetrating into and "living" in cells) agents may associate with *K*- or *D*-coded structures.

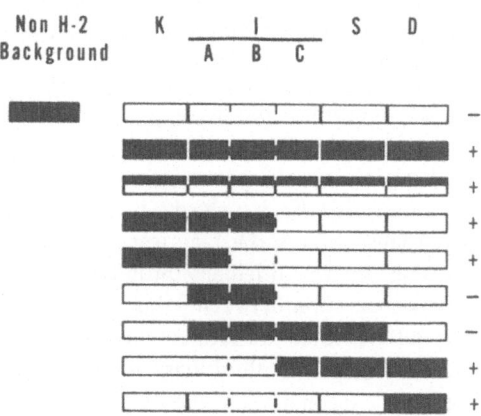

Fig. 9. Summary of the genetic requirement for the adoptive transfer of LCMV-specific DTH.

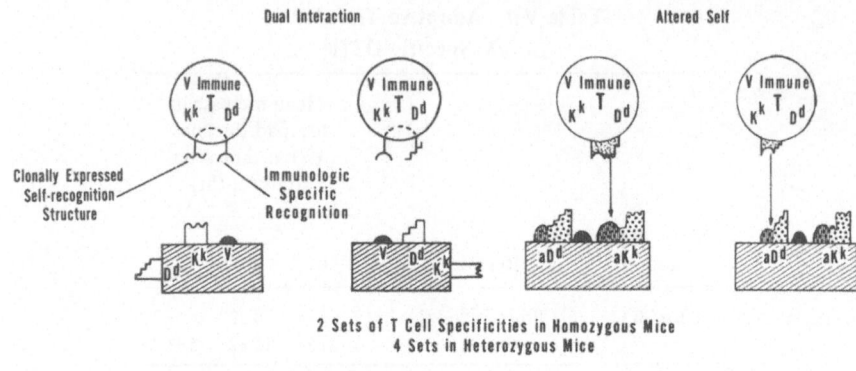

Fig. 10. Two hypotheses to explain the apparent H-$2K$ or D restriction of virus-specific cytotoxicity. (V) Viral antigen on cell surface; (K^k, D^d) structures coded in K or D region of H-2; (aD^d, aK^k) altered K- or D- coded structures.

IV. ANALYSIS OF THE *H-2* COMPATIBILITY REQUIREMENT FOR CYTOLYTIC T-CELL INTERACTIONS

The apparent compatibility requirement at *H-2K* or *H-2D* for virus-specific T-cell effector functions *in vitro* and *in vivo* has been explained by two mutually exclusive hypotheses (Fig. 10), which are described below.

1. The Intimacy and Dual Recognition Hypothesis

T cells interact specifically with viral antigens expressed on the cell surface. For lysis to occur, an additional physiological (self–selflike) interaction is necessary. Such interaction structures would have to be coded within *H-2K* or *H-2D*. That T cells from F_1 or *H-2* recombinants can apparently lyse both parental type targets could thus be explained with a minimal one set of T-cell specificities directed against viral surface antigens (Zinkernagel and Doherty, 1974c). Although this theory was originally proposed to explain the need of *H-2I* compatibility for cooperation between T helper cells and B cells (Katz and Benacerraf, 1975), it differs, since the interaction structures would have to be coded in *K* or *D*. This intimacy hypothesis has been modified to the dual recognition model in Fig. 10 to accommodate the data discussed in the subsequent paragraphs. Accordingly, T cells possess two separate but linked clonally expressed receptors for a viral antigen and for self.

2. Altered-Self Hypothesis

Virus-specific cytotoxic T cells are sensitized to virus-modified cell-surface structures coded for in *H-2K* or *H-2D* (probably major transplantation antigens) or by structures coded for very close to them. Altered-self could be envisaged as short- or long-range modification of self-structures or as biochemical alteration. Within this model, a minimum of two sets in homozygotes and four sets in heterozygotes of T-cell specificities directed against altered *H-2K* or *D* would have to exist to explain the fact that infected F_1 and *H-2* recombinants can generate T cells cytotoxic for either parental type of infected target. This model could easily embrace cytotoxic T-cell reactivity to alloantigens (being a form of altered-self) or to altered-self due to viral (or bacterial) infections or chemical modification (e.g., TNP; Shearer, 1974).

Quite speculatively, the theory of altered-self could be applied to explain the *H-2* restriction of T helper cells. T helper cells could be sensitized to antigen self-"altered" structures coded for in the *I* region of *H-2* (Zinkernagel, 1975, 1976a; Blanden *et al.*, 1975a; Doherty *et al.*, 1976a).

A trivial explanation for *H-2K* and *D* restriction *in vitro* of virus-immune cytotoxic T cells such as rejection or allogeneic inhibition (Hellström and Möller, 1965) is unlikely for the following reasons: cytotoxic lymphocytes from F_1 on (P), and P on F_1 work with comparable efficiency *in vitro* and *in vivo* (Doherty and Zinkernagel, 1975b; Zinkernagel, 1974; Blanden *et al.*, 1975b); addition of irrelevant virus-immune or normal allogeneic lymphocytes does not impair syngeneic interactions (Zinkernagel and Welsh, 1976). Compatibility at only one of four possible *K* plus *D* regions in addition to incompatibility of both *I*-region (except for *IC*) and non-*H-2* background results in excellent virus-specific cytolytic interactions, as shown for LCMV-immune B10.A×C57BL/6 ($H\text{-}2^{kId}\times$ $H\text{-}2^{bIb}$) assayed on infected P815 ($H\text{-}2^{dId}$, DBA/2) (Zinkernagel *et al.*, 1975).

Six different sets of experimental evidence impinge on these two hypotheses. These sets are discussed in Sections IV.A–F.

A. Antibody Blocking Experiments

Gardner *et al.* (1974a,b) showed that ectromelia virus-immune or hyperimmune sera were not very effective in blocking cytotoxicity *in vitro*, but anti-*H-2* sera of the relevant type inhibited ^{51}Cr release markedly. Although somewhat controversial, more detailed experiments by Koszinowski and Ertl (1975) with vaccinia virus and by Germain *et al.* (1975) and Schrader *et al.* (1975) with tumor viruses indicate that anti-*H-2* sera block only if they are directed against the *H-2* specificity that is common to killer and target cells. In the vaccinia virus model, however, antiviral antibody was reported to block very efficiently (Koszinowski and Thomssen, 1975). This finding contrasts with the LCMV system, in which only very moderate blocking was obtained with sera obtained 9–13 days after infection, but none occurred with mouse or rabbit hyperimmune antisera. These controversial results are as yet unexplained.

Anti-*H-2* sera thus block either directly or by sterically hindering the physiological interaction structure or alternatively the altered self-markers. The (controversial) failure of antiviral antibody to inhibit cytolytic interactions could be interpreted in favor of the altered-self hypothesis. It could quite generally mean, however, that secreted antibody and T cells do not react with the same antigenic entity.

Capping and cocapping studies of viral and *H-2* cell-surface antigen such as have been carried out by Schrader *et al.* (1975) with Rauscher leukemia virus will certainly yield more information, especially if these manipulations alone, or combined, should alter lysability of the target (Edidin and Henney, 1973).

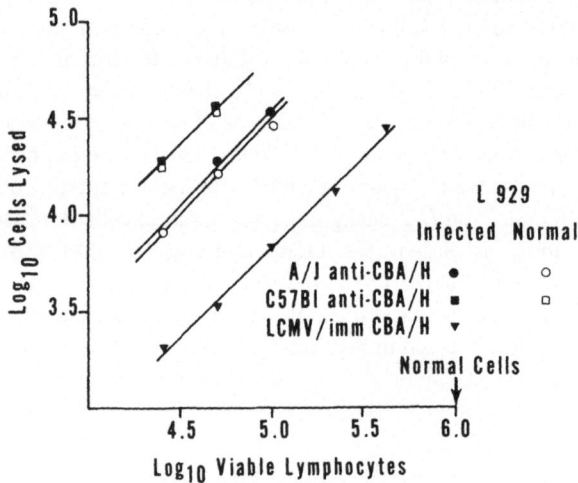

Fig. 11. Dose effect of cytotoxic activity generated *in vitro* by sensitizing in mixed lymphocyte reactions T cells A/J (●,○) and C57BL (■,□) against CBA/H (*H-2^k*) and assayed on LCMV-infected or uninfected L cells (*H-2^k*) as compared with the activity of 7 *d* LCMV-immune CBA/H spleen cells. Only the linear part is shown; at higher effector target ratios, plateaus were reached. No significant difference between antialloantigen-directed lysis of infected and uninfected targets was observed.

Table VIII. Antialloantigen *H-2^d*-Directed T-Cell-Mediated Cytotoxic Activity Against LCMV-Infected and Uninfected P815 (*H-2^d*) Target Cells

Cells	Immune cell/target cell ratio	^{51}Cr release from P815	
		LCMV-infected[a]	Uninfected[b]
LCMV-immune BALB/c[c]	30:1	82.7±1.5[d,e]	27.5±1.1
	6:1	48.0±0.9[e]	26.2±0.9
Normal BALB/c	30:1	26.5±1.6	26.4±2.1
CBA/H anti-BALB/c[f]	5:1	95.2±2.1[b]	98.4±1.8[b]
	1:1	75.6±1.6[b]	79.1±2.4[b]
CBA/H anti-CBA/H	5:1	28.1±0.8	29.2±1.2
Medium	–	27.5±1.2	25.1±1.0

[a]LCMV-infected P815 were from a continuously infected line (Doherty and Zinkernagel, 1975b).
[b]Significantly greater than syngeneic control, but no significant different between infected and uninfected targets.
[c]Mice were injected intravenously with 10^3 i.c. LD$_{50}$ 7 days previously.
[d]Means ± S.E.M. of triplicates; groups were compared by using the Student *t* test.
[e]Significantly greater than normal cells on infected or virus-immune or uninfected targets.
[f]CBA/H anti BALB/c cytotoxic T cells were generated in a mixed lymphocyte reaction *in vitro* for 4 days exactly as described by Lafferty *et al.* (1974).

Antialloantigen—which can be recognized by alloreactive cytotoxic T cells—decreases with time on ectromelia-infected fibroblasts (Gardner *et al.*, 1975). Vaccinia-infected target cells absorb less anti-*H-2* sera than uninfected ones (Koszinowski and Ertl, 1975). These facts may be interpreted as favoring the altered-self model; however, the results may be due to a quantitative rather than to qualitative changes (or both) of *H-2K* or *H-2D* structures. It is known that pox viruses stop cell protein synthesis completely. The rapidly overturning *H-2* cell-surface structures are thus not replaced, and their concentrations decrease rapidly. Mastocytoma P815 cells, which are very rich in *H-2* antigens, fail to show this decrease before the lytic effect of pox virus itself becomes obvious, i.e., during the 24–30 hr postinfection. Also, LCMV-infected target cells, which are metabolically functional carrier cells (Lehmann-Grube, 1971), and uninfected L cells are comparable in their susceptibilities to alloantigen-reactive cytotoxic T cells (Fig. 11 and Table VIII). Furthermore, L cells and other target cells infected for up to 24 hr with vaccinia virus did not prove to be drastically less susceptible to antialloantigen-reactive T cells (Table IX).

In summary, these results are controversial and are consistent with the altered-self idea, at least circumstantially, but do not contradict the dual recognition model.

Table IX. Susceptibility of Vaccinia-Virus-Infected Target Cells to Attack by Antialloantigen-Reactive T Cells

| | | ^{51}Cr release (%) from L cells ($H\text{-}2^k$) | | |
| | Lymphocyte target | | Infected with vaccinia virus | |
Cells	ratio	Uninfected	20 hr	6 hr
C57BL/6 anti-C3H ($H\text{-}2^k$)[a]	10:1	65[b]	61	51[c]
	3:1	30	36	27
	1:1	23	29	19
	0.3:1	16	27	13
C3H anti-C3H ($H\text{-}2^k$)	10:1	14	20	
C3H vaccinia immune[d]	10:1		75	
	3:1		39	

[a]Generated in mixed lymphocyte cultures (Lafferty et al., 1974).
[b]Means of triplicates; the S.E.M. were between 1.2 and 2.7.
[c]Statistically significant from uninfected targets, $P < 0.01$.
[d]For methods, see Zinkernagel (1976a).

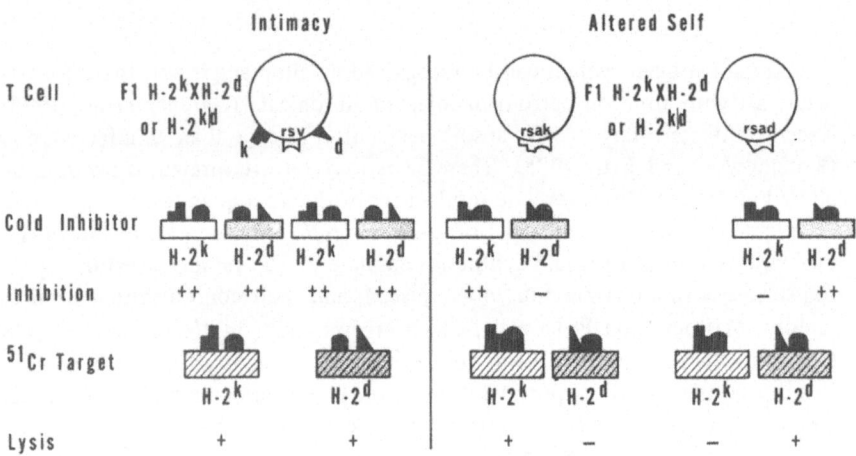

Fig. 12. Competitive inhibition experiments in vitro. If the physiological interaction model is correct, competitive inhibition should be observed when F_1 or H-2 recombinant immune T cells are exposed to either parental type LCMV-infected ^{51}Cr-labeled target and mixed with cold infected targets of either parental type. Experimentally, however, it was found that F_1 (or H-2 recombinant) immune T cells were competitively inhibited only by addition of cold infected targets compatible with both donor and ^{51}Cr-labeled infected targets.

B. Cold Target Competitive Inhibition
Experiments *in Vitro*

Specific ^{51}Cr release by LCMV-immune T cells can be competitively inhibited *in vitro* by the addition of excess unlabeled *H-2*-compatible LCMV-
infected target cells only. This approach was first used by Ortiz de Landazouri
and Herbermann (1972) in the murine sarcoma virus (MSV) system. If the
intimacy model is correct, ^{51}Cr release from each of the parental-type infected
targets by F_1 or *H-2* recombinant immune T cells should be inhibitable by
unlabeled infected targets of either parental type (Fig. 12), since the necessary
requirement for double recognition is fulfilled for both targets. However, ^{51}Cr
release could be inhibited only by adding cold infected targets that were
compatible with ^{51}Cr-labeled infected targets and donor immune cells (Fig. 12;
Zinkernagel and Doherty, 1975).

C. Selective Proliferation Experiments *in Vivo*

Seven-day LCMV-immune T cells proliferate further when transferred into
virus-infected, immunosuppressed, *H-2*-compatible recipient mice (Doherty and
Zinkernagel, 1974, 1975a). When F_1 or *H-2* recombinant immune cells are
transferred to such parental-type recipients, the intimacy model would predict
(Fig. 13) that cytotoxic T cells reactive with either parental type of infected
target will proliferate in either of the parental-type recipients; again, the conditions for double recognition occur in both combinations. As predicted within
the altered-self model, however, only T cells specific for the available parental-
type altered-self structures were found to proliferate. Thus, only T cells cytotoxic to infected targets compatible at *H-2K* or *H-2D* with both donors and
recipients expanded clonally (Zinkernagel and Doherty, 1974c, 1975).

Although the data so far discussed are much more readily reconciled with
the altered-self concept, a dual recognition model can still be invoked if three
assumptions are made:

1. The self-recognition structure is subject to allelic exclusion (to
   explain the data obtained with F_1 cells) (Gell, 1967).
2. If an interaction structure for *H-2K* or the self-marker itself is expressed,
   the interaction structure for *H-2D* or this marker itself cannot be
   expressed on the same cytotoxic T cell or target cell (to explain data
   obtained with *H-2* recombinant cytotoxic T cells).

There is no evidence that *H-2K*- and *H-2D*-coded structures (i.e., private

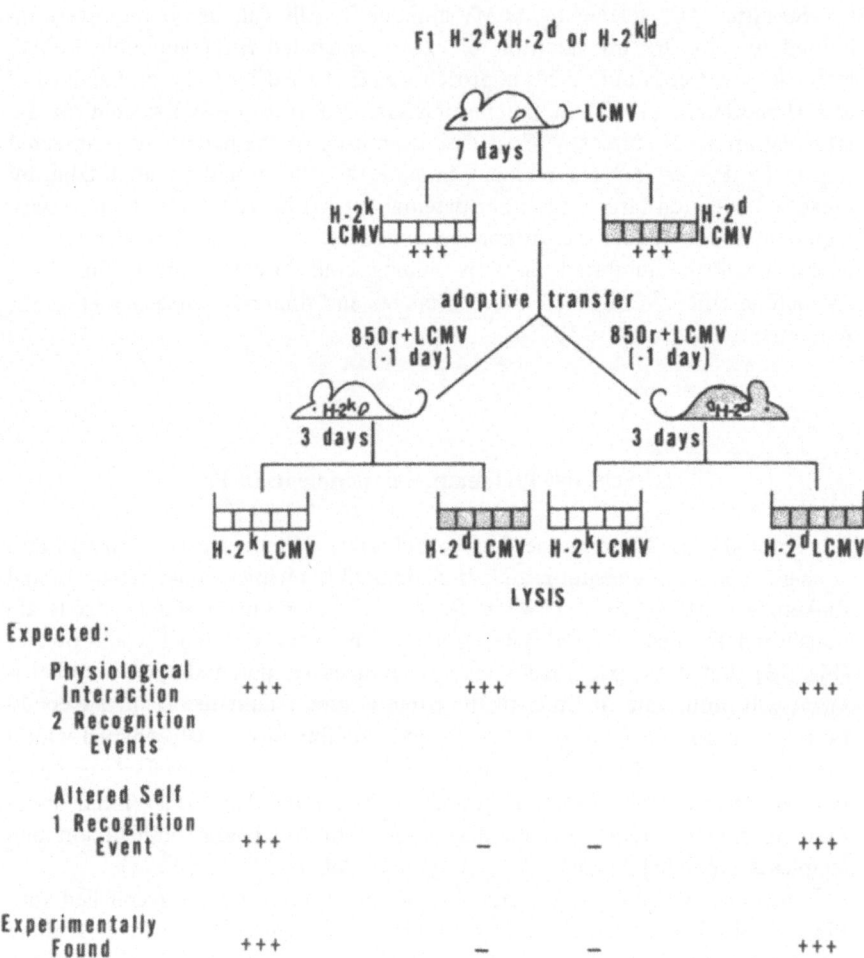

Fig. 13. Selective proliferation of cytotoxic T cells *in vivo*. F_1 or *H-2* recombinant immune T cells transferred for 3 days into infected and 850-rad-treated recipients are expected to proliferate. If the intimacy or physiological interaction model is correct, activity against both parental type infected targets is expected to expand in both parental-type recipients. However, only cytotoxicity against infected targets that are *H-2* compatible with both donors and recipients expanded.

specificity of major transplantation antigens) are subject to allelic or genic exclusion. Assumptions (1) and (2) would therefore have to apply to the structure "recognizing" or interacting with the self-marker.

3. Properties (1) and (2) are expressed clonally.

D. *H-2* Mutant Mice

The two hypotheses must also be viewed in light of the results with *H-2K* mutant mice, which define the gene(s) coding for the *H-2K* structure involved in the apparent restriction. Either this gene defines the alterable self-marker or—alternatively, according to the dual recognition model—this mutation affects (1) the self-marker for self-recognition or (2) the self-recognition structure, or (3) both, i.e., when self-marker and interaction structure are identical (e.g., in a mirror-type interaction) or on the same structure. Although these three propositions are complex and tortuous, the first could be envisaged easily if one assumed that physiological interaction structures could be evolutionarily ancient components. Then one could hypothesize that they are common to all mice and developed to fit the genetically determined self-marker during ontogeny. A great gene pool coding for all possibly evolving self-markers or a few genes undergoing somatic mutation, not necessarily located in *H-2K* or *D,* could represent its possible genetic basis (Jerne, 1971; Zinkernagel, 1976a).

If, second, the *H-2* mutation affects the interaction structure, then this must be coded in *K* or *D.* Besides implying allelic and genic exclusion, this possibility includes the difficult corollary (Bodmer, 1972) of a double mutation of self-marker and interaction structure for a permissive event. If, third, self-marker and interaction structures are on the same molecule or structure, the same corollary is requisite, unless one postulates that a mechanism such as somatic translocation associates the interaction structure and the self-marker (Doherty *et al.,* 1976a; Gally and Edelman, 1970). Also, the allelic and genic exclusion mechanisms would require that one part of this structure is phenotypically suppressed while the other part (self-marker) is apparently always expressed. For similar reasons, the hypothetical interaction structure and self-marker could not be identical.

A variation of the physiological interaction model proposed by Jan Klein, Shevach and Rosenthal, and others (in Katz and Benacerraf, 1976) suggests that not the antigen but the immunologically specific T-cell receptor is, on antigenic encounter, locked together with *K* or *D* structures or mutual interaction structures for *K* or *D.* However, this alternative would have to be subject to the same rules of genetic regulation, including allelic and genic exclusion and clonal expression, to remain compatible with the experimental data.

The results discussed so far can thus be explained by either the simpler idea that cytotoxic T cells are specific for altered-self, or the more complex alternative model of dual recognition.

E. Virus-Specific Cytotoxicity Across the *H-2* Barrier

If virus-specific cytotoxic T cells are specific for altered-self, it should be possible to sensitize T cells across the *H-2* barrier specifically to virus "altered alloantigen." To overcome the normally arising, very strong reactivity to alloantigens, which has made detection of cytotoxic T cells to altered alloantigen impossible, we used irradiated P→F$_1$ chimeras (von Boehmer *et al.*, 1975) reconstituted with bone marrow of one parent (P). C3H→C3HXDBA/2 F$_1$ chimeras infected with LCMV or vaccinia virus generated virus-specific cytotoxic T cells of exclusively *H-2^k* surface characteristics that could lyse virus-infected *H-2^d* targets, but did not lyse uninfected *H-2^b* targets (Fig. 14 and Table X). These T cells are thus tolerant for *H-2^d*, but react readily to virus-infected *H-2^d*

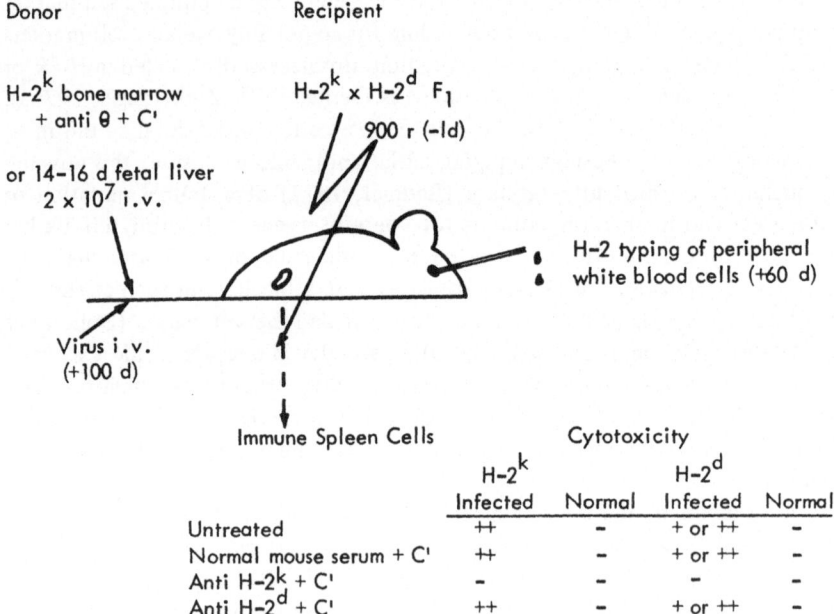

| | H-2^k | | H-2^d | |
	Infected	Normal	Infected	Normal
Untreated	++	–	+ or ++	–
Normal mouse serum + C'	++	–	+ or ++	–
Anti H-2^k + C'	–	–	–	–
Anti H-2^d + C'	++	–	+ or ++	–

Fig. 14. Experimental protocol for the preparation of irradiation P→F$_1$ bone marrow chimeras (von Boehmer *et al.*, 1975). Cytotoxicity against LCMV-infected *H-2^k* or *H-2^d* targets that was generated in *H-2^k→H-2^k×H-2^d* was caused by T cells of *H-2^k* surface characteristics.

Table X. Virus-Specific Cytotoxic Activity in Spleens of LCMV-Infected P→F₁ Bone Marrow Chimeras

Spleen cells from LCMV-infected mice (H-2 Type)[a]	Cell treatment (% dead cells after treatment)[b]	^{51}Cr release from target cells (%)[c]			
		L929 ($H\text{-}2^k$)		J774 ($H\text{-}2^d$)	
		LCMV-infected	Uninfected	LCMV-infected	Uninfected
C3H→C3HXDBA/2 F₁ ($H\text{-}2^k$) ($H\text{-}2^k$X$H\text{-}2^d$)	None	42	29	100	50
	Anti-$H\text{-}2^k$ + C'	29	–	62	–
	Anti-$H\text{-}2^d$ + C'	40	–	98	–
	Normal serum + C'	41	–	101	–
C3H ($H\text{-}2^k$)	None	79	29	64	63
	Anti-$H\text{-}2^k$ + C'	30	–	–	–
	Anti-$H\text{-}2^d$ + C'	78	–	–	–
	Normal serum + C'	76	–	–	–
C3H normal		29	–	–	–
BALB/c ($H\text{-}2^d$)	None	30	31	99	51
	Anti-$H\text{-}2^k$ + C'	–	–	97	–
	Anti-$H\text{-}2^d$ + C'	–	–	57	–
	Normal serum + C'	–	–	99	–
BALB/c normal		–	–	63	56

Cell treatment (% dead cells after treatment) values: (8), (>95), (7), (9); (8), (>98), (10), (11); (12), (10), (>97), (12).

[a] For antisera, complement, and treatment, see Zinkernagel (1976c).
[b] Mice were injected with 10³ i.c. LD₅₀ of WE LCMV i.v. and spleen cells assayed 7 days later.
[c] Release of ^{51}Cr was determined as described in Fig. 1. Spleen cell/target cell ratio, 10:1; 12 hr at 37°C. Anti-$H\text{-}2^k$ antiserum treatment abolished all cytotoxic activity of T cells from chimeras to background levels.

Table XI. Specificity of Cytotoxic T Cells of LCMV-Infected P→F$_1$ Irradiated Bone Marrow Chimeras[a]

Immune spleen cells and cell treatment[b]	Unlabeled LCMV targets added 6:1[c]	^{51}Cr release from target cell (%)[d]					
		L929 (H-2^k)		J774 (H-2^d)		C57BL Macrophage	
		LCMV	Uninfected	LCMV	Uninfected	LCMV	Uninfected
C3H–C3H×DBA/2 F$_1$	0	58[e,f]	35	47[f]	20	42[g]	41
Anti-H-2^k + C'	0	35[g]	N.T.[h]	19[g]	N.T.		
Anti-H-2^d + C'	0	56[f]	N.T.	54[f]	N.T.		
C' control	0	57[f]		56[f]	N.T.		
	L929 cells (H-2^k)	38[g]	N.T.	55[f]	N.T.		
	J774 (H-2^d)	54[f]	N.T.	20[g]	N.T.		
B10.BR anti-H-2^d + C'	0	78[f]	35	24[g]	22	42[g]	39
Anti-H-2^k + C'	0	37[g]	35	N.T.	N.T.	N.T.	N.T.
B10.D2 anti-H-2^k + C'	0	41[g]	42	51[f]	20	42[g]	38
Anti-H-2^d + C'	0	N.T.	N.T.	21[g]	N.T.	N.T.	N.T.
B10.	0	44	42	25	23	76[f]	38
Medium control	0	36	35	20	19		

[a] From Zinkernagel (unpublished results).
[b] See Table X.
[c] Unlabeled LCMV target cells were added to the ^{51}Cr-labeled targets at 6:1.
[d] Assay of ^{51}Cr release was for 12 hr at 37°C. Killer/target cell ratio, 10:1.
[e] Means of triplicates; S.E.M. were between 0.3 and 1.8.
[f] Significantly different than on normal targets or from release by allogeneic immune spleen cells (P<0.05).
[g] Not significantly different from spontaneous release (medium control).
[h] N.T.: Not tested.

targets (Zinkernagel, 1976c). Similar results were obtained by Pfizenmaier *et al.* (1976) for cytotoxicity against LCMV-infected and TNP-modified targets.

This result makes the parallels between reactivity to alloantigens and to virus-specific altered self-markers even more strikingly obvious. It suggests that altered-self, alloantigen, and altered alloantigen are comparable antigens in that they are all different from the "normal" self-marker, again negating the physiological interaction model, but not excluding a dual-recognition model (see below).

This conclusion is further supported by the results of cold target competitive inhibition experiments *in vitro*. Cytotoxic activity of LCMV-immune T cells from C3H→C3HXDBA/2 irradiated bone marrow chimeras could be inhibited only with cold LCMV targets that are compatible with the specific ^{51}Cr-labeled target (Table XI). Thus, there are at least two (and probably four) distinct sets of cytotoxic T cells of C3H type (H-2^k) generated in these chimeras; one set is specific for H-2^k infected targets, the other for altered H-2^d (Zinkernagel, 1976c, and unpublished results).

Similar findings have been obtained for the apparently H-$2I$-restricted T helper system. When T cells are tolerized to alloantigens, T helper cells can be readily sensitized to help allogeneic B cells across the H-2 barrier. This process was shown for T cells in zygote-fusion chimeras (tetraparental mice) *in vivo* (Bechtol *et al.*, 1974) and for P→F$_1$ irradiated bone marrow chimeras *in vivo* (von Boehmer *et al.*, 1975) and *in vitro* (Waldmann *et al.*, 1975). In general, if one attempts to evolve a unifying concept for T-cell reactivities, these results could be interpreted as discussed earlier to indicate that helper T cells may be sensitized to antigen "altered allogeneic" I-region structures under these conditions (Zinkernagel, 1975, 1976b).

The dual recognition model (as conceived for T–B cell interaction) has been extended to accommodate these findings (Katz and Benacerraf, 1976). Accordingly, the phenotypic expression of I-coded interaction structures differentiates according to the H-2 or H-$2I$ environment. Thus, T cells develop in these chimeras with interaction structures fitting the alloantigen that they are forced to accept as normal in their tolerant condition. To accommodate the crossing of the H-2 barrier by virus-specific T cells, a similar idea could be applied to the expression of interaction structures (coded in the K or D region) of virus-specific cytotoxic T cells, in addition to the aforementioned complicated genetic regulations. The results indicate, however, that self-recognition is most likely unidirectional and excludes like–like self-interactions.

F. The Nature of Altered-Self and Experimental Evidence from Other *H-2*-Restricted Cytotoxic T-Cell Models

In the virus models discussed, the molecular nature of altered-self is not easy to imagine and remains speculative as long as a biochemical characterization is missing. A hypothesis constructed by A. J. Hapel, D. Jackson, and R. V. Blanden involved mainly the carbohydrate part of cell-surface markers coded in *H-2*. Here, viruses may change the activities of glycosyl transferases, thus causing the expression of a different self-marker (Blanden *et al.*, 1976). A direct chemical alteration is more easily envisaged in another example. Shearer and colleagues (Shearer, 1974; Shearer *et al.*, 1975) showed that cytotoxic T cells generated *in vitro* against TNP-modified syngeneic irradiated spleen cells were cytotoxic only for *H-2K-* or *D*-compatible TNP-modified targets.

Another argument concerning the nature of altered-self is that virally specified cell-surface structures resemble *H-2* antigens (Invernizzi and Parmiani, 1975). The experimental evidence presented in favor of such an idea is rather weak, however, since tumor rejection could have been enhanced by other than immunologically specific factors in this model. Nonspecific macrophage activation could have been caused by the host-vs.-graft reaction.

More recently, it was emphasized that either chemical carcinogens or vaccinia virus may cause random mutation at the level of *H-2* (Invernizzi and Parmiani, 1975) or cause the depression of *H-2* or non-*H-2* antigen (Garrido *et al.*, 1976). Either model may imply that *H-2* polymorphism is regulatory rather than allelic (Bodmer, 1972, 1973). Such models could explain the differential expression of *H-2D* and TL antigens (reviewed in Klein, 1975), but are not readily reconciled with the virtual lack of cross-reactivity on the cytotoxic T-cell level for at least three different viruses (Doherty and Zinkernagel, 1976).

Recent experiments by Bevan (1975a,b) and Gordon *et al.* (1975) are difficult to explain with the altered-self idea. These authors have shown that cytotoxic activity generated against minor H antigens or male Y antigen is expressed only against targets sharing the same *H-2* type *in vitro*. The relevant restricting structures are apparently also coded for in *H-2K* or *H-2D*. It is possible but not readily imagined that these cell-surface antigens would influence the antigenicity of the self-marker as perceived by T cells.

The altered-self concept, in our opinion, seems to offer a simple explanation for the fact that T cells lyse only *H-2D-* or *K*-compatible virus-infected cells. Accordingly, T cells would be sensitized to specifically modified self-structures coded for by the *H-2* gene complex, in the *K* or *D* region for cytotoxic or "surveillance" T cells, in the *I* region for "helper" T cells. At the moment, however, the main appeal of the altered-self model is its simplicity. The dual recognition model may be correct and has the aura of appearing more "physiological" and causing fewer problems to molecular-minded biologists. Unless one or both models can be characterized biochemically, the issue will probably remain open. Most of the discussed results, however, appear to make a like–like self-interaction model very unlikely.

V. MAJOR TRANSPLANTATION ANTIGENS AND IMMUNOSURVEILLANCE

A. Enhanced Generation of Cell-Mediated Immunity in *H-2* Heterozygotes

From the foregoing arguments and results, *H-2* heterozygous mice evidently generate a broader spectrum of cell-mediated immunity than do mice homozygous at *H-2,* at least regarding specificities of cytotoxic T cells.

Cytotoxicity can be measured and compared semiquantitatively by determining lytic units (LU) (Cerottini and Brunner, 1974), i.e., the number of immune lymphocytes necessary to lyse a certain percentage of a standard number of target cells specifically. Also, lytic units generated per spleen (LU/spleen) can be compared. Based on these measurements, LU or LU/spleen generated in virus-infected heterozygous F_1 mice tested against each infected parental-type target were 70% to more than 100% of the amount generated in corresponding infected homozygous parental mice (Table XII). Thus, the total cytolytic activity generated in heterozygotes was between 140% and more than 200% of that found in homozygotes (Zinkernagel and Doherty, 1975; Doherty and Zinkernagel, 1975c). This result, however, may reflect summation of factors such as hybrid vigor. Furthermore, a much greater number of individual mice must be tested before the twofold difference becomes really significant. The concept that cytotoxic reactions are greater in heterozygotes is somehow strengthened by the

Table XII. Virus-Specific Cytotoxicity Generated in F_1 As Compared with Parental Strains[a]

Virus-immune spleen cell donors		Cytolytic activity (LU or LU/spleen) against infected target cells (%)		
		$\dfrac{K^k\,D^k}{K^k\,D^k}$	$\dfrac{K^d\,D^d}{K^d\,D^d}$	Sum
Parental 1	$\dfrac{K^k\,D^k}{K^k\,D^k}$	100	0–5	100
Parental 2	$\dfrac{K^d\,D^d}{K^d\,D^d}$	0–5	100	100
F_1 (P1×P2)	$\dfrac{K^k\,D^k}{K^d\,D^d}$	70–100	70–100	>140

[a]Modified from Doherty and Zinkernagel (1975c).

finding *in vivo* that over a wide range of virus doses infected intracerebrally, more heterozygous F_1 mice died and death occurred earlier than in corresponding homozygous parental strains (Doherty and Zinkernagel, 1975c; Zinkernagel, 1975). The use of LCMV is paradoxical for demonstrating the selective advantage of heterozygosity in generating a powerful cell-mediated immune response, since the consequences of the enhanced T-cell response to this particular virus injected intracerebrally kills more mice sooner after infection (Doherty and Zinkernagel, 1974; Cole and Nathanson, 1975). However, in models in which T-cell-mediated immunopathology is not induced, but antiviral protection, for example, is assayed, results that favor the idea of enhanced immunologic surveillance in *H-2* heterozygotes would be expected. Heterozygosity at *H-2* and duplication of *H-2* (Klein and Schreffler, 1971) could thus be of selective advantage. The great variety of alleles at *H-2K* or *H-2D* (genetic polymorphism) could partially serve to guarantee a maximal degree of heterozygosity at *H-2* and thus maximalize quality and the quantity of cell-mediated immune responses.

B. A Possible Explanation for Polymorphism of Major Antigens

The strong association of virus-specific immune T cells with loci of the *H-2* gene complex, which codes for the major transplantation antigens, may indicate a crucial role of these cell-surface antigens in signaling to T cells changes of their structural integrity. These surveillance T cells (monitored *in vitro* as cytotoxic T cells) would be functionally distinct from (noncytolytic) T helper cells for T−B collaboration, or some DTH-effector T cells (J. F. A. P. Miller *et al.*, 1975), which are associated with structures coded within *H-2I*. Also, these two T-cell populations express different cell-surface antigens (Cantor and Boyse, 1975). Surveillance T cells may be essential in immunosurveillance, whereby this altered-self concept would embrace reactivity not only to tumor antigens, but also to all kinds of antigens (Burnet, 1971).

It is not understood why T-cell-mediated cytotoxicity seems to be associated mostly (if not exclusively) with structures coded in *H-2K* or *D*. Several explanations are possible: structural damage resulting in ^{51}Cr release is most easily caused at the site of *H-2K* or *D*, or generation of cells reactive to these structures is enhanced, or both. Bretscher (1974) and Lafferty and Cunningham (1975) proposed the latter because of their special association of *K* and *D* with a second signal, mitogenic signal, or stimulatory capacity expressed only on immunocompetent "stimulator" cells. That LCMV, ectromelia, and vaccinia viruses seem to infect lymphoid tissue (Mims and Tosolini, 1969) is consistent with this idea.

For reasons not yet understood, some self-structures may fail to be altered immunogenically by, for example, certain viruses. If only one locus for major transplantation antigens possessing only one to a few alleles existed, the consequences could be disastrous for the whole population. Failure to generate surveillance T cells could result in death of a species. Genetic polymorphism of major transplantation antigens could have evolved under this evolutionary pressure. A wide variety of alterable self-markers would minimize the danger of any particular virus being able to escape immune surveillance (Doherty and Zinkernagel, 1975d; Zinkernagel and Doherty, 1975).

By not altering *H-2K* or *D* structures, viruses associated with tumors may well be agents that have evolved to escape effective surveillance (Burnet, 1971). That cytotoxic T cells have been found so far only in a few tumor models (Herbermann *et al.*, 1973) (in regressor mice) could be compatible with this idea. One could similarly explain the empirical association between susceptibilities to certain diseases and certain major transplantation antigen types (summarized in Morris, 1974; McDevitt and Bodmer, 1974). In pathophysiological processes, susceptibility to diseases would be due to decreased immunogenicity of possibly involved self-markers; in immunopathological processes, susceptibility to diseases would be due to enhanced immunogenicity (Doherty and Zinkernagel, 1975d). There are, however, many other possible mechanisms, e.g., *Ir* genes, which may be of equal importance (Bodmer, 1972; McDevitt and Bodmer, 1974).

VI. CONCLUSIONS

Whether the altered self hypothesis or alternatively the dual recognition model truly explains the association of *K*- or *D*- region-coded cell-surface markers with virus specificity for cytotoxic T cells remains unresolved. In this review we have emphasized the altered self-concept although the dual recognition model is a viable alternative. At the moment circumstantial evidence seems to favor the altered-self idea. Thus, virus-specific cytotoxic T cells appear to be specific for altered structures coded within *H-2K* or *H-2D*, probably major transplantation antigens or structures coded very close to them. This functional T-cell population (surveillance T cells) is distinct from T helper cells associated with *H-2I*. Monitoring of major transplantation antigens for structural integrity by surveillance T cells may be crucial to immunosurveillance. Infectious agents, not altering those relevant self-markers, may escape the cell-mediated immune defense system. *H-2* duplication and *H-2* heterozygosity, together with genetic polymorphism of major transplantation antigens, could protect a species from extinction caused by a virus not altering the host's only self-marker. The association of surveillance T cells with major transplantation antigens may explain some aspects of the empirical finding that susceptibility to disease relates to certain *HL-A* types.

Several practical implications may arise from the altered-self concept:

- If cell-mediated effector functions can be shown to be restricted by the *H-2* gene complex, this is a very strong indication that it is a direct

T-cell-mediated function. This may be a quite generally applicable functional T-cell marker.

- Thus, on the other side, any attempt to demonstrate virus-specific direct T-cell-mediated immunity on non-*H*-compatible infected targets must fail.
- The *H-2* restriction phenomenon can be used for tissue typing of random bred populations, since only major *H* antigens are involved, the non-*H* background being irrelevant.
- T-cell-mediated immunity can be adoptively transferred for a short period of time against the rules of transplantation immunology, as long as the transferred T cells are sensitized to at least one altered self-marker that is expressed in the recipient.

ACKNOWLEDGMENTS

This is Publication No. 1097 from the Department of Immunopathology, Scripps Clinic and Research Foundation, La Jolla, California 92037. Part of the experimental work has been supported by U.S. Public Health Service Grant AI-07007. We would like to thank Miss Gail Essery, Mrs. Cathy Woodhams, and Ms. Alana Althage for expert technical assistance; Mrs. Jeanine Gouveia and Mrs. Phyllis Minick for the preparation of the manuscript; and the Schweizerische Stiftung für Biologisch Medizinische Stipendien for partial financial support (R. M. Zinkernagel).

VII. REFERENCES

Allison, A.C., 1974, The immune response to infectious disease, *Transplant. Rev.* **19**:3.

Bailey, D.W., Snell, G.D., and Cherry, M., 1971, Complementation and serological analysis of *H-2* mutant mice, in: *Immunogenetics of the H-2 System,* p. 155 (A. Lengerova and M. Vojtiskova, eds.), State Publishing House, Prague.

Bechtol, K.B., Freed, J.H., Herzenberg, L.A., and McDevitt, H.O., 1974, Genetic control of the antibody response to POLY-L(TYR, GLU)-POLY-D,L-ALA-POLY-L-LYS in C3H↔CWB tetraparental mice, *J. Exp. Med.* **140**:1660.

Benacerraf, B., and McDevitt, H.O., 1972, Histocompatibility-linked immune response genes, *Science* **175**:273.

Bevan, M.J., 1975a, Interaction antigens detected by cytotoxic T cells with the major histocompatibility complex as modifier, *Nature (London)* **256**:419.

Bevan, M.J., 1975b, The major histocompatibility complex determines susceptibility to cytotoxic T cells directed against minor histocompatibility antigens, *J. Exp. Med.* **142**:1349.

Blanden, R.V., 1971, Mechanism of recovery from a generalized viral infection: Mouse pox II. Passive transfer of recovery mechanisms with immune lymphoid cells, *J. Exp. Med.* **133**:1074.

Blanden, R.V., 1974, T cell response to viral and bacterial infection, *Transplant. Rev.* 19:56.

Blanden, R.V., Doherty, P.C., Dunlop, M.B.C., Gardner, I.D., Zinkernagel, R.M., and David, C.S., 1975a, Genes required for T cell-mediated cytotoxicity against virus infected target cells are in the *K* or *D* regions of the *H-2* gene complex, *Nature (London)* 254:269.

Blanden, R.V., Bowern, N.A., Pang, T.E., Gardner, I., and Parish, C.R., 1975b, Effects of thymus-independent (B) cells and the *H-2* gene complex on antiviral function of immune thymus-derived (T) cells, *Aust. J. Exp. Biol. Med. Sci.* 53:187.

Blanden, R.V., Hapel, A.J., Doherty, P.C., and Zinkernagel, R.M., 1975c, Lymphocyte–macrophage interactions and macrophage activation in the expression of antimicrobial immunity *in vivo,* in: *Immunobiology of the Macrophage* (D. Nelson, ed.), p. 367, Academic Press, New York.

Blanden, R.V., Hapel, A.J., and Jackson, D., 1976, Mode of action of Ir genes and the nature of T cell receptors for antigen, *Immunochemistry* 13:179.

Blank, K.J., Freedman, H.A., and Lilly, F., 1976, T lymphocyte response to Friend virus-induced tumor cell lines in mice of strains congenic at H-2, *Nature (London),* in press.

Bodmer, W.F., 1972, Evolutionary significance of the *HLA* system, *Nature (London)* 237:139.

Bodmer, W.F., 1973, New genetic model for allelism at histocompatibility and other complex loci: Polymorphism for control of gene expression, *Transplant. Proc.* 5:147.

Bretscher, P.A., 1974, On the control between cell-mediated IgM and IgG immunity, *Cell. Immunol.* 13:171.

Brunner, K.T., Mauel, J., Cerottini, J.C., and Chapuis, B., 1968, Quantitative assay of the lytic action of immune lymphoid cells on ^{51}Cr-labeled alloantigeneic target cells *in vitro;* inhibition by isoantibody and by drugs, *Immunology* 14:181.

Brunner, K.T., Mauel, J., Rudolf, H., and Chapuis, B., 1970, Studies of allograft immunity in mice. I. Induction, development and *in vitro* assay of cellular immunity, *Immunology* 18:501.

Burnet, M., 1971, *Immunological Surveillance,* Pergamon Press, Sidney, Australia.

Cantor, H., and Boyse, E.A., 1975, Functional subclasses of T lymphocytes bearing different *Ly* antigens. II. Cooperation between subclasses of Ly+ cells in the generation of killer activity, *J. Exp. Med.* 141:1390.

Cerottini, J.C., and Brunner, K.T., 1974, Cell-mediated cytotoxicity, allograft rejection and tumor immunity, *Adv. Immunol.* 19:67.

Cerottini, J.C., Nordin, A.A., and Brunner, K.T., 1970, Specific *in vitro* cytotoxicity of thymus-derived lymphocytes sensitized to alloantigens, *Nature (London)* 228:1308.

Cole, G.A., and Nathanson, N., 1975, Lymphocytic choriomeningitis: Pathogenesis, *Prog. Med. Virol.* 18:94.

Cole, G.A., Nathanson, N., and Prendergast, R.A., 1972, Requirement for Θ-bearing cells in lymphocytic choriomeningitis virus-induced central nervous system disease, *Nature (London)* 238:335.

Cole, G.A., Prendergast, R.A., and Henney, C.S., 1973, *In vitro* correlates of lymphocytic choriomeningitis (LCM) virus-induced immune response, *Fed. Proc. Fed. Amer. Soc. Exp. Biol.* 32:964.

Crowle, A.J., 1975, Delayed hypersensitivity in the mouse, *Adv. Immunol.* 20:197.

Delovitch, T.L., and McDevitt, H.O., 1975, Isolation and characterization of murine Ia antigens, *Immunogenetics* 2:39.

Doherty, P.C., and Zinkernagel, R.M., 1974, T cell mediated immunopathology in viral infections, *Transplant. Rev.* 19:89.

Doherty, P.C., and Zinkernagel, R.M., 1975a, Capacity of sensitized thymus derived lymphocytes to induce fatal lymphocytic choriomeningitis is restricted by the *H-2* gene complex, *J. Immunol.* **114**:30.

Doherty, P.C., and Zinkernagel, R.M., 1975b, *H-2* compatibility is required for T cell mediated lysis of target cells infected with lymphocytic choriomeningitis virus, *J. Exp. Med.* **141**:502.

Doherty, P.C., and Zinkernagel, R.M., 1975c, Enhanced immunological surveillance in mice heterozygous at the *H-2* complex, *Nature (London)* **256**:50.

Doherty, P.C., and Zinkernagel, R.M., 1975d, Immune surveillance and the role of major histocompatibility antigens, *Lancet* **1**:1406.

Doherty, P.C., and Zinkernagel, R.M., 1976, Specific immune lysis of paramyxovirus-infected cells by *H-2* compatible thymus-derived lymphocytes, *Immunology* **31**:27.

Doherty, P.C., Zinkernagel, R.M., and Ramshaw, I.A., 1974, Specificity and development of cytotoxic thymus-derived lymphocytes in lymphocytic choriomeningitis, *J. Immunol.* **112**:1548.

Doherty, P.C., Blanden, R.V., and Zinkernagel, R.M., 1976a, Specificity of virus-immune effector T cells for *H-2K* or *H-2D* compatible interactions: Implications for H-antigen diversity, *Transplant. Rev.* **29**:89.

Doherty, P.C., Dunlop, M.B.C., Parish, C., and Zinkernagel, R.M., 1976b, Inflammatory process in murine lymphocytic choriomeningitis is maximal in *H-2K* or *H-2D* compatible interactions, *J. Immunol.,* in press.

Edidin, M., and Henney, C.S., 1973, The effect of capping *H-2* antigens on the susceptibility of target cells to humoral and T cell mediated lysis, *Nature (London) New Biol.* **246**:47.

Erb, P., and Feldman, M., 1975, The role of macrophages in the generation of T helper cells. II. The genetic control of the macrophage–T-cell interaction for helper cell induction with soluble antigens, *J. Exp. Med.* **142**:460.

Festenstein, H., 1973, Immunogenetic and biological aspects of *in vitro* lymphocyte allo-transformation (MLR) in the mouse, *Transplant. Rev.* **15**:62.

Forman, J., 1975, On the role of the *H-2* histocompatibility complex in determining the specificity of cytotoxic effector cells sensitized against syngeneic trinitrophenyl-modified targets, *J. Exp. Med.* **142**:403.

Gally, J.A., and Edelman, G.M., 1970, Somatic translocation of antibody genes, *Nature (London)* **277**:341.

Gardner, I., Bowern, N.A., and Blanden, R.V., 1974a, Cell-mediated cytotoxicity against ectromelia virus-infected target cells. I. Specificity and kinetics, *Eur. J. Immunol.* **4**:63.

Gardner, I., Bowern, N.A., and Blanden, R.V., 1974b, Cell-mediated cytotoxicity against ectromelia virus-infected target cells. II. Identification of effector cells and analysis of mechanism, *Eur. J. Immunol.* **4**:68.

Gardner, I., Bowern, N.A., and Blanden, R.V., 1975, Cell-mediated cytotoxicity against ectromelia virus-infected target cells. III. Role of the *H-2* gene complex, *Eur. J. Immunol.* **5**:122.

Garrido, F., Schirrmacher, V., and Festenstein, H., 1976, *H-2*-like specificities of foreign haplotypes appearing on a mouse sarcoma after vaccinia virus infection, *Nature (London)* **259**:228.

Gell, P.G.H., 1967, Restrictions on antibody production by single cells, *Cold Spring Harbor Symp. Quant. Biol.* **32**:441.

Germain, R.N., Dorf, B., and Benacerraf, B., 1975, *J. Exp. Med.* **142**:547.

Gilden, D.H., Cole, G.A., Monjan, A.A., and Nathanson, N., 1972, Immunopathogenesis of acute central nervous system disease produced by lymphocytic choriomeningitis virus. I. Cyclophosphamide-mediated induction of the virus-carrier stage in adult mice, *J. Exp. Med.* **135**:860.

Gordon, R.D., Simpson, E., and Samelson, L.E., 1975, *In vitro* cell-mediated immune responses to the male specific (H-Y) antigen in mice, *J. Exp. Med.* **142**:1108.

Gorer, P.A., 1937, The genetic and antigenic basis of tumor transplantation, *J. Pathol. Bacteriol.* **44**:691.

Hämmerling, G.J., Mauve, G., Goldberg, E., and McDevitt, H.O., 1975, Tissue distribution of Ia antigens: Ia on spermatozoa, macrophages and epidermal cells, *Immunogenetics* **1**:428.

Häyry, P., Anderson, L.C., Nordling, S., and Virolainen, M., 1972, Allograft response *in vitro, Transplant. Rev.* **12**:91.

Hëllstrom, K.E., and Möller, G., 1965, Immunological and immunogenetic aspects of tumor transplantation, *Prog. Allergy* **9**:158.

Henney, C.S., 1971, Quantitation of the cell-mediated immune response. I. The number of cytolytically active mouse lymphoid cells induced by immunization with allogeneic mastocytoma cells, *J. Immunol.* **107**:1558.

Herbermann, R.B., Nunn, M.E., Lavrin, D.H., and Asofsky, R., 1973, Effect of antibody to Θ-antigen on cell-mediated immunity induced in syngeneic mice by murine sarcoma virus, *J. Natl. Cancer Inst.* **51**:1509.

Hotchin, J., 1971, Persistent and slow virus infections, *Monogr. Virol.* **3**:1.

Invernizzi, G., and Parmiani, G., 1975, Tumor-associated transplantation antigens of chemically induced sarcoma cross reacting with alloantigeneic histocompatibility antigens, *Nature (London)* **254**:713.

Jerne, N.K., 1971, The somatic generation of immune recognition, *Eur. J. Immunol.* **1**:1.

Katz, D.H., and Benacerraf, B., 1975, The function and interrelationship of T cell receptors, Ir genes and other histocompatibility gene products, *Transplant. Rev.* **22**:175.

Katz, D.H., and Benacerraf, B. (eds.), 1976, *The Role of Products of the Histocompatibility Gene Complex in Immune Responses,* Academic Press, New York.

Katz, D.H., Hamaska, T., Dorf, M.E., and Benacerraf, B., 1973, Cell interactions between histoincompatible T and B lymphocytes. The *H-2* gene complex determines successful physiologic lymphocyte interactions, *Proc. Natl. Acad. Sci. U.S.A.* **70**:2624.

Katz, D., Graves, M., Dorf, M.E., Dimuzio, H., and Benacerraf, B., 1975, Cell interactions between histoincompatible T and B lymphocytes. VII. Cooperative responses between lymphocytes are controlled by genes in the *I* region of the *H-2* complex, *J. Exp. Med.* **141**:263.

Kindred, B., and Schreffler, D.C., 1972, *H-2* dependence of cooperation between T and B cells *in vivo, J. Immunol.* **109**:940.

Klein, J., 1975, *Biology of the Mouse Histocompatibility-2 Complex,* Springer-Verlag, New York.

Klein, J., 1976, An attempt at an interpretation of the mouse *H-2* complex, in: *Contemporary Topics in Immunobiology,* Vol. 5, p. 297 (W.O. Weigle, ed.), Plenum Press, New York.

Klein, J., and Schreffler, D.C., 1971, The *H-2* model for the major histocompatibility systems, *Transplant. Rev.* **6**:3.

Koszinowski, U., and Ertl, H., 1975, Lysis mediated by T cells and restricted by *H-2* antigen of target cells infected with vacinia virus, *Nature (London)* **255**:552.

Koszinowski, U., and Thomssen, R., 1975, Target cell-dependent T cell-mediated lysis of vaccinia virus-infected cells, *Eur. J. Immunol.* **5**:245.

Lafferty, K.J., and Cunningham, A.J., 1975, A new analysis of allogeneic interactions, *Aust. J. Exp. Biol. Med. Sci.* **53**:27.

Lafferty, K.J., Ryan, M., and Misko, I.S., 1974, An improved system for the assay of stimulation in mouse mixed leukocyte cultures, *J. Immunol. Methods* **4**:263.

Lehmann-Grube, F., 1971, Lymphocytic choriomeningitis virus, *Virol. Monogr.* **10**:1.

MacDonald, H.R., Phillips, R.A., and Miller, R.G., 1973, Allograft immunity in the mouse. I. Quantitation and specificity of cytotoxic effector cells after *in vitro* sensitization, *J. Immunol.* 111:565.

Mackaness, G.B., 1969, The influence of immunologically committed lymphoid cells on macrophage activity *in vivo, J. Exp. Med.* 129:973.

Marker, O., and Volkert, M., 1973, Studies on cell-mediated immunity to lymphocytic choriomeningitis virus in mice, *J. Exp. Med.* 137:1511.

Mauel, J., Rudolf, H., Capuis, B., and Brunner, K.T., 1970, Studies of allograft immunity in mice. II. Mechanism of target cell inactivation *in vitro* by sensitized lymphocytes, *Immunology* 18:517.

McDevitt, H.O., and Bodmer, W., 1974, *HLA,* immune-response genes and disease, *Lancet* 1:1269.

Miller, J.F.A.P., Vadas, M.A., Whitelaw, A., and Gamble, J., 1975, *H-2* gene complex restricts transfer of delayed-type hypersensitivity in mice, *Proc. Natl. Acad. Sci. U.S.A.* 72:5095.

Miller, R.G., and Dunkley, M., 1974, Quantitative analysis of the ^{51}Cr release cytotoxicity assay for cytotoxic lymphocytes, *Cell. Immunol.* 14:284.

Mims, C., and Blanden, R.V., 1972, Antiviral action of immune lymphocytes in mice infected with lymphocytic choriomeningitis virus, *Infect. Immun.* 6:695.

Mims, C., and Tosolini, F.A., 1969, Pathogenesis of lesions in lymphoid tissue of mice infected with lymphocytic choriomeningitis (LCM) virus, *Br. J. Exp. Pathol.* 50:584.

Morris, P.J., 1974, Histocompatibility systems, immune response and disease in man, *Contemp. Top. Immunobiol.* 3:141.

Nabholz, M., Vives, J., Young, H.M., Meo, T., Miggiano, V., Rijnbeck, A., and Schreffler, D.C., 1974, Cell-mediated cell lysis *in vitro*: Genetic control of killer cell production and target specificities in the mouse, *Eur. J. Immunol.* 4:378.

Oldstone, M.B.A., 1976, Relationship between major histocompatibility antigens and disease: Possible associations to human adenovirus diseases, International Symposium on Adrenoviral Infections of Public Health Importance, Atlanta, Georgia, *WHO Bull.* 52:479.

Oldstone, M.B.A., and Dixon, F.J., 1970, Tissue injury in lymphocytic choriomeningitis viral infection: Virus-induced immunologically specific release of cytotoxic factor from immune lymphoid cells, *Virology* 112:805.

Oldstone, M.B.A., Habel, E., and Dixon, F.J., 1969, The pathogenesis of cellular injury associated with persistent LCM viral infection, *Fed. Proc. Fed. Amer. Soc. Exp. Biol.* 28:429.

Oldstone, M.B.A., Dixon, F.J., Mitchel, G.F., and McDevitt, H.O., 1973, Histocompatibility linked genetic control of disease susceptibility: Murine lymphocytic choriomeningitis virus infection, *J. Exp. Med.* 137:1201.

Ortiz de Landozouri, M., and Herbermann, R.B., 1972, Specificity of cellular immune reactivity to virus-induced tumors, *Nature (London) New Biol.* 238:18.

Pfizenmaier, K., Starzinski-Powitz, A., Rodt, H., Rollinghoff, M., and Wagner, H., 1976, Virus and TNP-hapten specific T cell mediated cytotoxicity against *H-2* incompatible target cells, *J. Exp. Med.* 143:999.

Rosenau, W., and Moon, H.D., 1966, Studies on the mechanism of the cytotoxic effect of sensitized lymphocytes, *J. Immunol.* 96:80.

Rosenthal, A.S., and Shevach, E.M., 1973, Function of macrophages in antigen recognition by guinea pig T lymphocytes. I. Requirement for histocompatible macrophages and lymphocytes, *J. Exp. Med.* 138:1194.

Rosenthal, A.S., and Shevach, E.M., 1976, in: *The Role of Products of the Histocompati-*

bility Gene Complex in Immune Responses, p. 335 (D.H. Katz and B. Benacerraf, eds.), Academic Press, New York.

Schrader, J.W., Cunningham, B.A., and Edelman, G.M., 1975, Functional interactions of viral and histocompatibility antigens at tumor cell surfaces, *Proc. Natl. Acad. Sci. U.S.A.* **72**:5066.

Shearer, G.M., 1974, Cell-mediated cytotoxicity to trinitrophenyl-modified syngeneic lymphocytes, *Eur. J. Immunol.* **4**:257.

Shearer, G.M., Rehn, G.R., and Garbarino, C.A., 1975, Cell-mediated lympholysis of trinitrophenyl-modified autologous lymphocytes. Effector cell specificity to modified cell surface components controlled by the *H-2K* and *H-2D* regions of the murine major histocompatibility complex, *J. Exp. Med.* **141**:1348.

Shreffler, D.C., and David, C.S., 1975, The *H-2* major histocompatibility complex and the *I* immune response region: Genetic variation, function and organization, *Adv. Immunol.* **20**:125.

Snell, G., 1974, Immunogenetics: Retrospect and prospect, *Immunogenetics* **1**:1.

Stimpfling, J.H., 1971, Recombination within a histocompatibility locus, *Annu. Rev. Genet.* **5**:121.

Unanue, E.R., Dorf, M.E., David, C.S., and Benacerraf, B., 1974, The presence of *I*-region-associated antigens on B cells in molecules distinct from immunoglobulin and *H-2K* and *H-2D, Proc. Natl. Acad. Sci. U.S.A.* **71**:6014.

von Boehmer, H., Hudson, L., and Sprent, J., 1975, Collaboration of histoincompatible T and B lymphocytes using cells from tetraparental bone marrow chimeras, *J. Exp. Med.* **142**:989.

Wainberg, M.A., Markson, Y., Weiss, D.W., and Donjanski, F., 1974, Cellular immunity against Rous sarcoma of chickens. Preferential reactivity against autochthonous target cells as determined by lymphocyte adherence and cytotoxicity tests *in vitro, Proc. Natl. Acad. Sci. U.S.A.* **71**:3565.

Waldmann, H., Pope, H., and Munro, A.J., 1975, Cooperation across the histocompatibility barrier, *Nature (London)* **258**:730.

Widmer, M.B., Alter, B.J., Bach, F.H., Bach, M.L., and Bailey, D.W., 1973, Lymphocyte reactivity to serologically undetected components of the major histocompatibility complex, *Nature (London) New Biol.* **242**:239.

Zinkernagel, R.M., 1974, Restriction by the *H-2* gene complex of the transfer of cell-mediated immunity to *Listeria monocytogenes, Nature (London)* **251**:230.

Zinkernagel, R.M., 1975, The role of the *H-2* gene complex in cell-mediated immunity to viral and bacterial infections in mice, Ph.D. thesis, Australian National University, Canberra, Australia.

Zinkernagel, R.M., 1976a, *H-2* compatibility requirement for virus-specific T cell mediated cytolysis. The *H-2K* structure involved is coded by single cistron defined by *H-2K^b* mutant mice, *J. Exp. Med.* **143**:437.

Zinkernagel, R.M., 1976b, T helpers may be sensitized by antigen-specifically altered structures which are coded by the *I* region of the *H-2* gene complex, in: *Proceedings of the 5th Congress on Germinal Centers and Lymphatic Tissue,* 527 (M. Feldmann and A. Globerson, eds.), Academic Press, New York.

Zinkernagel, R.M., 1976c, Virus specific T cell-mediated cytotoxicity across the *H-2* barrier to "virus-altered alloantigen," *Nature (London)* **261**:139.

Zinkernagel, R.M., 1976d, *H-2* compatibility requirements for virus-specific T cell mediated effector functions *in vivo.* II. Adoptive transfer of delayed type hypersensitivity to murine lymphocytic choriomeningitis virus is restricted by the *K* and *D* regions of *H-2, J. Exp. Med.* **144**:776.

Zinkernagel, R.M., and Doherty, P.C., 1973, Cytotoxic thymus-derived lymphocytes in cerebrospinal fluid of mice with choriomeningitis, *J. Exp. Med.* **138**:1266.

Zinkernagel, R.M., and Doherty, P.C., 1974a, Characteristics of the interaction *in vitro* between cytotoxic thymus derived lymphocytes and target monolayers infected with lymphocytic choriomeningitis virus, *Scand. J. Immunol.* **3**:287.

Zinkernagel, R.M., and Doherty, P.C., 1974b, Restriction of *in vitro* T cell mediated cytotoxicity in lymphocytic choriomeningitis within a syngeneic or semiallogeneic system, *Nature (London)* **248**:701.

Zinkernagel, R.M., and Doherty, P.C., 1974c, Activity of sensitized thymus derived lymphocytes in lymphocytic choriomeningitis reflects immunological surveillance against altered self components, *Nature (London)* **251**:547.

Zinkernagel, R.M., and Doherty, P.C., 1975, *H-2* compatibility requirement for T cell mediated lysis of targets infected with lymphocytic choriomeningitis virus. Different cytotoxic T cell specificities are associated with structures coded in *H-2K* or *H-2D, J. Exp. Med.* **141**:1427.

Zinkernagel, R.M., and Welsh, R., 1976, *H-2* compatibility requirement for virus-specific T cell-mediated effector functions *in vivo*. I. Specificity of T cells conferring antiviral protection against lymphocytic choriomeningitis virus is associated with *H-2K* and *H-2D, J. Immunol.* **117**:1495.

Zinkernagel, R.M., Dunlop, M.B.C., and Doherty, P.C., 1975, Cytotoxic T cell activity is strain specific in outbred mice infected with lymphocytic choriomeningitis virus, *J. Immunol.* **115**:1613.

Zinkernagel, R.M., Dunlop, M.B.C., Blanden, R.V., Doherty, P.C., and Shreffler, D.C., 1976, *H-2* compatibility requirement for virus-specific T cell-mediated cytolysis. Evaluation of the role of *H-2I* region and non *H-2* genes in regulating immune response, *J. Exp. Med.* **144**:519.

Chapter 6

Significance of the Major Histocompatibility Complex As Assessed by T-Cell-Mediated Lympholysis Involving Syngeneic Stimulating Cells

Gene M. Shearer, Anne-Marie Schmitt-Verhulst, and Terry G. Rehn

Immunology Branch, National Cancer Institute
Bethesda, Maryland

I. THE MURINE MAJOR HISTOCOMPATIBILITY COMPLEX

The major histocompatibility complex (MHC), which is known to code for cell-surface antigens responsible for allograft rejection (Gorer et al., 1948; Shreffler and David, 1975), has also been shown to play an essential role in a number of functions associated with the immune systems of several animal species (Benacerraf and McDevitt, 1972; McDevitt and Bodmer, 1974). The murine MHC, which is known as the *H-2* complex, has been divided into four major regions, which include two serologic regions known as *H-2K* and *H-2D,* or *K* and *D,* separated by two other regions designated *I* and *S* (Shreffler and David, 1975). The *K* and *D* regions determine the strong serologically detectable transplantation antigens of the mouse, which appear to be important as the target antigens for thymus-derived-(T-)cell-mediated lympholysis generated by culturing lymphocytes with *H-2*-incompatible stimulating cells (Alter *et al.,* 1973; Abbasi *et al.,* 1973; Schendel *et al.,* 1973; Nabholz *et al.,* 1974; Bevan, 1975a). Cytotoxic effector cells can be generated without inducing strong proliferation by culturing mixtures of cells differing only at the *K* or *D* region or both, whereas cell mixtures differing only at the *I* region induce strong proliferative responses in the absence or presence of only weak cytotoxic responses (Widmer *et al.,* 1973; Plate, 1974; Wagner *et al.,* 1975; Hodes *et al.,* 1976). The

S region is positioned adjacent to and to the left of the *D* region with respect to the centromere. It determines the level of a serum α-globulin known as Ss, as well as a sex-linked allotypic variant of Ss designated Slp (Shreffler and Passmore, 1971), and appears to have functional relevance in the complement system (Lachman *et al.*, 1975; Hansen *et al.*, 1975). Genes mapping within the *I* region designated *Ir*, or immune response, genes are located between *K* and *S*, and control immune response potential to a number of immunogens (for a review, see Benacerraf and Katz, 1975), as well as the expression of *Ia* antigens on the surfaces of certain cell types (David *et al.*, 1973; Hauptfeld *et al.*, 1973; Götze *et al.*, 1973; Sachs and Cone, 1973). Recent *Ir*-gene (Lieberman *et al.*, 1972; Melchers *et al.*, 1973; Lozner *et al.*, 1974) and *Ia*-antigen (Sachs *et al.*, 1975) studies in B10.A recombinant mouse strains have led to the division of the *I* region into three subregions designated *I-A*, *I-B*, and *I-C* (Sachs *et al.*, 1975). At present, the *H-2* complex is clearly divisible into at least six regions: *K*, *I-A*, *I-B*, *I-C*, *S*, and *D*.

One of the most recent functions associated with the murine MHC has been the discovery that cell-mediated lympholysis (CML) reactions can be generated *in vivo* or *in vitro* to virally infected or chemically modified cells only when the target cells are *H-2*-matched with the infected or modified stimulating or responding cells or both (Zinkernagel and Doherty, 1974a; Doherty and Zinkernagel, 1975a; Gardner *et al.*, 1975; Koszinowski and Thomssen, 1975; Shearer *et al.*, 1975; Rehn *et al.*, 1976; and see other chapters of this volume). Similar requirements for *H-2* homology have been demonstrated for sensitization and lysis of cells expressing a number of weak transplantation antigens (Gordon *et al.*, 1975; Bevan, 1975a,b). The studies that have been carried out in this laboratory with the chemically modified autologous system, as well as the virally infected and weak transplantation antigen models of others, introduce new functional significance for the MHC in autologous cytotoxic reactions and raise interesting evolutionary possibilities for MHC polymorphism (Doherty and Zinkernagel, 1975b; Schmitt-Verhulst and Shearer, 1975; Shearer *et al.*, 1975; Shearer *et al.* 1976).

II. REQUIREMENT OF SEROLOGICALLY DETECTABLE REGION HOMOLOGY FOR CYTOTOXICITY IN CHEMICALLY MODIFIED AUTOLOGOUS SYSTEMS

A. Generation of Cytotoxic Effector Cells to Chemically Modified Autologous Cells

Thymus-derived cytotoxic effector cells have been generated *in vitro* in primary 5-day culture systems for sensitization of responding splenic lympho-

Table I. Target-Cell Characteristics Required for Lysis by
Effectors Sensitized with Chemically Modified Autologous Cells

Responding cells	Modified stimulating cells	Target cells		Lysis of target cells	
		Non H-2 genetic "background"	H-2 haplotype	Unmodified	Modified[a]
A	A	a	a	−	+
A	A	b	a	−	+
A	A	b	b	−	−
A	A	a	b	−	−
B	B	b	b	−	+
B	B	a	b	−	+
B	B	a	a	−	−
B	B	b	a	−	−

[a]The same modifying agent is used for treatment of stimulating and target cells.

cytes with chemically modified autologous stimulating spleen cells. The modifying agents thus far used include trinitrobenzene sulfonate (TNBS) (for TNP-modified cells) (Shearer, 1974), N-(3-nitro-4-hydroxy-5-iodophenyl acetyl)-β-alanylglycylglycylazide (for N-modified cells) (Koren *et al.*, 1975), and NaIO$_4$ (for sodium periodate-modified cells) (Schmitt-Verhulst and Shearer, 1976). The initial observations indicated that effector cells generated by sensitization with TNP-modified autologous cells were capable of lysing only target cells that were both TNP-modified and shared the H-2 haplotype with the cells of the sensitization phase (i.e., responder or stimulating cells or both) (Shearer, 1974). These same general observations have been made with N-modified cells (Rehn *et al.*, 1976) and to some extent with NaIO$_4$-treated cells (Schmitt-Verhulst and Shearer, 1976; and see Section II.C.2). A summary of these initial findings is presented in Table I. These results indicated that the respective modifying agent is necessary but not sufficient in order to obtain lysis, and raised the possibility that one or more regions of the H-2 complex are important in the sensitization or lytic phases, or both phases, of the response (Shearer, 1974; Shearer *et al.*, 1975).

B. Intra-H-2 Mapping of the Homology Required

To verify that the H-2 complex does play an important role in CML reactions against chemically modified autologous cells and to determine which regions within H-2 are important for such cytotoxicity. C57BL/10 congenic resistant lines of mice (i.e., mouse strains on a C57BL/10 genetic background that differ only at H-2) as well as B10.A congenic recombinant mouse strains

Table II. Intra-*H-2* Mapping of the Homology Required Between Stimulating or Effector and Target Cells

Responding and TNP-modified stimulating cells	Strain or origin of target cells	Modified target cell *H-2* region common to responding and stimulating cells	Specific lysis[a]
B10.A *kkkddd*[b]	B10.A (*kkkddd*)	All of *H-2*	++
	B10.A(4R) (*kkbbbb*)	*K, I-A*	++
	B10.D2 (*ddddd*)	*I-C, S, D*	−
	A.TL (*skkkkd*)	*I-A, I-B, D*	−
B10.D2 *ddddd*	B10.D2 (*ddddd*)	All of *H-2*	+
	B10.A (*kkkddd*)	*I-C, S, D*	+
	B10.A(2R) (*kkkddb*)	*I-C, S*	−
	A.TL (*skkkkd*)	*D*	+
	C3H.OH (*dddddk*)	*K, I-A, I-B, I-C, S*	+

[a](++)>25%; (+) 15–20%; (−) <5%. Effector/target cell ratio, 20:1.
[b]Indicates alleles at *k, Ia, Ib, Ic, S,* and *D* regions of *Hz*.

(which exhibit intra-*H-2* genetic recombination) were used as donors of responder, modified stimulator, and modified target cells. It was necessary that the responding and modified stimulating cell be from the same mouse strain, since effector cells generated by a strong allogeneic sensitization (even in the absence of TNP) lysed any TNP-modified target cell to a significant extent (Shearer *et al.*, 1976; and see Section II.C.2). Thus, splenic responding lymphocytes were always sensitized against modified autologous stimulating cells, and the effector cells generated 5 days later were assayed on a series of modified target cells, sharing all, some, or no *H-2* regions with the cells of the sensitization phase. Results typical of such an experiment are summarized for the B10.A and B10.D2 strains in Table II. Similar results were obtained irrespective of whether the experiment involved stimulating cells that were TNP- or N-modified, although the specific lysis obtained using N-modified cells was generally slightly lower than that obtained for TNP-modified cells (Shearer *et al.*, 1975; Rehn *et al.*, 1976). These studies indicated that B10.A effector cells appreciably lysed only modified target cells sharing at least *K* and *I-A* regions with the cells of the stimulating phase, whereas these effectors did not lyse TNP-modified targets having either *I-C, S, D* or *I-A, I-B, D* regions. Thus, *H-2* homology was required only at *K* or *K* plus I-A between target cells and stimulating or effector cells in the B10.A strain. In contrast, Table II shows that B10.D2 effector cells were able to lyse TNP-modified target cells sharing either the *D* region only or all other *H-2* regions except *D* (targets sharing *I-C, S* only were not lysed). These findings indicated that in some strains of mice (e.g., B10.D2), effector cells can be generated in the TNP-autologous CML system when either an *H-2D* or a non-*H-2D* region (presumed to be *H-2K*) are shared by target cells and cells of the sensitization phase (Shearer *et al.*, 1975). This contrasts with the TNP-autologous CML responses in some other C57BL/10 congenic strains (e.g., B10.A), in which there is exclusive or preferential reactivity against targets matched at *K* or *K* plus *I-A* (Shearer *et al.*, 1975, 1976). (This differential reactivity against *H-2D*-modified targets can be accounted for by *Ir* genes and will be considered in Section III.) Similar specificity requirements have been demonstrated for N-modified autologous CML reactions (Rehn *et al.*, 1976). The use of mouse strains involving recombination between the *K* and *I-A* regions (i.e., A.TL and A.TH; Shreffler and David, 1975) has localized the homology requirement to the *K* region only. Similar to the findings in allogeneic and xenogeneic CML models (Lindahl, 1975), these results indicate that also in the autologous modified systems, the cell-surface products coded for by genes mapping in or near the *K* and *D* serologically detectable regions are intimately associated with the antigenic structures recognized by cytotoxic effector cells.

C. Analysis of the Mechanisms of the *H-2* Homology Requirement

1. Models

Two basic models have been proposed that can account for the *H-2* homology requirements observed for the virally infected, chemically modified, and weak antigen-associated autologous CML (Zinkernagel and Doherty, 1974b). These two models essentially differ in that one involves a single receptor recognizing self-*H-2* products (either altered or unaltered) in close association with the infecting (viral) or modifying (chemical) agent, whereas the other involves two distinct receptors—one specific for the agent and the second specific for self *H-2K-* or *H-2D*-associated cell-surface products (see Fig. 1). In the single-receptor model, the agent (e.g., virus, chemical, or weak antigen) could be modifying cell-surface products coded for by *K* and *D* region genes, making them appear as non-self-recognition structures (altered-self). Alternatively, a model involving a single receptor recognizing unaltered self-*H-2* products in close association with the infecting or modifying agent is possible. For the two-receptor, or dual recognition, model, one receptor would be specific for the "hapten" or infecting agent only. The second receptor would be a responder-and/or effector-cell receptor that would function as a responder–stimulator and/or effector–target interaction structure recognizing syngeneic K- or D-region products. Such a hypothetical recognition structure might function through a like–like or a complementary interaction.

Experiments have been performed in the virally infected (Zinkernagel and Doherty, 1974b, 1975), chemically modified (Shearer *et al.,* 1975; Forman, 1975; Rehn *et al.,* 1976), and weak antigen (Gordon and Simpson, 1976; Bevan, 1975c) systems in an attempt to distinguish between the one- and two-receptor models. In such studies, lymphocytes from various F_1 hybrid mouse strains were sensitized with infected or modified cells of one parental H-2 haplotype. The effector cells generated lysed ^{51}Cr-labeled infected or modified target cells of the same parental haplotype used for sensitization, but not targets of the other parental type (Table III). These findings are compatible with the single-receptor model and incompatible with the dual-receptor model as presented in their simplest forms. In the single-receptor model, clones of responding lymphocytes sensitized to parental cells of a given H-2 haplotype would lyse modified target

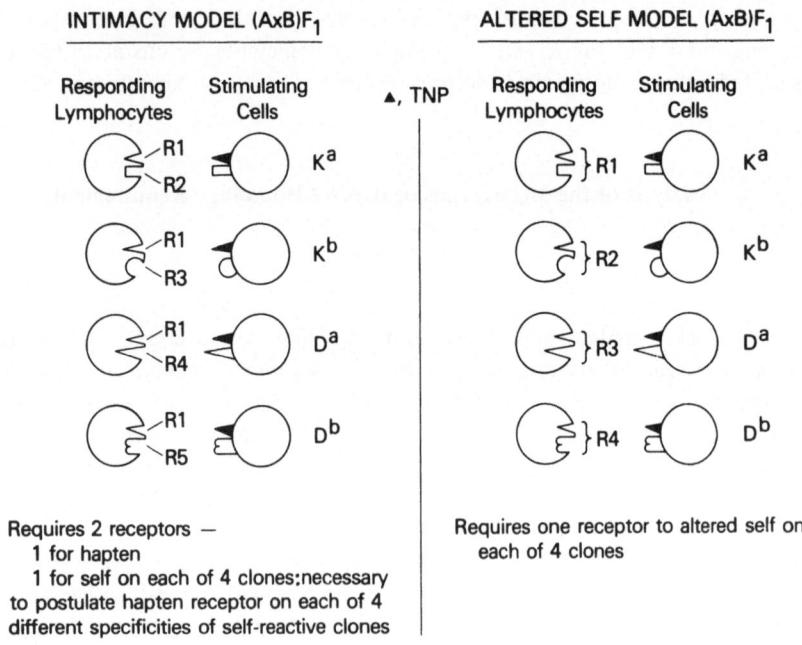

Fig. 1. Diagram of the cell clones and receptors required to postulate the dual- and single-receptor models. The self-recognition antigens and receptors are shown as complementary rather than identical structures.

Table III. Demonstration That the *H-2* Homology Required Is Between Modified Stimulating and Modified Target Cells

Responding cells	Stimulating cells[a]	Target cells[a]	Specific lysis[b]
(A×B)F$_1$	A′	A′	+
(A×B)F$_1$	A′	B′	−
(A×B)F$_1$	B′	B′	+
(A×B)F$_1$	B′	A′	−

[a]The modifying agent (denoted by the prime sign) is either TNP or N.
[b](+) >20%; (−) <5%. Effector/target cell ratio, 20:1.

cells sharing K or D products or both with the parental stimulating cells. These F$_1$ results are incompatible with the two-receptor model in its simplest form. This model predicts that modified parental cells of either haplotype would be lysed, since there is *H-2* homology both between responding and stimulating cells through one haplotype and between effector and target cells through the other parental haplotype. The F$_1$ data would be compatible with a dual-receptor model, however, if the following restrictions were imposed: First, it must be assumed that receptors for each parental haplotype are clonally expressed in the F$_1$ hybrid responding lymphocytes, and that this expression is subject to allelic exclusion; i.e., a given clone of F$_1$ lymphocytes can interact with only a single parental haplotype, both at the responder–stimulator and at the effector–target cell levels. Second, if the *H-2* receptor in the dual recognition is required for cell–cell interaction, then this interaction must occur via complementary and not between like–like structures, since a like–like interaction through *H-2* antigens would necessitate allelic exclusion of *H-2* cell-surface products on the F$_1$ cells. It is known that serologically detectable region *H-2* antigens are codominantly expressed on F$_1$ cell surfaces (Cullen *et al.*, 1972). Distinct clones of cells have been shown to react against K and D regions of allogeneic cells (Nabholz *et al.*, 1974; Bevan, 1975a) and autologous modified cells (see Section II.C.2). Thus, in order for a two-receptor model to be valid, it is necessary to postulate four distinct clones, each expressing a receptor for virus, "hapten," or weak antigens, plus a complementary receptor for a single parental K- or D-region product to account for full F$_1$ cytotoxic potential.

Since it has been demonstrated that F$_1$ hybrid anti-parental-cell-mediated cytotoxicity can be generated *in vitro* against uninfected or unmodified parental hemopoietic histocompatibility determinants mapping in or near *H-2D* (Shearer and Cudkowicz, 1975), such experiments should be controlled using unmodified target cells or by using F$_1$ cells homozygous at *H-2D*.

2. *Specificity of Recognition*

If TNP served as a "hapten" as postulated in the two-receptor model, one would expect that nonradioactive TNP-modified target cells of any *H-2* type would block the lytic phase. To test this possibility, nonradioactive TNP-modified spleen cells of various *H-2* haplotypes were mixed with effector cells 30 min prior to the addition of ^{51}Cr-labeled, TNP-modified target cells that were *H-2*-matched with the effector and stimulating cells in the lytic assay. Results typical of such experiments are outlined in Table IV. Only spleen cells that were both TNP-modified and *H-2*-matched with effectors, stimulators, and target cells were effective in blocking the CML, indicating that the same specificity requirements are necessary for blocking lysis s for recognition leading to lysis. Similar blocking results were obtained in the N-modified autologous CML system. In a two-receptor model, it might have been predicted that either an *H-2*-matched, unmodified or a TNP-modified, non-*H-2*-matched cell could have bound to the relevant effector-cell receptor strongly enough to have sterically inhibited the interaction of effectors with modified, *H-2*-matched ^{51}Cr-labeled target cells. The failure of such blocking suggests that either (1) the two-receptor model is not valid and specificity is via a single receptor recognizing TNP and self (either altered or unaltered), or (2) the dual-receptor model is valid, but the binding energy of a single receptor is insufficient for competitive blocking to occur; i.e., effective inhibition requires binding at both receptors.

The similarities observed in the TNP- and N-modified autologous systems with respect to both the *H-2* homology requirements and the response patterns observed to modified *K*- and *D*-end products raised the possibility that TNP and N were modifying the same cell-surface components in an identical manner, such that the responding lymphocytes recognized the same specificity. To test this

Table IV. Inhibition by Unlabeled Syngeneic and Allogeneic Spleen Cells of the Lysis of TNP-Modified Target Cells by C57BL/10 Effector Cells Sensitized by TNP-Modified Autologous Cells

Responding and TNP-modified stimulating cells	Specific lysis (%) ± S.E. in the presence of blocking cells[a]				
	None[b]	C57BL/10 (*bbbbbb*)	C57BL/10-TNP (*bbbbbb*)	B10.BR (*kkkkkk*)	B10.BR-TNP (*kkkkkk*)
C57BL/10 *bbbbbb*	67.8±6.1	46.9±2.9	9.7±3.6	51.8±2.0	42.8±0.9

[a]Effector/target cell ratio, 20:1.
[b]C57BL/10-TNP (*bbbbbb*) spleen target cells.
[c]blocker/target cell ratio, 40:1.

Table V. Specificity of Cytotoxicity
As a Function of TNP- or N-Modification of
the Autologous Sensitizing Spleen Cells

Responding cells	Stimulating cells	Target cells	Specific lysis[a]
C57BL/10	C57/10-TNP	EL-4-TNP	+
C57BL/10	C57BL/10-TNP	EL-4-N	−
C57BL/10	C57BL/10-N	EL-4-TNP	−
C57BL/10	C57BL/10-N	EL-4-N	+

[a](+) >20%; (−) <5%. Effector/target cell ratio, 20:1.

possibility, experiments were performed in the C57BL/10 congenic mouse strains, in which splenic lymphocytes from each strain were sensitized to either TNP- or N-modified autologous spleen cells. The effector cells generated were assayed separately on both TNP- and N-modified, H-2-matched target cells (see Table V). Effector cells generated by sensitization with autologous stimulating cells modified with either agent lysed only H-2-matched target cells modified with the same agent. This demonstrates that no detectable cross-reactive specificities were generated by TNP or N modification (Rehn et al., 1976). These findings are compatible with the hypothesis that the modifying agents are themselves involved in the specificity—either as one component of the dual-receptor model or as an integral part of the single-receptor model. It is not excluded, however, that these modifying agents are inducing specific conformational changes in cell-surface proteins without themselves being integrally involved in the recognition unit.

Studies are currently in progress in this laboratory to further investigate the specificity requirements associated with the modifying agent. The specificities of the effector cells generated by sensitization with autologous cells modified with either trinitrobenzene sulfonate (for TNP-modified cells) or with N-(2,4,6-trinitrophenyl)-β-alanylglycylglycyl-acyl azide [for TNP—(AGG)-modified cells] were compared. In the TNP—(AGG) modification, the TNP variety is separated from the cell surface by an alanylglycylglycyl tripeptide spacer. Both reagents would be expected to react predominantly with ε-amino groups of exposed lysines on the cell surface. If the two-receptor model were valid, effector cells sensitized to TNP should be capable of lysing TNP—(AGG)-modified target cells, since such a target cell would fulfill the requirements of having both TNP and self-H-2 on its surface. One cannot predict, however, whether effector cells sensitized with TNP—(AGG)-modified autologous cell would lyse TNP-modified, H-2-matched target cells, since the "haptenic unit" recognized could be TNP alone, AGG alone, TNP—(AGG), or any combination of TNP and AGG. It is not possible to

**Table VI. Specificity of Cytotoxicity As a Function of TNP- or
TNP–(AGG)-Modification of the Autologous Sensitizing Cells**

Responding cells	Stimulating cells	Target cells	Specific lysis[a]
C57BL/10	C57BL/10-TNP	L5M-22-TNP	+++
C57BL/10	C57BL/10-TNP	L5M-22-(AGG)-TNP	−
C57BL/10	C57BL/10-(AGG)-TNP	L5M-22-(AGG)-TNP	++
C57BL/10	C57BL/10-(AGG)-TNP	L5M-22-TNP	+ or −

[a](+++) 30–50%; (++) 20–30%; (+) 5–15%; (−) <5%. Effector/target cell ratio, 80:1.

make such predictions for the single-receptor model, since cross-reactivity between TNP and TNP–(AGG) might depend on the size of the receptor and its
affinity for the hapten [i.e., a receptor for TNP–(AGG)-H-2 product might
interact with TNP-H-2 product]. The observations outlined in Table VI indicate
that effector cells generated by sensitization with TNP-modified autologous cells
never lysed TNP–(AGG)-H-2-matched targets. Effector cells generated by sensitization with TNP–(AGG)-modified autologous cells lysed H-2-matched target
cells modified with TNP–(AGG) consistently. Target cells modified with TNP
were either not lysed by such effectors or were lysed to a lesser extent. Other
studies have tested the ability of H-2-matched, nonradioactive TNP- and TNP–
(AGG)-modified spleen cells to block the lytic phase of a TNP-autologous CML.
Competitive inhibition of lympholysis was obtained using the TNP-modified but
not using TNP–(AGG)-modified spleen cells. These observations verify that
effectors generated in a TNP-modified autologous CML do not recognize
H-2-matched, TNP–(AGG)-modified cells. Such results argue against the dual-
receptor model in which the "hapten" recognition unit is assumed to be a single
chemical determinant such as the TNP group.

It has been observed that effector cells generated by sensitization with
TNP-modified allogeneic tumor cells can lyse to some extent TNP-modified
tumor target cells H-2-matched with the responding rather than the stimulating
cell type (Dennert and Hatlen, 1975). These results have been presented as
evidence suggesting "hapten-specific" CML reactions. Experiments have been
performed in this laboratory to further explore the possibility that TNP-specific
(hapten-specific) effector cells can be detected in the primary *in vitro* CML
(Table VII). Effector cells generated by allogeneic sensitization of
C57BL/10(H-2^b) splenic lymphocytes with TNP-modified P-815(H-2^d) tumor
cells were capable of lysing EL-4 target cells only when modified with TNP (i.e.,
H-2-matched with the responders and effectors but not with the stimulator
cells). It was found, however, that the allogeneic sensitization of C57BL/10
lymphocytes with unmodified P-815 cells generated effectors giving the same
pattern of lysis. Furthermore, the differences in optimal numbers of stimulator

Table VII. Failure of Effector Cells Generated by Sensitization
to TNP-Modified Allogeneic Tumor Cells to Demonstrate
"Hapten Specificity"

Responding cells	Stimulating cells	Stimulating cell dose	Target cell[a]			
			L5M22 (*bbbbbb*)	L5M22-TNP (*bbbbbb*)	P815 (*dddddd*)	P815-TNP (*dddddd*)
C57BL/10 (*bbbbbb*)	C57BL/10-TNP (*bbbbbb*)	3×10^6	1.0±0.5	42.7±1.2	5.4±1.0	0.6±0.9
C57BL/10 (*bbbbbb*)	P815 (*dddddd*)	3×10^3	0.6±0.8	1.9±1.3	13.4±0.9	8.8±1.4
C57BL/10 (*bbbbbb*)	P815 (*dddddd*)	3×10^4	2.3±0.3	17.9±1.3	41.8±1.7	37.8±1.2
C57BL/10 (*bbbbbb*)	P815 (*dddddd*)	3×10^5	0.4±0.7	3.3±0.9	13.3±1.2	11.0±0.9
C57BL/10 (*bbbbbb*)	P815-TNP (*dddddd*)	3×10^3	−0.6±0.2	2.1±0.6	10.3±1.6	7.5±1.3
C57BL/10 (*bbbbbb*)	P815-TNP (*dddddd*)	3×10^4	2.2±0.8	18.4±1.3	40.0±2.4	34.6±1.3
C57BL/10 (*bbbbbb*)	P815-TNP (*dddddd*)	3×10^5	0.9±0.7	16.4±0.9	26.8±0.8	17.1±2.3

[a]Effector/target cell ratio for L5M22 and L5M22-TNP, 40:1; for P815 and P815-TNP, 10:1. Effector cells were generated by incubation in Linbro culture plates in 2 cc of media at a concentration of 3.5×10^6 cells/ml. All tumors were irradiated with 5000 rads.

cells in the sensitization, depending on whether they were or not TNP-modified, necessitates the use of a series of responder/stimulator ratios for proper interpretation of such data. At present, there is no evidence to unequivocally support "hapten-specific" CML in the TNP-modified system. From the studies cited above, it is a possibility that allogeneically sensitized effector cells can interact with TNP-modified target cells in a nonspecific manner to effect lysis.

Oxidation of target cells with sodium periodate provides another example of nonspecific interaction between allogeneically generated effector cells and modified target cells leading to lysis (Schmitt-Verhulst and Shearer, 1976). In this case, it was shown that the effector cells leading to nonspecific lysis of periodate-modified targets (syngeneic with the effectors) were the relevant effectors resulting from specific allogeneic sensitization, since their nonspecific lysis of periodate-modified ^{51}Cr-labeled targets was competitively blocked only with unmodified nonradioactive cells *H-2*-matched with the stimulating cells (Schmitt-Verhulst and Shearer, 1976). The observation that there is an increase in nonspecific interaction between TNP-modified target cells and cytotoxic effectors suggests that an apparent lack of specificity could result from such an effect either when there is a strong allogeneic sensitization detected on any

TNP-modified targets or with effectors sensitized against TNP-modified autologous cells and assayed on sensitive TNP-modified tumor targets at high effector/target cell ratios.

3. Association Between TNP and H-2K and H-2D Products

It has been demonstrated that the lytic phase of an allogeneic CML can be blocked by antisera directed against the serologic region antigens of the target cells used for sensitization (Nabholz *et al.*, 1974). A similar approach has been used in the TNP autologous system. Antisera directed against *K-*, *D-*, or *I*-region specificity of unmodified target cells were used to test their ability to inhibit the lytic phase of the TNP autologous CML (Schmitt-Verhulst *et al.*, 1976). The results of such studies are outlined in Table VIII. The lysis of B10.A effector

Table VIII. Selective Inhibition by Specifically Directed Anti-*H-2* Sera and Anti-TNP-KLH Serum of the Lysis of TNP-Modified Target Cells by Effector Cells Sensitized with TNP-Modified Autologous Stimulating Cells

Section	Responding cells	Stimulating cells	Target cells	Antiserum directed against	Inhibition of lytic phase[a]
A	B10.A (*kkkddd*)	B10.ATNP (*kkkddd*)	B10.A-TNP (*kkkddd*)	K^k	++
				$(I\text{-}C, S, D)^d$	−
				$(I\text{-}A, I\text{-}B)^k$	−
B	B10.D2 (*dddddd*)	B10.D2-TNP (*dddddd*)	B10.D2-TNP (*dddddd*)	All $H\text{-}2^d$	++
				$(K, I\text{-}A, I\text{-}B)^d$	+
				$(I\text{-}C, S, D)^d$	+
				Ia-8	−
C	B10.D2 (*dddddd*)	B10.D2-TNP (*dddddd*)	B10.A-TNP (*kkkddd*)	$(K, I\text{-}A, I\text{-}B)^k$	−
				$(I\text{-}C, S, D)^d$	++
D	B10.BR (*kkkkkk*)	B10.BR-TNP (*kkkkkk*)	B10.BR-TNP (*kkkkkk*)	TNP-KLH	++
		C57BL/10 (*bbbbbb*)	C57BL/10-TNP (*bbbbbb*)	TNP-KLH	++
		C57BL/10 (*bbbbbb*)	C57BL/10 (*bbbbbb*)	TNP-KLH	−

[a](++) Complete inhibition of lysis; (+) partial inhibition of lysis; (−) no inhibition of lysis.

cells sensitized by TNP-modified B10.A spleen cells, assayed on B10.A targets, was blocked by antiserum directed against K^k, but not by antiserum directed against D^d or $(I\text{-}A, I\text{-}B)^k$). Effector cells generated against the entire $H\text{-}2^d$ and partially blocked by anti-$(K, I\text{-}A, I\text{-}B)^d$ and anti-$I\text{-}C, S, D)^d$, but not by anti-Ia-8,* when assayed on B10.D2-TNP targets. Lysis by the same effectors assayed on B10.A-TNP targets (sharing only $I\text{-}C, S, D$ with the cells of the stimulating phase) was inhibited by antiserum directed against $(I\text{-}C, S, D)^d$, but not by anti-$(K, I\text{-}A, I\text{-}B)^d$. Furthermore, anti-TNP-KLH antibodies were found to block either effector cells generated by a TNP-modified autologous or an allogeneic sensitization when assayed on TNP-modified targets. These observations indicate that some TNP groups are closely associated with unmodified $H\text{-}2$ serologically detectable region specificities (see Table VII, Section D), and that reactivity against or associated with D-end specificities in the TNP-autologous CML is blocked only by anti-$H\text{-}2D$-end reagents, but not by anti-$H\text{-}2K$-end reagents (Table VIII, section C). The latter results suggest that some TNP groups are more closely associated with K- and D-region products than the K- and D-region antigens are to each other. The observation that in the B10.A CML, antiserum directed against K^k completely blocked lympholysis, whereas antiserum directed against D^d did not block lysis (Table VIII, Section A), suggests that the reactivity in this strain is directed exclusively or preferentially against TNP-modified or TNP-associated K-end products. In contrast, the pattern of blocking shown in Sections B and C of Table VIII demonstrates that B10.D2 effector populations are generated specific for both the K-end and D-end regions of TNP-modified target cells. This differential response pattern seen by the B10.A and B10.D2 responding lymphocytes (also see Table II) raised the possibility that $H\text{-}2$-linked immune response (Ir) genes control response potential to TNP-modified or TNP-associated $H\text{-}2$ serologically detectable region products.

III. ROLE OF $H\text{-}2$-LINKED IMMUNE RESPONSE GENES

As was summarized in Table II and verified in the latter part of the preceding section, effector cells generated by sensitization of B10.A splenic lymphocytes with TNP-modified, autologous cells lysed TNP-modified targets $H\text{-}2$-matched at the K-end, but not TNP-modified targets $H\text{-}2$-matched at the D-end (Shearer et al., 1975; Schmitt-Verhulst and Shearer, 1975). This observation contrasts with that made using B10.D2 splenic lymphocytes, since the latter effectors lysed TNP-modified targets $H\text{-}2$-matched at D as well as those matched

---

*Ia-8 is a specificity expressed by the $H\text{-}2^d$ haplotype. See Schmitt, Verhulst et al. (1976) for additional details.

at K (Shearer *et al.*, 1975; Schmitt-Verhulst and Shearer, 1975). The possibility was raised that H-2-linked immune response (*Ir*) genes control responder-cell potential to TNP-modified or TNP-associated self-H-2 products. H-2-linked *Ir* genes controlling antibody production are characteristically expressed as dominant traits for responsiveness (Benacerraf and Katz, 1975), and have been mapped in the *I-A* or *I-B* region of the murine MHC (Lieberman *et al.*, 1972; Melchers *et al.*, 1973; Lozner *et al.*, 1974). To test whether high responder potential is dominant for this system, spleen cells from (B10.A×B10.D2)F$_1$ donors were sensitized with TNP-modified F$_1$, B10.A, or B10.D2 stimulating cells, and the effectors generated were assayed on TNP-modified F$_1$, B10.A, and B10.D2 target cells. In this case, no F$_1$ antiparent cytotoxicity attributed to hemopoietic histoincompatibility was generated, since the F$_1$ expresses homozygous *d* alleles at *H-2D* (Shearer and Cudkowicz, 1975). The results are schematically diagrammed in Table IX. Effector cells generated by sensitizing B10.A responder lymphocytes with B10.A-TNP stimulating cells did not lyse B10.D2-TNP targets, whereas F$_1$ effector cells sensitized with the same stimulating cells lysed TNP-modified, *D*-end-matched target cells as well as the B10.D2 high-responder effectors did. Thus, the results summarized in Table IX demon-

Table IX. Dominant Genetic Expression of Cytotoxicity by
(B10.A×B10.D2)F$_1$ Responding Cells to TNP-Modified
Product of *H-2D^d*

Responding cells	Stimulating cells	Target cells	Target cell *H-2* region common to responding and stimulating cells	Specific lysis[a]
B10.A (*kkkddd*)	B10.A-TNP (*kkkddd*)	B10.A-TNP (*kkkddd*)	All of *H-2^a*	++
		B10.D2-TNP (*dddddd*)	(*I-C, S, D*)^d	−
(B10.A×B10.D2)F$_1$ *kkkddd* *dddddd*	B10.A-TNP (*kkkddd*)	B10.A-TNP (*kkkddd*)	All of *H-2^a*	++
		B10.D2-TNP (*dddddd*)	(*I-C, S, D*)^d	+
	B10.D2-TNP (*dddddd*)	B10.A-TNP (*kkkddd*)	(*I-C, S, D*)^d	+
		B10.D2-TNP (*dddddd*)	All of *H-2^d*	+
B10.D2	B10.D2-TNP	B10.A-TNP (*kkkddd*)	(*I-C, S, D*)^d	+
		B10.D2-TNP (*dddddd*)	All of *H-2^d*	+

[a](++) >30%; (+) 10–20%; (−) <5%. Effector/target cell ratio, 20:1.

Table X. Intra-*H-2* Mapping of Cytotoxic Response Potential
to TNP-Modified Syngeneic *K* and *D* Serologic Region Specificities

Mouse strain strain	*K*- and *I*-region alleles				TNP-modified *K*-end products		TNP-modified *D*-end products	
	K	*I-A*	*I-B*	*I-C*	Probable serologically defined allele	Response range	Probable serologically defined allele	Response range
C57BL/10 (*bbbbbb*)	*b*	*b*	*b*	*b*	*b*	25–35%	*b*	25–35%
B10.D2 (*dddddd*)	*d*	*d*	*d*	*d*	*d*	15–25%	*d*	15–25%
B10.BR (*kkkkkk*)	*k*	*k*	*k*	*k*	*k*	25–35%	*k*	0–10%
B10.A (*kkkddd*)	*k*	*k*	*k*	*d*	*k*	25–35%	*d*	0–10%
B10.A(2R) (*kkkddb*)	*k*	*k*	*k*	*d*	*k*	25–35%	*b*	0–10%
B10.A(4R) (*kkbbbb*)	*k*	*k*	*b*	*b*	*k*	25–50%	*b*	0–30%

strate that responsiveness to TNP-modified or associated H-$2D^d$ is expressed as a dominant genetic trait. Studies are in progress to map this genetic control of responsiveness in the *K* or *I* regions using the A.AL, A.TL, and A.TH recombinant mouse strains. This type of genetic control appears not to be restricted to antigenic complexes involving only *d* alleles of *H-2D*, since B10.BR, B10.A(2R), and B10.A(4R) show weak reactivity to TNP-modified or -associated products of their respective *H-2D* alleles (i.e., *k*, *b*, and *b*) (see Table X). Furthermore, *Ir* genes of this type may also exist for CML responses to *H-2K* and *H-2D* products associated or modified with other agents, such as N, since B10.A and B10.BR effector cells both exhibit weaker reactivity against N-modified, *D*-end than against N-modified, *K*-end autologous products (Rehn *et al.*, 1976). Thus, the type of *H-2*-linked *Ir* gene described here appears to be influencing CML responses associated with *H-2D*-region autologous products, but does not seem to be immunogen-specific, since its effects are detected (whenever *k* alleles are expressed in the *K* end of *H-2*) irrespective |of |whether| the |*H-2D* allele expressed is *d*, *k*, or *b*, or of whether the modifying agent is TNP or N. However, another type of *Ir* gene that appears to be immunogen-specific may be detected in the CML response of C57BL/10 cells to N-modified H-$2D^b$ products, since responding cells from this strain respond well to TNP-modified H-$2D^b$, but poorly to N-modified H-$2D^b$ (Rehn *et al.*, 1976).

Since synergy has been demonstrated between subpopulations of cells generating CML to TNP-modified autologous *H-2* products (Hodes *et al.*, 1975), *Ir* genes could be expressed in either or both of the collaborating cell types. The lack of immune response potential to a specific immunogen (e.g., differential responsiveness of C57BL/10 lymphocytes to TNP- and N-modified *D*-end autologous products) could be a defect either in the specific clone of CML precursors or in accessory cells. The weak responsiveness observed to different haplotypes of TNP- and N-modified *H-2D* products might be accounted for by a genetic defect in the interaction between accessory and precursor cells, rather than by the absence of multiple specific clones for cytotoxic precursors.

IV. CONCLUSIONS AND SPECULATION

Two basic models have been proposed to account for *H-2K-* or *H-2D*-region homology requirements in the chemically modified, virally infected, and minor transplantation antigen CML systems. The simpler of the two models assumes that the chemical or infectious agent modifies *H-2* products, and that the relevant clones of lymphocytes recognize and respond to the altered *H-2* cell-surface proteins via a single receptor. In this model, therefore, the *H-2* homology requirements are exclusively between the altered stimulating and altered target cells. An alternate single-receptor model is that responding lymphocytes and their descendent effector cells recognize the chemical agent or virus and unaltered cell-surface MHC products as a single recognition structure or unit. Such a model might imply a special role for *H-2* serologically detectable region products in autologous CML reactions, as well as in allogeneic and xenogeneic cytotoxic responses. In allogeneic and xenogeneic reactions, the *H-2K-* and *H-2D*-associated proteins represent the antigens themselves, whereas in the autologous reaction, a non-self determinant must be closely associated with these self proteins in order to generate lympholysis.

In the two-receptor model, it is assumed that the relevant responding lymphocytes possess two receptors—one expressing specificity for a determinant containing the infectious (virus) or modifying (TNP) agent. It has been postulated in this dual-receptor model that the antigenic structure would be virus or hapten, whereas additional *H-2* homology might be required for "physiological" cell–cell interaction between effector and target cells (Zinkernagel and Doherty, 1974b). The results obtained using F_1 responding cells (see Table III) place some complicating restrictions on the dual recognition model. First, if *H-2* homology is required for efficient cell–cell interaction, this interaction must occur via the same *H-2* haplotype both between responder lymphocytes and stimulator cells and between effector cells and target cells. Thus, it is necessary to postulate that such interacting structures are noncodominantly expressed in distinct clones, all of the clones having the same specificity for the antigen (i.e., TNP, virus, or weak transplantation antigen). These hypothetical interaction structures are therefore necessarily distinct from serologically defined *H-2* antigens, since the latter are known to be codominantly expressed on the cell surface (Cullen *et al.*, 1972; Neauport-Sautes *et al.*, 1973). Such a dual-receptor model involving syngeneic *H-2* products for efficient cell interactions would more easily account for the observations that *H-2K* or *H-2D* homology is also required for lysis against weak transplantation antigens (Bevan, 1975b,c; Gordon *et al.*, 1975). In these cases, the genes controlling expression of these weak antigens map outside the *H-2* complex. There is no evidence that modification of *H-2* products naturally occurs in such weak antigen models.

Recent evidence that favors the single-receptor model involving altered autologous *H-2* products is the finding by Pfizenmaier *et al.* (1976) that parental lymphocytes taken from an F_1 chimera are incapable of generating a cytotoxic reaction against the unmodified *H-2* antigens of the other parental haplotype. Lymphocytes from the chimera, however, are able to respond against virally infected or chemically modified cells of the other parental type. This study provides an example (in the absence of allogeneic sensitization) in which efficient sensitization and lysis against virally infected or chemically modified cells can occur in the absence of *H-2* homology between responding and stimulating cells or between effector and target cells. Although unlikely, it is possible that the parental cells growing in the chimeras have acquired a hypothetical interaction structure concomitantly with the acquisition of tolerance to the second parental antigens. Such an interaction structure would be different from the *H-2* serologically detectable antigens, since the responding lymphocytes express their original *H-2* serologic antigens (Pfizenmaier *et al.*, 1976). Furthermore, a model not involving the requirement for homologous *H-2* interaction structures would permit a unitarian model for lympholysis in autologous-modified, allogeneic, and xenogeneic systems.

The cellular interactions involved in the chemically modified autologous CML can be further analyzed by investigating the specificity of recognition at the sensitization and lytic phases. As was shown in Table IV, inhibition of the lysis of TNP-modified target cells by syngeneic effector cells could be obtained only when the blocking cells were *both* TNP-modified *and H-2*-matched. These results indicate that (1) the "hapten" present on a cell surface and (2) unmodified syngeneic *H-2*-matched targets are not efficient in blocking effector-cell lysis of TNP-modified, *H-2*-matched target cells. Such results imply that the recognition involves both *H-2* and the agent (TNP) as a single antigenic unit. If the "haptenic moiety" is recognized by a "hapten-specific" receptor on the lymphocyte, one would have expected that effector cells generated by TNP-modified autologous stimulating cells would have lysed TNP–(AGG)-modified, *H-2*-matched targets (see Table VI), or that TNP–(AGG)-modified *H-2*-matched cells would have blocked lysis of TNP-modified, *H-2*-matched targets. For the dual-receptor model, this would have been predicted, since the stimulating and target cells both meet the requirements of *H-2* homology and presentation of the TNP group. The lack of cross-reactivity between TNP- and TNP–(AGG)-modified cells implies, however, that the antigenic structure is larger than the TNP hapten, and must include some self-components. Such self components could be modified *H-2* serologically detectable region products, but could also be other autologous cell-surface components. Furthermore, blocking of the target-cell lysis with anti-TNP-KLH antibodies and antisera directed against unmodified *K*- and *D*-region products demonstrates that there is an intimate association between unmodified *K*- or *D*-region products and TNP groups on the cell surface (Schmitt-Verhulst *et al.,* 1976), although *K*- and *D*-region products behave independently of each other on the cell surface (Cullen *et al.,* 1972; Neuport-Sautes *et al.,* 1973).

If all these results are considered together, one cannot prove whether recognition occurs via a single- or a dual-receptor model. Nevertheless, it is clear that the T lymphocyte relevant for generating cytotoxic responses recognizes more than just the "hapten" by that receptor in which the "hapten" is recognized. Therefore, the cytotoxic T cell and its precursor recognize more than is required for the interaction between hapten and antibody combining site (see Table VI and Janeway *et al.,* 1975). Since this receptor appears to be specific for more than just the "haptenic moiety," it is possible that it could include *H-2* serologically detectable region products that might serve as cell interaction structures. If such interaction structures are involved, it need not be via a homologous interaction between responding and stimulating cells or between effector and target cells, as the results of Pfizenmaier *et al.* (1976) indicate, and as occurs in the generation of allogeneic and xenogeneic CML.

Genes mapping within the *I* regions of the *H-2* complex are known to control antibody response potential to a number of natural and synthetic thymus-dependent antigens (Benacerraf and Katz, 1975). The same *I* regions also control the expression of cell-surface structures known as *Ia* antigens. These same *Ia* structures are found on soluble T-cell factors involved in the stimulation of bone-marrow-derived precursors for antibody-forming cells (B lymphocytes) by T helper cells (Munro *et al.*, 1974; Armeding *et al.*, 1974). Furthermore, these *Ia* determinants also appear to be associated with suppressor function for antibody production (Takemori and Tada, 1975). For the generation of secondary antibody responses, there seems to be some *I*-region homology required between interacting B and T cells (Katz *et al.,* 1975). Thus, it would appear that the genes controlling antibody responsiveness in mice and the antigenic determinants controlling cell–cell interaction leading to secondary antibody responses both map within the same area of the *H-2* complex. It should be noted, however, that although *Ia* structures are present on the soluble mediators of T–B cell interaction, these structures need not necessarily be homologous to the structures on the B-cells (Munro and Taussig, 1975). This would be in keeping with the observations of others that under certain experimental conditions, T and B lymphocytes need not be *H-2*-matched in order to generate antibody responses (Shearer *et al.*, 1972; Lichtenberg *et al.*, 1974; Heber-Katz and Wilson, 1975; von Boehmer *et al.*, 1975). Such discordant findings could be accounted for if it is assumed that subpopulations of T helper and B precursor cells exist, some of which require *I*-region homology for interaction and some of which do not, and whether primary or secondary responses are involved.

In T-cell-mediated immune reactions such as delayed hypersensitivity to soluble antigens (Miller *et al.*, 1975), T-cell-mediated stimulation (Meo *et al.*, 1973) and suppression (Rich and Rich, 1975) of mixed lymphocyte reactions, T-cell proliferative response to soluble antigens (Schwartz *et al.*, 1976), and for the interaction between T cells and macrophages in guinea pigs (Rosenthal and Shevach, 1973; Lipsky and Rosenthal, 1975) and mice (Erb and Feldmann, 1975), *I*-region products appear to be involved in the cellular interactions leading to these immune responses. By analysis with anti-*Ly* sera, different subpopulations of T lymphocytes have been identified (Cantor and Boyse, 1975). These studies indicated that helper and MLR-responsive lymphocytes express different *Ly* antigens than do CML precursors and effectors (Cantor and Boyse, 1975). The possibility can be raised that different *H-2*-controlled interaction structures could be important in the activation and differentiation of such T-cell subpopulations. Thus, for T-cell-mediated cytotoxic functions (Ly-2,3 positive), the relevant interaction structures could be coded for by genes mapping in the serologically detectable regions of *H-2*, rather than in the *Ir* regions, which would code, in turn, for cell interaction structures relevant for at least some functions associated with Ly-1-positive cells.

For T-cell-dependent immune reactions in which *Ia* structures are involved for cellular interactions, it has been shown that genes mapping in the *I* regions also control immune responsiveness (Benacerraf and Katz, 1975; Schwartz *et al.*, 1976). The murine MHC plays an important role in T-cell-mediated lympholysis against TNP- or N-modified autologous cells at two distinct levels: (1) the antigenic unit involving *H-2K*- or *H-2D*-region products, which is associated with stimulator and target cells; and (2) *H-2*-linked immune response genes expressed in responding lymphocytes. The level of cytotoxic activity against TNP-modified or -associated *D*-region products (irrespective of the *D* alleles and modifying agents thus far studied) is controlled by gene(s) mapping in the left half of *H-2*. From mapping studies of *Ir* genes controlling antibody production, one might have predicted that the *Ir* genes controlling CML responses will map in one or more of the *I* regions. However, in view of the fact that serologically detectable region antigens may serve as interaction structures necessary for the generation of cytotoxic effector cells, the prediction could be made that these *Ir* genes controlling cytotoxic responses at the effector-cell level to these K- and D-region structures will also map in the *same* serologically detectable regions rather than in the I regions. Thus, it might be speculated that the genes controlling recognition and response potential for a given immune function will map in the same region as the structural genes coding for the cell-surface proteins functioning as interaction structures in the expression of that particular immune function.

V. REFERENCES

Abbasi, K., Demant, P., Festenstein, H., Holmes, J., Huber, B., and Rychlikova, M., 1973, Mouse mixed lymphocyte reaction and cell mediated lympholysis: Genetic control and relevance to antigenic strength, *Transplant. Proc.* **5**:1329.

Alter, B.J., Schendel, D.J., Bach, M.L., Bach, F.H., Klein, J., and Stimpfling, J.H., 1973, Cell-mediated lympholysis. Importance of serologically defined *H-2* regions, *J. Exp. Med.* **137**:1303.

Armeding, D., Sachs, D.H., and Katz, D.H., 1974, Activation of T and B lymphocytes *in vitro*. III. Presence of *Ia* determinants on allogeneic effect factor, *J. Exp. Med.* **140**:1717.

Benacerraf, B., and Katz, D.H., 1975, The histocompatibility linked immune response genes, *Adv. Cancer Res.* **21**:121.

Benacerraf, B., and McDevitt, H.O., 1972, The histocompatibility linked immune response genes, *Science* **175**:273.

Bevan, M.J., 1975a, Alloimmune cytotoxic T cells: Evidence that they recognize serologically defined antigens and bear clonally restricted receptors, *J. Immunol.* **114**:316.

Bevan, M.J., 1975b, Interaction antigens detected by cytotoxic T cells with the major histocompatibility complex as modifier, *Nature (London)* **256**:419.

Bevan, M.J., 1975c, The major histocompatibility complex determines susceptibility to cytotoxic T cells directed against minor histocompatibility antigens, *J. Exp. Med.* **142**:1349.

Cantor, H., and Boyse, E.A., 1975, Functional subclasses of T lymphocytes bearing different Ly antigens. II. Cooperation between subclasses of Ly^+ cells in the generation of killer activity, *J. Exp. Med.* **141**:1390.

Cullen, S.E., Schwartz, B.D., Nathenson, S.G., and Cherry, M., 1972, The molecular basis of codominant expression of the histocompatibility-2 genetic region, *Proc. Natl. Acad. Sci. U.S.A.* **69**:1394.

David, C.S., Shreffler, D.C., and Frelinger, J.A., 1973, New lymphocyte antigen system (Lna) controlled by the *Ir* region of the mouse *H-2* complex, *Proc. Natl. Acad. Sci. U.S.A.* **70**:2509.

Dennert, G., and Hatlen, L.E., 1975, Induction and properties of cytotoxic T cells specific for hapten-coupled tumor cells, *J. Immunol.* **114**:1705.

Doherty, P.C., and Zinkernagel, R.M., 1975a, *H-2* compatibility is required for T-cell-mediated lysis of target cells infected with lymphocytic choriomeningitis virus, *J. Exp. Med.* **141**:502.

Doherty, P., and Zinkernagel, R.M., 1975b, A biological role for the major histocompatibility antigens, *Lancet* **1**:1406.

Erb, P., and Feldmann, M., 1975, The role of macrophages in the generation of T-helper cells. II. The genetic control of the macrophage–T-cell interaction for helper cell induction with soluble antigens, *J. Exp. Med.* **142**:460.

Forman, J., 1975, On the role of the *H-2* histocompatibility complex in determining the specificity of cytotoxic effector cells sensitized against syngeneic TNP-modified targets, *J. Exp. Med.* **142**:403.

Gardner, I.D., Bowern, N.A., and Blanden, R.V., 1975, Cell-mediated cytotoxicity against ectromelia virus-infected target cells. III. Role of the *H-2* gene complex, *Eur. J. Immunol.* **5**:122.

Gordon, R.D., and Simpson, E., 1976, *H-2* restricted T-cell cytotoxicity responses to H-Y antigens, in: *Proceedings of the Tenth Leukocyte Culture Conference*, p. 521 (V.P. Eijsvoogel, D. Roos, and W.P. Zeylemaher, eds.), Academic Press, New York.

Gordon, R.D., Simpson, E., and Samuelson, L.E., 1975, *In vitro* cell-mediated immune responses to the male specific (H-Y) antigen in mice, *J. Exp. Med.* **142**:1108.

Gorer, P.A., Lyman, S., and Snell, G.D., 1948, Studies on the genetic and antigenic basis of tumour transplantation. Linkage between a histocompatibility gene and "fused" in mice, *Proc. R. Soc. London Ser. B.* **135**:499.

Götze, D., Reisfeld, R.A., and Klein, J., 1973, Serologic evidence for antigen controlled by the *Ir* region in mice, *J. Exp. Med.* **138**:1003.

Hansen, T.H., Shin, H.S., and Shreffler, D.C., 1975, Evidence for the involvement of the Ss protein of the mouse in the hemolytic complement system, *J. Exp. Med.* **141**:1216.

Hauptfeld, V., Klein, D., and Klein, J., 1973, Serological identification of an *Ir*-region antigen, *Science* **181**:167.

Heber-Katz, E., and Wilson, D.B., 1975, Collaboration of allogeneic T and B lymphocytes in the primary antibody response to sheep erythrocytes *in vitro*, *J. Exp. Med.* **142**:928.

Hodes, R.J., Schmitt-Verhulst, A.-M., Hathcock, K.S., and Shearer, G.M., 1976, Mixed lymphocyte reactivity and cell-mediated lympholysis to *D*-end differences of the murine major histocompatibility complex. Comparison of *in vitro* responses to exclusive *D*-end or more extensive MHC differences, *Scand. J. Immunol.* **5**:369.

Janeway, C.A., Jr., Cohen, B.E., Ben-Sasson, S.Z., and Paul, W.E., 1975, The specificity of cellular immune responses in guinea pigs. I. T cells specific for 2,4-dinitrophenyl-0-tyrosyl residues, *J. Exp. Med.* **141**:42.

Katz, D.H., Graves, M., Dorf, M.E., Dimuzio, H., and Benacerraf, B., 1975, Cell interactions between histoincompatible T and B lymphocytes. VII. Cooperative responses between lymphocytes are controlled by genes in the *I* region of the *H-2* complex, *J. Exp. Med.* **141**:263.

Koren, H.S., Wunderlich, J.R., and Inman, J.K., 1975, *In vitro* development of cytotoxic T cells specific for hapten-associated antigens on syngeneic cells, *Transplant. Proc. VII, Suppl.* **1**:169.

Koszinowski, U., and Thomssen, R., 1975, Target cell-dependent T cell-mediated lysis of vaccinia virus-infected cells, *Eur. J. Immunol.* **5**:245.

Lachmann, P.J., Grennan, D., Martin, A., and Demant, P., 1975, Identification of Ss protein as murine C4, *Nature (London)* **258**:242.

Lichtenberg, L., Mozes, E., Shearer, G.M., and Sela, M., 1974, The role of thymus cells in the immune response to poly(Tyr,Glu)-poly DL Ala-poly Lys as a function of the genetic constitution of the mouse strain, *Eur. J. Immunol.* **4**:430.

Lieberman, R., Paul, W.E., Humphrey, W., and Stimpfling, J.H., 1972, *H-2* linked immune response (*Ir*) genes. Independent loci for *Ir-IgG* and *Ir-IgA*, *J. Exp. Med.* **136**:1231.

Lindahl, K.F., 1975, Specificity of xenograft reactions *in vitro*, Ph.D. thesis, University of Wisconsin, Madison.

Lipsky, P.E., and Rosenthal, A.S., 1975, Macrophage–lymphocyte interaction. II. Antigen-mediated physical interactions between immune guinea pig lymph node lymphocytes and syngeneic macrophages, *J. Exp. Med.* 141:138.

Lozner, E.C., Sachs, D.H., and Shearer, G.M., 1974, Genetic control of the immune response to staphylococcal nuclease. I. *Ir*-Nase; control of the antibody response to nuclease by the *Ir* region of the mouse *H-2* complex, *J. Exp. Med.* 139:1204.

McDevitt, H.O., and Bodmer, W.F., 1974, *HL-A* immune-response genes, and disease, *Lancet* 1:1269.

Melchers, I., Rajewsky, K., and Shreffler, D.C., 1973, Ir-LDH$_B$: Map position and functional analysis, *Eur. J. Immunol.* 3:754.

Meo, T., Vives, J., Miggiano, V., and Shreffler, D.C., 1973, A major role for the *Ir-1* region of the mouse *H-2* complex in the mixed leukocyte reaction, *Transplant. Proc.* 5:377.

Miller, J.F.A.P., Vodar, M.A., Whitelaw, A., and Gamble, J., 1975, *H-2* gene complex restricts transfer of delayed-type hypersensitivity in mice, *Proc. Natl. Acad. Sci. U.S.A.* 72:5095.

Munro, A.J., and Taussig, M.J., 1975, Two genes in the major histocompatibility complex control immune response, *Nature (London)* 256:103.

Munro, A.J., Taussig, M.J., Campbell, R., Williams, H., and Lawson, Y., 1974, Antigen-specific T-cell factor in cell cooperation: Physical properties and mapping in the left-hand (*K*) half of *H-2*, *J. Exp. Med.* 140:1579.

Nabholz, M., Vives, J., Young, H.M., Meo, T., Miggiano, V., Rijnbeek, A., and Shreffler, D.C., 1974, Cell-mediated cell lysis *in vitro*: Genetic control of killer cell production and target specificities in the mouse, *Eur. J. Immunol.* 4:378.

Neauport-Sautes, C., Lilly, F., Silvestre, D., and Kourilsky, F., 1973, Independence of *H-2K* and *H-2D* antigenic determinants on the surface of mouse lymphocytes, *J. Exp. Med.* 139:511.

Pfizenmaier, K., Starzinski-Powitz, A., Rodt, H., Röllinghoff, H., and Wagner, H., 1976, Virus and TNP-hapten specific T cell mediated cytotoxicity against *H-2* incompatible target cells, *J. Exp. Med.* 143:999.

Plate, J., 1974, Mixed lymphocyte culture responses of mice, *J. Exp. Med.* 139:851.

Rehn, T.G., Shearer, G.M., Koren, H.S., and Inman, J.K., 1976, Cell-mediated lympholysis of *N*-(3-nitro-4-hydroxy-5-iodophenylacetyl)-β-alanylglycylglycyl-modified autologous lymphocytes, *J. Exp. Med.* 143:127.

Rich, S.H., and Rich, R.R., 1975, Regulatory mechanism in cell-mediated immune responses. II. A genetically restricted suppressor of mixed lymphocyte reactions released by alloantigen-activated spleen cells, *J. Exp. Med.* 142:1391.

Rosenthal, A.S., and Shevach, E.M., 1973, Function of macrophages in antigen recognition by guinea pig T lymphocytes. I. Requirement for histocompatible macrophages and lymphocytes, *J. Exp. Med.* 138:1194.

Sachs, D.H., and Cone, J.L., 1973, A mouse B-cell alloantigen determined by gene(s) linked to the major histocompatibility complex, *J. Exp. Med.* 138:1289.

Sachs, D.H., David, C.S., Shreffler, D.C., Nathenson, S.G., and McDevitt, H.O., 1975, Ir associated antigens (workshop summary), *Immunogenetics* 2:301.

Schendel, D.J., Alter, B.J., and Bach, F.H., 1973, The involvement of LD- and SD-region differences in MLC and CML: A three cell experiment, *Transplant. Proc.* 5:1651.

Schmitt-Verhulst, A.-M., and Shearer, G.M., 1975, Bifunctional major histocompatibility-linked genetic regulation of cell-mediated lympholysis to trinitrophenyl-modified autologous lymphocytes, *J. Exp. Med.* 142:914.

Schmitt-Verhulst, A.-M., and Shearer, G.M., 1976, The effects of sodium periodate modification of lymphocytes on the sensitization and lytic phases of T-cell mediated lympholysis, *J. Immunol.* 116:947.

Schmitt-Verhulst, A.-M., Sachs, D.H., and Shearer, G.M., 1976, Cell-mediated lympholysis of trinitrophenyl-modified autologous lymphocytes. Confirmation of genetic control of response to TNP-modified *H-2* antigens by the use of anti-*H-2* and anti-*Ia* antibodies, *J. Exp. Med.* **143**:211.

Schwartz, R.H., David, C., Sachs, D.H., and Paul, W., 1976, T lymphocyte-enriched murine peritoneal exudate cells. III. Inhibition of antigen-induced lymphocyte proliferation with antihistocompatibility antisera, *J. Immunol.* in press.

Shearer, G.M., 1974, Cell-mediated cytotoxicity to trinitrophenyl-modified syngeneic lymphocytes, *Eur. J. Immunol.* **4**:527.

Shearer, G.M., and Cudkowicz, G., 1975, Induction of F_1 hybrid antiparent cytotoxic effector cells, *Science* **190**:890.

Shearer, G.M., Mozes, E., and Sela, M., 1972, Contribution of different cell types to the genetic control of immune response as a function of the chemical nature of the polymeric side chains (poly-L-prolyl and poly-DL-alanyl) of synthetic immunogens, *J. Exp. Med.* **135**:1009.

Shearer, G.M., Rehn, T.G., and Garbarino, C.A., 1975, Cell-mediated lympholysis of trinitrophenyl-modified autologous lymphocytes, *J. Exp. Med.* **141**:1348.

Shearer, G.M., Rehn, T.G., and Schmitt-Verhulst, A.-M., 1976, Role of the murine major histocompatibility complex in the specificity of *in vitro* T-cell-mediated lympholysis against chemically modified autologous lymphocytes, *Transplant. Rev.* **29**:222.

Shreffler, D.C., and David, C.S., 1975, The *H-2* major histocompatibility complex and the *I* immune response region. Genetic variation, function, and organization, *Adv. Immunol.* **20**:125.

Shreffler, D.C., and Passmore, H.C., 1971, *Immunogenetics of the H-2 System*, S. Karger, Basel.

Takemori, T., and Tada, T., 1975, Properties of antigen-specific suppressive T-cell factor in the regulation of antibody response of the mouse. I. *In vivo* activity and immunochemical characterizations, *J. Exp. Med.* **142**:1241.

von Boehmer, H., Hudson, L., and Sprent, J., 1975, Collaboration of histoincompatible T and B lymphocytes using cells from tetraparental bone marrow chimeras, *J. Exp. Med.* **142**:989.

Wagner, H., Götze, D., Ptschelinzew, L., and Röllinghoff, M., 1975, Induction of cytotoxic T lymphocytes against *I*-region-coded determinants: *In vitro* evidence for a third histocompatibility locus in the mouse, *J. Exp. Med.* **142**:1477.

Widmer, M.B., Peck, A.B., and Bach, F.H., 1973, Genetic mapping of *H-2* LD loci, *Transplant. Proc.* **5**:1501.

Zinkernagel, R.M., and Doherty, P.C., 1974a, Restriction of an *in vitro* T cell-mediated cytotoxicity in lymphocytic choriomeningitis within a syngeneic or semiallogeneic system, *Nature (London)* **248**:701.

Zinkernagel, R.M., and Doherty, P.C., 1974b, Immunological surveillance against altered self components by sensitized T lymphocytes in lymphocytic choriomeningitis, *Nature (London)* **251**:547.

Zinkernagel, R.M., and Doherty, P.C., 1975, *H-2* compatibility requirement for T cell-mediated lysis of target cells infected with lymphocytic choriomeningitis virus, *J. Exp. Med.* **141**:1427.

Chapter 7

T-Cell-Mediated Cytolysis:
An Overview of Some Current Issues

Christopher S. Henney

Departments of Medicine and Microbiology
Johns Hopkins University School of Medicine
and
O'Neill Memorial Research Laboratories
Good Samaritan Hospital
Baltimore, Maryland

I. INTRODUCTION

It is the purpose of this brief review to summarize some recent developments in our understanding of the mechanism of T-cell-mediated cytolysis. As is customary in this series, the account will be a rather personal one, and the "developments" to be discussed will center principally on observations made in this laboratory during the course of the last two years.

Much of our current understanding of how cytolytically active T cells function comes from *in vitro* studies on the destruction of mouse tumors. One widely used system, first described by Brunner *et al.* (1968), raises killer cells in C57BL/6 mice by intraperitoneal injection with an allogeneic tumor (P815 of the DBA/2 strain). Lymphoid cells are assayed for lytic activity by culturing with a ^{51}Cr-labeled sample of the immunizing tumor. In this system, the lytically active cell is exclusively a thymus-derived (T) lymphocyte (Cerottini *et al.*, 1970a,b).

T-cell-mediated cytolysis requires intimate contact between the effector cell and its homologous target (Wilson, 1965; Rosenau, 1968). When killer and target cell are separated either by a semipermeable membrane or by suspension in a viscous medium such as agarose or dextran, cytolysis does not occur (Cerottini and Brunner, 1974; Henney, 1974). Cytolysis results from single collisions between effector and target cell and is dependent on a viable killer cell (Berke *et al.*, 1969; Henney, 1971).

T-cell-induced target-cell destruction is probably independent both of antibody and of the complement system. Although it is currently impossible to rule out totally a role for these proteins in T-cell-mediated lysis, the evidence weighs heavily against their participation. For example, lymphoid-cell populations in which antibody cannot be detected, even by the most sensitive methods, often mediate cytolysis (Berke *et al.*, 1972). Similarly, T-cell-mediated lysis can take place in the absence of serum, and neither the rate nor the extent of lysis is affected by the addition of a fresh serum source. Perhaps even more incisively, the addition of antibodies directed against the C_2, C_3, and C_5 components of the complement cascade is without effect on cell-mediated cytolysis (Henney and Mayer, 1971).

Except for an early observation that the effector cell must be viable, little is known of precise metabolic requirements for cytolysis. The reason lies in the problem of interpretating drug inhibition studies. Since a viable cell is required for cytolysis, any drug that compromises the metabolism of the cell may eventually suppress its lytic performance. This does not necessarily imply that the metabolic pathway inhibited is directly involved in the lytic event; it may simply reflect that the effector cell is dying. On the other hand, *failure* to inhibit lysis with a number of drugs has enabled delineation of a number of metabolic pathways that are unrelated to lytic expression. For example, the effector T cell does not need to proliferate in order to lyse target cells, nor does it need to synthesize RNA (Brunner *et al.*, 1968) or protein (Thorn and Henney, 1976a). The latter conclusion has been reached only of late, for earlier experiments designed to evaluate the role of protein synthesis in cytolysis yielded ambiguous results. In a series of studies both from this laboratory and from that of Brunner, a number of inhibitors of protein synthesis were assayed for their effects on cytolysis (Henney, 1973a; Brunner *et al.*, 1968). In all cases, some diminution of lytic activity was observed when amino acid incorporation was suppressed. Indeed, pactamycin employed at concentrations of 10^{-5} M inhibited cytolysis completely (Henney, 1973a). These studies led to the conclusion that cytolysis was dependent on protein synthesis. When dose–response curves were established for the drug-induced inhibition of lysis and protein synthesis, however, a different answer was forthcoming. For example, pactamycin and emetine totally inhibited protein synthesis in lymphocyte populations at concentrations that had no effect whatsoever on the cells' lytic activity (Henney *et al.*, 1974). These findings would argue that *de novo* protein synthesis is not required for cytolysis, and that inhibition of lysis seen at higher drug concentrations was related to effects other than on protein synthesis (Thorn and Henney, 1976a). Perhaps the

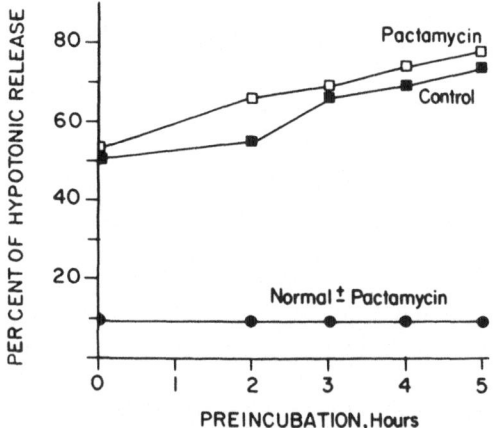

Fig. 1. Effect of prolonged incubation on the lytic activity of pactamycin-treated effector cells. Normal C57BL/6 spleen cells were cultured for 7 days in the presence of mitomycin-C-treated P815 cells (Thorn, 1974; Wagner and Feldman, 1972). The resulting effector population was treated with either 10^{-7} M pactamycin (□———□) or RPMI 1640 (■———■) for 1 hr, washed, and preincubated at 37°C for various lengths of time. Uncultured spleen cells from normal C57BL/6 animals were treated identically(●———●). ^{51}Cr-labeled target cells were added to the cultures to give a viable spleen cell/target cell ratio of 2:1. ^{51}Cr-release was determined after 5 hr. The hypotonic release was 81% of the incorporated ^{51}Cr. Reproduced from *Journal of Immunology* **116**:146 (1976) by the kind permission of the Williams and Wilkins Company, Baltimore, Maryland.

most emphatic denial of a role for *de novo* protein synthesis in T-cell-mediated lysis is shown in the experiment recorded in Fig. 1. Killer cells treated with 10^{-7} M pactamycin and then cultured for extended periods were subsequently found capable of killing target cells as efficiently as were untreated effector cells, even though the drug-treated cells synthesized no protein.

Killer T cells display an exquisite immunologic specificity *in vitro;* they can, for example, distinguish cells haptenated with TNP from those bearing DNP (Forman and Kettman, 1976). This specificity has led to a continuing quest not only for the effector cell's antigen receptor, but also to define that series of events that follow antigen "recognition" by the killer cell and that lead to target-cell lysis.

To discuss our current appreciation of these complex events, I would like to consider three separate aspects of the lytic cycle: (1) cell–cell interaction and (2) events following interaction and leading to (3) the cytolytic event.

II. STAGES IN THE LYTIC CYCLE

A. Cell–Cell Interactions

Clearly, the key to the expression of lytic activity by effector T cells lies in the interaction between killer and target cell. When the close apposition of effector and target cell is prevented by the use of a semipermeable membrane or a viscous medium, or by coating the target cell with antibody, lysis does not take place.

Studies with a number of plant agglutinins have led some investigators to suggest that proximity of the interacting cells is the sole requirement for lysis. It has been shown, for example, that the specificity of effector-cell populations is lost when the plant lectins Concanavalin A (Con A) or phytohemagglutinin (PHA) are added to the cultures (Möller, 1965; Bevan and Cohn, 1975; Waterfield et al., 1975). In the presence of these lectins, cytolytically active lymphocyte populations from alloimmunized animals have been shown to kill syngeneic target cells. How do these findings relate to the exquisite immunologic specificity that effector T cells exhibit in vitro in the absence of lectins?

It has long been argued that the immunologic specificity of T-cell-mediated lysis is attributable to antigen receptor sites associated with the membrane of the effector cell. Although the biochemical nature of such receptors remains the subject of controversy (see, for example, Crone et al, 1972; Binz and Wigzell, 1975), it has proved relatively simple to define the existance of such structures on killer T cells. Thus, the lytic activity of an immune lymphoid-cell population is readily adsorbed when lymphocytes are incubated on cell monolayers that bear antigens against which the effector cells are directed. No such depletion occurs when the same lymphocytes are added to syngeneic cell monolayers (Werkele et al., 1972; Stulting and Berke, 1973; Henney and Bubbers, 1973a).

If cell agglutinins render effector T cells capable of nonspecific cytotoxicity, one could argue that the antigen receptor site associated with the membrane of the killer cell plays only a passive role in cytolysis, i.e., that it serves merely to bring target cells close enough to subject them to the lytic action of the effector cell. Although this simple "bridging" function for the receptor site would account for the specificity of the lytic event, it would dictate that the differentiated killer cell is an intrinsically lytic cell, which needs only target-cell proximity to express its lytic activity.

There is, however, an alternative viewpoint: that the killer cell, although possessing the potentiality for lytic expression, cannot kill unless its antigen receptor is accommodated by antigen. In this model, there would be direct linkage between the antigen receptor site and the lytic mechanism. Antigen would be viewed as a "trigger" for the metabolic machinery associated with lysis.

We have recently carried out experiments designed to define more clearly the role of the antigen receptor in cytolysis (Kuppers and Henney, 1976). Our experimental approach was based on the observation of Golstein (1974) that killer cells can themselves serve as targets for lytic attack. We asked a rather simple question: if one mixes effector cells of two specificities, selected so that antigen recognition could occur only in one direction, does killing occur in both directions? We argued that if the antigen receptor served only to bring cells into proximity, then both effector cells would exert their lytic activity, and there would be a mutual destruction of effector cells. If, however, antigen insertion into the killer cell's antigen receptor was required to "trigger" the lytic event, then killing would proceed only in the direction of antigen recognition. These arguments are depicted schematically in Fig. 2. Two populations of killer cells were raised in congenic mice by mixed lymphocyte culture: one effector population was raised by culturing B.10.A spleen cells with B.10.D2 lymphocytes and was designated the *a anti d* population; the other was raised by coculturing B.10.D2 and C57BL/10 spleen cells and was referred to as *d anti b*.

The effect of coculturing these two effector populations was assessed by incubating the cells together for 6 hr at 37°C at a multiplicity of 1:1 or 1:0.25

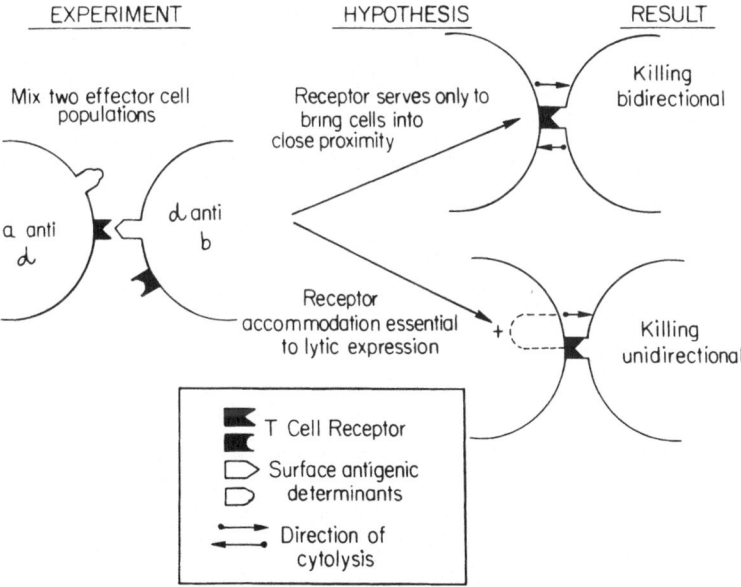

Fig. 2. Schematic representation of possible roles of the antigen receptor in T-cell-mediated lysis. Reproduced from *Journal of Experimental Medicine* **143**: 684 (1976) by the kind permission of the Rockefeller University Press, New York, New York.

Table I. Effect of Coculturing Effector-Lymphocyte Populations on Their Subsequent Lytic Activity[a]

Spleen cells cocultured		Ratio a:d	Residual specific activity after coculture			
B.10.A	B.10.D2		Specific ^{51}Cr release against H-2^d cells (%)	Reduction in a anti d activity (%)	Specific ^{51}Cr release against H-2^b cells (%)	Reduction in d anti b activity (%)
a anti d	–		43.8	–	1.3	–
–	d anti b		1.2	–	58.0	–
a anti d	d		17.6	0	0	–
a	d anti b	1:1	0.8	–	63.7	0
a anti d	$anti$ b		16.3	7	39.1	39
a anti d	d		27.2	0	3.8	–
a	d anti b	1:0.25	0	–	53.0	0
a anti d	d anti b		31.4	0	4.9	98

[a] The a anti d populations were B.10.A spleen cells raised in mixed lymphocyte culture against B.10.D2 spleen cells. The d anti b populations were B.10D2 spleen cells raised against C57BL/10 spleen cells. 2×10^6 B.10.A spleen cells were cultured (6 hr, 37°C) with either normal or immune B.10.D2 spleen cells at a ratio of 1:1 or 1:0.25. Lytic activity was then assessed in a 4-hr assay using 10^4 ^{51}Cr target cells of either H-2^b (EL4) or H-2^d (P815) specificities, and 4×10^5 lymphoid cells. These multiplicities were based on the total number of "a" lymphoid cells initially added to the cultures. Spontaneous release of ^{51}Cr from EL4 target cells was 13.1%, and from P815 cells 8.2%. In both cases freeze-thawing cells released 80±1% of the incorporated ^{51}Cr.

"a" cells to "d" cells. Control cultures contained either normal a or normal d spleen cells instead of the effector populations. At the end of incubation, the cell cultures were added to either ^{51}Cr-labeled EL4 or ^{51}Cr-P815 target cells, and the residual lytic activity was assessed.

As can be seen from Table I, the a anti d effector cells maintained comparable levels of activity after incubation with either normal d or effector d cell populations (17.6 vs. 16.3% after incubation at 1:1 ratio, 27.2 vs. 31.4% at 1:0.25 ratio).

In contrast, the d anti b effector cells lost considerable activity on culture with a anti d effector cells, but not when cultured with normal a cells. At a ratio of 1:1, there was a 39% fall in the lytic activity of the d anti b population and a 98% loss when cocultured at a ratio of 1:0.25.

Similar experiments using effector cells of different specificities gave comparable results (Table II). In all cases, the inactivation of effector cells proceeded only in the direction of antigen recognition. Reciprocal effector-cell death

Table II. Further Experiments on the Effect of
Coculturing Effector-Cell Populations

Effector-cell combination in coculture		Ratio effector I:II	Reduction in lytic activity following coculture (%)	
Effector population I	Effector population II		Effector population I	Effector population II
B.10.A anti B.10.D2	B.10.D2 anti C57BL/10	1:1	4	39
B.10.A anti B.10.D2	B.10.D2 anti C57BL/10	1:0.25	0	94
C57BL/6 anti P815	A/J anti Chang	1:1	6	85
C57BL/6 anti P815	DBA/2 anti L	1:2	15	98
C57BL/6 anti P815	DBA/2 anti L	1:0.25	0	91
DBA/2 anti EL4	C57BL/6 anti L	1:0.25	0	96
BALB/c anti EL4	C57BL/6 anti P815	0.5:1	22	20

occurred only when recognition could take place in both directions (Table II, bottom row).

It is clear, therefore, that when two lytically active cell populations are mixed in circumstances in which antigen recognition can occur in only one direction, then the activity of that population exhibiting the antigen is lost, while cells bearing receptors for the antigen retain their lytic function. Antigen recognition, then, is intimately associated with lytic expression, a demonstration that insists that cytolysis is more than a simple collision between effector and target cells.

If antigen recognition is required for lytic expression, how is one to interpret the findings, earlier alluded to, that lytically active cell populations lose their specificity in the presence of cell agglutinins? Two possibilities seem deserving of consideration: (1) the agglutinins bind to cell-surface receptors, which, like the antigen receptor, are linked to the killing mechanism, or (2) those cells that kill in the presence of lectins are not the T killer cells. Our preliminary experiments (Rubens and Henney, 1977) lead us to favor the latter possibility, but the alternatives may be neither mutually exclusive nor the sole possibilities.

1. Use of Cell Monolayers To Define Metabolic Requirements
for Cell–Cell Interactions

A relatively simple assay system has aided in definition of some of the metabolic requirements for antigen insertion into the killer cell's antigen receptor site. As earlier stated, killer cells bind rapidly and specifically to homologous allogeneic monolayers; the efficacy of this binding can be measured simply by following the lytic activity of nonadherent cells. By altering the culture conditions under which binding takes place, a number of investigators have established that killer cell–target cell interaction is an active process, inhibited at low temperatures, by azide, and by dinitrophenol (Werkele *et al.*, 1972; Todd, 1975; Berke and Gabison, 1975). Using a similar system, we observed that binding of killer cells to homologous targets was also inhibited by cytochalasin B (Henney and Bubbers, 1973b), indicating, perhaps, a role for microfilamentlike structures in the interaction (Table III), [These conclusions have also been reached by Martz (1975) using the ingenious, but technically more cumbersome, approach of centrifuging the effector and target cells together for brief periods in the presence of drug, followed by dispersal of the cells in dextran solutions.]

The requirement of divalent cations in the binding of killer to target cell has also been probed by following the extent of adhesion of lytically active cells to allogeneic monolayers in media of defined cation content (Stulting and Berke, 1973; Plaut *et al.*, 1976). The results obtained suggest two distinct roles for divalent cations in the lytic cycle: a requirement for Mg^{2+} in the binding of a

Table III. Effect of Various Drugs on the
Adsorption of Killer T Cells onto
Allogeneic Fibroblast Monolayers[a]

Effector lymphocytes	Adsorbing monolayer	Drug present during adsorption	Depletion of lytic activity (%)
C57BL/6 anti	C57BL/6	None	0
	DBA/2	None	87
DBA/2	DBA/2	Cytochalasin B (5 µg/ml)	8
	DBA/2	PGE 1 (10^{-5} M)	78
	DBA/2	$PGF_{1\alpha}$ (10^{-5} M)	81

[a]Spleen cells harvested from C57BL/6 mice 10 days after the mice received 10^7 P815 mastocytoma cells of the DBA/2 strain were used as effector cells. The adsorbing monolayers used were primary embryonic fibroblasts. Adsorption was carried out for 45 min at 37°C in the presence or absence of drug; the nonadherent cells were then washed to remove drug, and the lytic activity of this population was assayed using a constant number of viable cells. Depletion of lytic activity is relative to that of unfractionated spleen cells.

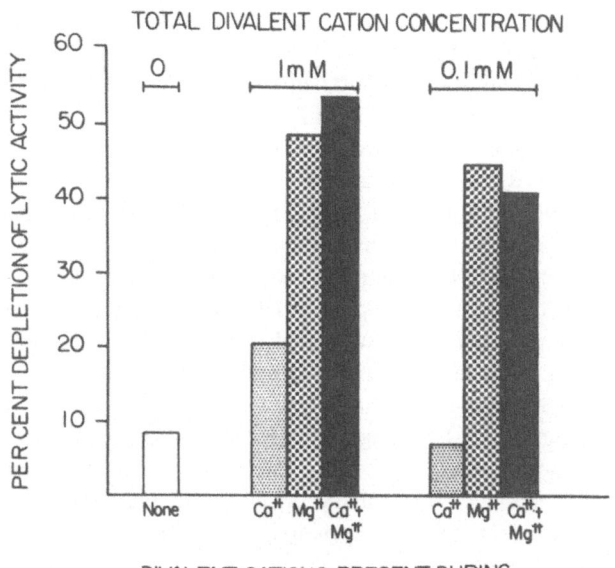

Fig. 3. Effect of Ca^{2+} and Mg^{2+} on the interaction of cytolytically active T cells with homologous targets. Spleen cells obtained from C57BL/6 mice 10 days after intraperitoneal injection with 10^7 DBA/2 mastocytoma cells (P815) were incubated for 45 min at 37°C on poly-L-lysine-induced monolayers of P815 cells. The incubation was performed in Ca^{2+}-, and Mg^{2+}-free HBSS to which was added Ca^{2+}, Mg^{2+}, or both. Adsorption in the presence of both cations was performed in a medium containing equimolar amounts of each cation (the numbers above the bar graphs are total cation concentrations). After incubation, non-adsorbed cells were collected, and their lytic activity was assessed. Depletion of effector cells by the monolayer procedure was calculated relative to the lytic activity of unfractionated cells. Reproduced from *Journal of Immunology* **116**:150 (1976) by the kind permission of the Williams and Wilkins Company, Baltimore, Maryland.

killer cell to its target and a later, absolute, requirement for Ca^{2+} probably in the lytic event itself.

When lymphocytes from C57BL/6 mice immune to DBA/2 alloantigens were adsorbed to P815 cell monolayers in the absence of divalent cations, an insignificant depletion of lytic activity was observed (Fig. 3) (Plaut *et al.*, 1976). No binding of killer cells to targets occurred in the presence of 0.1 mM Ca^{2+}, but a small amount of binding was seen in the presence of 1 mM Ca^{2+}. In contrast, effector cell–target cell interaction occurred readily in the presence of even low concentrations of Mg^{2+}. The binding observed in the presence of Mg^{2+} was not increased when Ca^{2+} was added (Fig. 3). Thus, in keeping with the earlier observations of Stulting and Berke (1973), these studies confirm that lymphocyte–target cell interactions occur readily in the presence of Mg^{2+}, that Ca^{2+} is much less effective, and that in the absence of cations, no binding takes place (Plaut et al., 1976; Golstein and Smith, 1975).

Interestingly, while Mg^{2+} supports interactions between lymphocytes and target cells, in the absence of Ca^{2+} such liasons do not lead to lysis. As mixtures of Ca^{2+} and Mg^{2+} have been shown to have synergistic effects on the overall rate of cytolysis, it appears that Ca^{2+} is required to initiate target-cell destruction (Henney and Bubbers, 1973b). Further evidence supporting this interpretation was obtained by following the kinetics of target-cell destruction in Mg^{2+} containing cultures to which Ca^{2+} was later added. Cultures containing lymphocytes and target cells were preincubated at 37°C in cation-free medium and were then centrifuged and resuspended in fresh medium. Target cells were found to be killed to the identical extent observed when lymphocytes and target cells were mixed without preincubation. On the other hand, cultures preincubated in the presence of 10^{-3} M Mg^{2+} showed, on addition of fresh medium as a Ca^{2+} source, much more rapid ^{51}Cr release than did those cultures not preincubated (Table IV). This enhanced cell death was not observed when lymphocytes and target cells were preincubated with Mg^{2+} at 0°C before addition of Ca^{2+} (Plaut et al., 1976).

The mechanism(s) by which Mg^{2+} and Ca^{2+} produce their effects in T-cell-

Table IV. Effect of Preincubating Lymphocytes and Target Cells in the Absence of Ca^{2+} on Subsequent T-Cell-Mediated Lysis[a]

		Specific lysis after addition of 10^{-3} M Ca^{2+} (%)	
Preincubation	Cation content of medium	30 min	110 min
Lymphocytes and target cells	None	1.0	14.8
Lymphocytes and target cells	10^{-3} M Mg^{2+}	6.8	28.5
Lymphocytes alone	10^{-3} M Mg^{2+}	0.0	13.6

[a]Lymphocytes from C57BL/6 mice immunized 10 days earlier with P815 cells were incubated for 2 hr at 37°C with P815 cells (ratio 80 Ly:1 target cell) in either cation-free medium or in medium containing 10^{-3} M Mg^{2+}. The cell suspensions were then centrifuged, the supernatants discarded, and medium containing 10^{-3} M Ca^{2+} added. Specific cytolysis was assayed 30 and 110 min later.

mediated lysis remains unknown. The cell—cell contact required to initiate lysis is presumably made in the face of repulsive charges between the interacting cell membranes. Because of the considerably greater effectiveness of Mg^{2+} in allowing lymphocyte—target cell interaction (Mauel *et al.*, 1970; Henney and Bubbers, 1973b), it is unlikely that the role of divalent cations is simply to overcome the charge repulsion. It seems much more likely that cations play a specific receptor role in interaction, e.g., as an enzyme cofactor.

In addition to providing considerable insight into the role of divalent cations in cytolysis, monolayer depletion studies have also provided useful information on the inhibitory action of a number of drugs that suppress T-cell-mediated killing. Specifically, it has been determined that some drugs that inhibit cytoloysis have little or no effect on lymphocyte—target cell interactions (Henney and Bubbers, 1973a). The most interesting of these agents are those that elevate levels of cyclic $3'5'$-adenosine monophosphate (cAMP) in lymphocytes (see pp. 258–259).

Although effector cells are efficiently depleted by incubation on allogeneic monolayers, such tactics have, disappointingly, not enabled one to prepare homogeneous populations of killer cells. The reason is simple: although killer cells are specifically depleted on such monolayers, a large number of other cells (some 25–35% of the total spleen-cell population) adhere nonspecifically. The degree of enrichment for killer cells obtained by harvesting adherent cells from the monolayer is thus usually only of the order of two- to threefold. We have not yet found any agent that will selectively interfere with the nonspecific binding of spleen cells to the monolayer; those agents that do prevent such interactions (e.g., cytochalasin B) also prevent the specific adhesion of killer cells. The key event in the cell—cell interaction leading to cytolysis, therefore, is the binding of antigen into the antigen receptor site on the effector cell's membrane. Berke and Fishelson (1975) have suggested that such interactions are accompanied by a polar localization of target-cell-surface components to the site of binding with the effector cell. Whether this phenomenon is germane to the subsequent lysis of the target cell is unknown, but seems unlikely, since glutaraldehyde-fixed cells, which presumably could not "cap" their surface antigens, can still be lysed by effector T cells (Bubbers and Henney, 1975a).

The demonstration that lymphocyte—target cell interactions take place in the presence of Mg^{2+}, but do not lead to cytolysis unless Ca^{2+} is added, has enabled us to look again at an old question: what is the incidence of killer cells in an immune lymphoid-cell population?

2. Enumeration of Killer T Cells

To date, two factors have hampered the enumeration of the killer cells in cytolytically active lymphoid-cell populations: (1) the effector T cell can kill more than one target cell (Zagury *et al.,* 1975; Martz, 1976a), and (2) the number of effector cells cannot be distinguished from their intrinsic lytic efficiency. The latter factor is presumably a complex function composed of the mobility of effector cells, their avidity for target cells, and their ability to lyse and disengage from targets. Standard assay conditions for *in vitro* cytotoxicity enable comparisons between the lytic activities of different "immune" lymphoid-cell populations, but these comparisons may bear little relationship to the relative numbers of effector cells if there is wide variation in killing efficiency.

By incubating lymphocytes with target cells in medium containing Mg^{2+} but not Ca^{2+}, interactions occur that do not lead to lysis. If Ca^{2+} is now added to such cultures together with cytochalasin A, those target cells that have functionally engaged with effector cells during the preincubation period will go on to lyse. The presence of cytochalasin A will, however, prevent any new interactions to proceed to a Ca^{2+}-dependent stage (Bubbers and Henney, 1975b); thus, if new liasons are formed after the addition of Ca^{2+}, they will not lead to lysis. Assuming each effector cell becomes bound to one target cell during the preincubation period, the subsequent number of target cells that lyse when Ca^{2+} is added to the cultures is equivalent to the number of effector cells present.

In a typical experiment, cytolytically active lymphoid-cell populations were generated by immunizing adult C57BL/6 mice with the DBA/2 mouse mastocytoma P815. Ten million P815 cells were given intraperitoneally, and the lymphoid-cell populations were harvested 10–12 days later.

Specific cytolysis was totally inhibited when lymphocytes and target cells were incubated in the presence of 5 μg/ml (6×10^{-6} M) cytochalasin A. Lymphoid cells preincubated for 10 min with cytochalasin A and then washed did not recover their lytic activity, but target cells treated in an identical manner were as susceptible to lysis as untreated cells. The drug did not increase the rate of spontaneous release of ^{51}Cr from target cells.

The experimental protocol used to enumerate effector T cells was as follows:

Lymphocytes	Mg^{2+} No Ca^{2+}		Ca^{2+}	Target cell death
+				measured
^{51}Cr target cells	1 min	Cytochalasin A		1–6 hr later
	200 g			

(Cytochalasin A was added 10 min before Ca^{2+} in order to allow a finite time for the drug to exert its effect.)

No cytolysis occurred when lymphocytes were incubated with target cells in a medium containing Mg^{2+} but not Ca^{2+} (Fig. 4). On the addition of Ca^{2+}, however, ^{51}Cr release readily occurred (Fig. 4). Two features of the target-cell

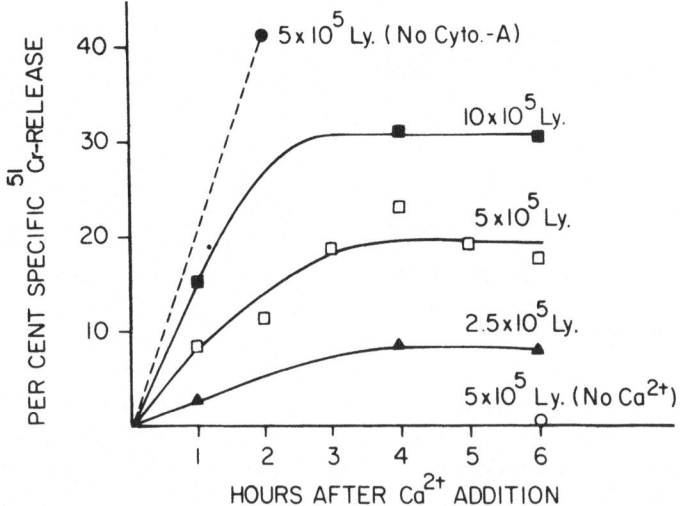

Fig. 4. Spleen and ^{51}Cr-labeled tumor cells were washed twice in Ca^{2+}-free medium containing 5×10^{-5} M ethyleneglycol-*bis*-(β-aminoethyl ether) *N,N'*-tetraacetic acid to remove trace amounts of Ca^{2+} just prior to use. Spleen and target cells were then centrifuged 1 min at 200g and incubated for 1 hr at 37°C. Cytochalasin A in Ca^{2+}-free medium was then added, followed 10 min later by Ca^{2+}-containing medium (MEM-Earle's Salts) with 5% fetal calf serum. Spleen cells from uninjected C57BL/6 mice were identically treated as controls. The following numbers of spleen cells were used: ($\blacktriangle$——$\blacktriangle$) 2.5×10^5; ($\square$———$\square$) 5×10^5; ($\blacksquare$——$\blacksquare$) 10×10^5; ($\bullet$) 5×10^5 (no cytochalasin A added); ($\circ$) 5×10^5 (no Ca^{2+}-containing medium added).

destruction following the addition of Ca^{2+} are worthy of note: (1) the number of target cells killed was proportional to the number of spleen cells present in the culture; (2) a period of about 3 hr in Ca^{2+}-containing medium was necessary to allow maximal ^{51}Cr release.

If the maximum amount of target-cell destruction depicted in Fig. 4 is equivalent to the number of effector cells present in the lymphocyte population, several provisions must hold:

1. For a given effector-cell population, the target-cell destruction 3 hr after the addition of Ca^{2+} to the cultures should be directly proportional to the number of lymphocytes present. The data in Fig. 4 show this to be the case.
2. Increasing the size of the target-cell pool above the minimum required to engage all effector cells should not affect the number of target cells killed. In other experiments, we showed that when 5×10^5 immune spleen cells were incubated with between 5×10^4 and 20×10^4 target cells, the number of target cells killed after the addition of Ca^{2+} was constant (Thorn and Henney, 1976b).

3. The number of target cells killed should not be increased if the incubation period in Ca^{2+}-free medium is extended (i.e., a maximum number of interactions had occurred in the preincubation time chosen). The number of functional engagements between lymphocyte and target cell was found not to increase significantly over the period 30 min to 2 hr, in keeping with previous studies (Zagury et al., 1975; Berke et al., 1975).

Since these criteria were fulfilled, the number of target cells maximally killed was equated with the number of effector cells. This approach was used on several occasions to enumerate effector cells in C57BL/6 spleen-cell populations at the peak of the primary immune response (10–12 days) after immunization with P815 cells. The data, shown in Table V, indicate that at this time, 0.7–2.2% of the total spleen-cell population was specific anti-P815 T effector cells (Thorn and Henney, 1976b).

There are two principal assumptions necessary for our calculations to be valid:

1. All effector cells must functionally interact with a target cell during the preincubation period (obviously, if some effector cells do not engage a target cell, the number of effector cells calculated will be an underestimate).
2. Each effector cell must not functionally engage more than one target during preincubation in the Mg^{2+}-containing medium (or else the calculated value would be an overestimate of the effector-cell incidence).

The first of these assumptions appears warranted, for preincubation times between 30 min and 120 min led to the same amount of lysis following the addition of cytochalasin A and Ca^{2+}. Indeed, we have found no difference in the subsequent ^{51}Cr release whether cytochalasin A was added after 5 or 120 min. In all cases, however, cytochalasin A added at the same time as the target cells completely inhibited cytolysis. It would thus seem that functional engagements between lymphocyte and target cell occur rapidly, and, under the conditions used, were complete within 30 min.

The same arguments would seem to dictate that an effector cell does not functionally engage more than one target cell during the preincubation period. If such were the case, then extending the preincubation period would be expected to increase the number of such engagements. In fact, preincubation periods between 30 and 120 min showed an identical number of functional interactions. It would seem unlikely that an effector cell undergoes multiple nonlytic interactions in the period 0–30 min but not thereafter, although admittedly this remains a faint possibility. It is also not likely that each effector engages several target cells simultaneously, for if this were the case, increasing the size of the target-cell pool should increase the likelihood of such interactions.

Table V. Frequency of Specific Cytolytic T Cells in the Spleens of Alloimmunized Mice

Experiment No.	Days after immunization	Maximum number ($\times 10^{-3}$) of target cells lysed per 5×10^5 viable cells[a]	Frequency of effector cells $(\%)$[b]
1	10	11.0	2.2
2	10	9.0	1.8
3	10	7.0	1.4
4	10	5.0	1.0
5	10	3.5	0.7
6	11	8.0	1.6
7	11	6.0	1.2
8	11	4.5	0.9
9	12	4.0	0.8
10	12	4.0	0.8

[a]The number of effector cells in each spleen cell suspension was determined using the experimental approach shown in Fig. 4 (Thorn and Henney, 1976b).
[b]The frequency equals the maximum number of target cells killed divided by 5×10^4 spleen cells.

Two methods of estimating effector cells have been used previously. One approach has been to equate the frequency of cytolytic T cells with the number of target cells specifically lysed in the presence of a great excess of target cells (Henney, 1971; Wilson, 1965). The possibility that the effector cells "recycle" (i.e., that one lymphocyte kills more than one target cell) was largely ignored in these studies, and it is therefore likely that those calculated frequencies were overestimates. Indeed, I have earlier reported (Henney, 1971) the incidence of effector cells in the system reevaluated here as approximately 4% of splenic lymphocytes, a number 2–3 times higher than that estimated in the present study. The higher number presumably reflects the destruction of several target cells by individual killers.

The frequency of cytolytically active cells has also been measured by counting lymphocytes that adhere to target cells (Zagury et al., 1975; Berke et al., 1975; Martz, 1975). The critical assumption in this approach is that each lymphocyte that binds to a target cell is a specific effector cell. This is almost certainly not the case; indeed, both precursor (Mage and McHugh, 1975) and memory cells (Kamat and Henney, 1975) have been shown to have an affinity for homologous allogeneic cells, but neither of these T-cell populations is cytolytic (Kamat and Henney, 1975; Cerottini et al., 1974). The contribution of noncytotoxic lymphocytes to the overall frequency of target binding cells remains to be established.

B. Events Following Cell—Cell Interaction

This is the least well defined of the three divisions of the lytic cycle that I have chosen to discuss. I will use this section principally to outline the effects of agents that inhibit cytolysis, but that apparently do not affect cell—cell interaction. Principal among the drugs in this category are those that augment cellular cAMP levels.

1. Relationships Between Effector-Cell cAMP Levels and Cytotoxic Expression

An inverse relationship between lymphocyte cAMP levels and cytolytic activity was first observed during studies with a stimulator of adenylate cyclase, isoproterenol, and a phosphodiesterase inhibitor, theophylline (Henney and Lichtenstein, 1971). The relationship was strengthened considerably by studies involving a number of prostaglandin congeners (Lichtenstein *et al.*, 1972). These drugs, which exhibited a wide range of adenylate-cyclase-stimulatory activities, showed a great variability in their inhibitory activity in lytic assays. There was a close correlation between the increased cAMP levels seen in the presence of the prostaglandins and the inhibition of cytolysis observed. Thus, prostaglandins E_1 and E_2 were found to be potent adenylate-cyclase-stimulating agents and important inhibitors of cytolysis. Prostaglandins F 1α and F 2α, on the other hand, caused little or no rise in the cAMP content of spleen cell suspensions, and interfered only very poorly with cytolysis (Lichtenstein *et al.*, 1972).

It appears that increased cAMP levels in lymphocyte populations, resulting from adenylate cyclase stimulation, are mediated via specific membrane-associated hormone receptors closely linked to the enzyme. This inference is drawn from the exquisite specificity shown by hormone antagonists. Thus, propranolol, a β-adrenergic antagonist, specifically reversed the augmentation of cAMP and the inhibition of cytolysis caused by isoproterenol, but had no effect on activities mediated by prostaglandin E_1 (PGE_1) (Henney *et al.*, 1972). Similarly, we have shown that the ability of histamine to increase cAMP levels, and to inhibit the cytolytic activity of spleen cells, was reversed by the anti-histamines burimamide and metiamide (but not, interestingly enough, by other antihistamines, e.g., diphenhydramine or pyrilamine, which antagonize different histamine-receptor-site specificities) (Plaut *et al.*, 1973). Neither burimamide nor metiamide had effects on the augmentation of lymphocyte cAMP levels or on the inhibition of cytolysis caused by PGE_1 (Plaut *et al.*, 1973).

These earlier studies were all made with drugs that inhibited cytolysis, and increased cAMP levels, in a reversible manner. It was thus difficult to decide whether the inhibition of cytolysis was mediated via the effector or target cell. In investigations employing cholera enterotoxin, which stimulates adenylate cyclase in a very protracted manner, we were able to show that augmented cAMP levels in the effector-cell population were associated with a depressed cytolytic activity (Lichtenstein *et al.*, 1973). On the other hand, cholera-toxin treatment of target cells had no effect on their susceptibility to lymphocyte-induced lysis (Lichtenstein *et al.*, 1973). These findings clearly strengthen the evidence relating lymphocyte cAMP levels to the expression of cytolytic activity. Perhaps the only weak link to date in this chain of association lies in the cell populations employed for cyclic nucleotide assays. The cells used for cAMP measurements have invariably been extremely heterogeneous, and include only a small proportion of effector cells. To equate increased cAMP levels in this population with changes in the biological activity of a small fraction of the cells is thus clearly a questionable practice. The isolation of purified effector-cell populations would obviously be useful in resolving the validity of these suppositions.

Recently, Goldberg and his colleagues (George *et al.*, 1970; Hadden *et al.*, 1972) have demonstrated that events mediated by augmented cAMP levels are often antagonized by agents that augment intracellular guanosine cyclic $3'5'$-monophosphate (cGMP). Thus, while elevation of cAMP levels had an anti-mitotic role in various cell types, a rise in cGMP was reported to have a proliferative effect (Hadden *et al.*, 1972). In an apparent confirmation of this phenomenon in cytolytically active rat-lymphocyte populations, Strom *et al.* (1973) showed that while β-adrenergic agents suppressed cytolysis (presumably by augmenting cAMP levels), cholinergic agents (which augment cGMP in some tissues) increased the cytolytic activity of lymphocyte populations. This finding was not reproducible using murine effector cells (Cerottini and Brunner, 1974; Henney, 1974b). Indeed, the existence of cholinergic receptors on T lymphocytes has been questioned by some (Wedner *et al.*, 1975). Despite our current inability to implicate cGMP in T-cell-mediated cytolysis, interrelationships between this cyclic nucleotide and cAMP seem worthy of further study.

The stage in the cytolytic pathway inhibited by increased cAMP levels awaits definition. We have previously argued that the inhibitory effects of the cAMP-active drugs, cytochalasin B, and colchicine collectively suggest that the T cell must be able to secrete in order to kill (Henney, 1973a). The evidence for this assertion is, of course, circumstantial, but is based on the antisecretory effects of these drugs in a wide variety of cell types. I will consider the implications of such T-cell "secretion" during discussion of the lytic event.

2. *"Late" Requirement for Ca²⁺ During Cytolysis*

Our earlier discussions on the role of divalent cations in the lytic process alluded to a requirement for Ca^{2+} in events following cell–cell interaction. This requirement is an intriguing one. There does not appear to be a "universal" requirement for these cations in cell-mediated cytotoxicity, because Golstein and collaborators (Golstein and Gomperts, 1975; Golstein and Fewtrell, 1975) have recently demonstrated that the lysis of antibody-coated sheep erythrocytes by both mouse and human effector cells occurs independently of Ca^{2+}.*

It is possible that Ca^{2+} may be involved in a mechanism analogous to the "stimulus–secretion coupling" (Rasmussen, 1970; Forman et al., 1973; Rubin, 1974) observed in many other cell types, although we, among others, have been unable to demonstrate a secreted lytic substance during T-cell-mediated cytolysis (Brunner and Cerottini, 1971; Henney, 1975).

C. The Lytic Event: Destruction of the Target-Cell Membrane

The terminal stages of the lytic cycle are perhaps the best understood. As a result of the collision with an effector T lymphocyte, the target cell undergoes a progressive series of membrane permeability changes ending in rupture of the cell membrane (Henney, 1973b). During these changes, the presence of the lymphocyte is no longer required (Martz and Benacerraf, 1973; Wagner and Rollinghoff, 1974). The progressive changes in the target-cell membrane that herald lysis of the cell have perhaps been most clearly demonstrated using markers of varying molecular size as indicators of target-cell destruction (Henney, 1973b; Martz et al., 1974). Typical results from our own studies are shown in Fig. 5.

Using the P815 mastocytoma as target cell and effector lymphocytes from alloimmunized C57BL/6 mice, changes in the permeability of the target cell membrane (as measured by ATP and ^{86}Rb efflux) were specifically induced within 10 min of lymphocyte addition. Protein-bound ^{51}Cr or $[^3H]$thymidine-DNA effluxed from target cells only later, after lag periods that were related to the effective molecular size of the indicator (Fig. 5). These findings, later confirmed by Martz et al. (1974), suggest that the initial lesion allows rapid exchange of inorganic ions and small molecules, but not of macromolecules. It seems likely that the latter become able to pass the cell membrane only after secondary effects on the cell, resulting from disordered osmotic regulation. The eventual demise of the target cell appears to be caused by colloid osmotic forces

---

*Martz (1976b) has suggested that there may be no "late" requirement for Ca^{2+}. He asserts that those cell–cell interactions that occur in the presence of Mg^{2+} and absence of Ca^{2+} are "unphysiological," that they are abnormal adhesions, not compatible with lysis. He argues that Ca^{2+} is necessary only for the formation of "appropriate" adhesions, and is not needed elsewhere. While conceptually possible, it would be difficult for this hypothesis to explain data such as those shown in Table IV, which argue that adhesions formed in the presence of Mg^{2+} do indeed lead to lysis.

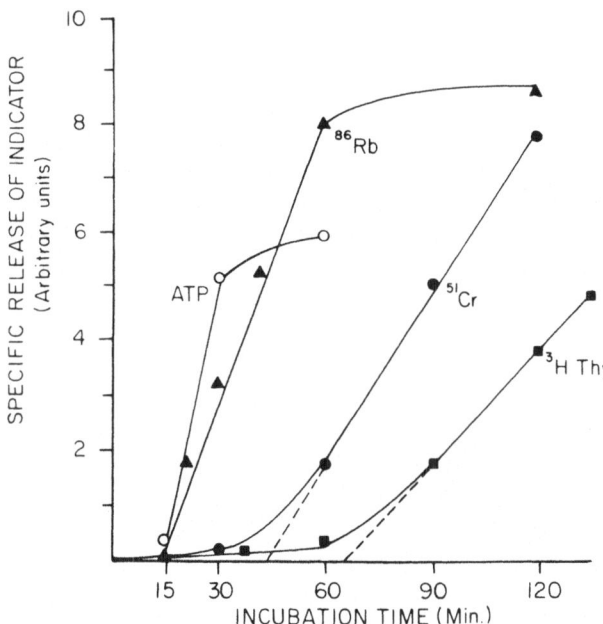

Fig. 5. Lymphocyte-mediated release of various indicators from target cells. 10^5 DBA/2 mastocytoma cells internally labelled with [^{86}Rb], [^{51}Cr], or [^{3}H]thymidine were incubated with 10^7 splenic lymphocytes derived from a pool of C57BL/6 mice that had been immunized 10 days earlier with 10^7 mastocytoma cells intraperitoneally. The specific release of each indicator was calculated by subtraction of the amount of indicator released in the presence of 10^7 normal C57BL/6 splenic lymphocytes. Reproduced from *Journal of Immunology* 110:73, (1973) by the kind permission of Williams and Wilkins Company, Baltimore, Maryland.

resulting from water influx. This conclusion is based on observations that both macromolecular efflux from the damaged target cell and plasma-membrane destruction can be prevented by the addition of exogenous high-molecular-weight dextrans (Henney, 1974a; Ferluga and Allison, 1974). The minimum size of dextran molecules that we found to afford such protection was approximately 40,000 mol. wt., leading us to suggest that the initial T-cell-induced lesion was approximately 90 Å in diameter (Henney, 1974a).

The progressive nature of the lytic lesion induced by T cells, the suppression of its development by solutions of high osmotic pressure, and the apparent initial size of the lesion all parallel remarkably the nature of the complement-induced membrane-permeability changes in tumor cells (Green *et al.*, 1959a,b). As stated earlier, however, it seems unlikely that T-cell-induced lesions can be attributed to complement components (Henney and Mayer, 1971).

III. OVERVIEW AND SOME POSSIBLE FUTURE DIRECTIONS

In sum, we have a fairly good overall appreciation of the events involved in T-cell-mediated cytolysis, which are summarized in Fig. 6. It will be noted that Fig. 6 adds an additional dimension to the issues discussed so far: the effector cell itself survives the interaction that results in the demise of the target cell and can interact with other target cells. T-cell-mediated lysis is thus a lytic *cycle*. This conclusion has been most elegantly established by micromanipulative proce-

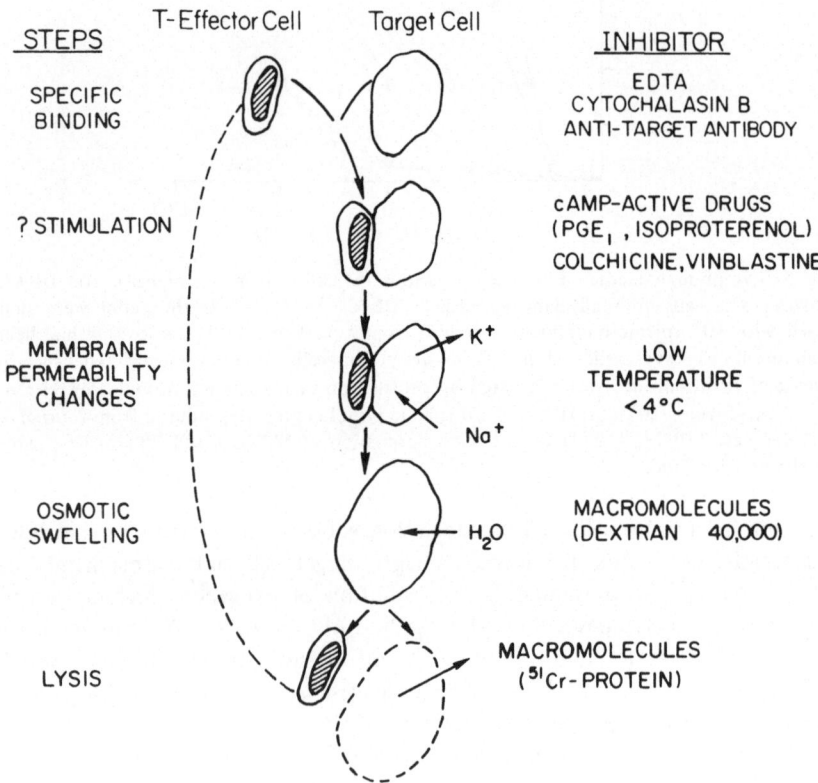

Fig. 6. Sequence of events in direct T-cell-mediated cytotoxic reactions. The phase described as stimulatory is largely of conceptual significance, and is offered here as an explanation of the inhibition of cytolysis by adenylate-cylase-stimulating drugs, which do not appear to affect cell–cell interaction. Reproduced from *Annals of the New York Academy of Sciences* **256**:141 (1975) by the kind permission of the New York Academy of Sciences, New York, New York.

dures in which a single effector T cell has been identified, isolated with a micropipette, and transferred to a new target cell (Zagury *et al.*, 1975). In such maneuvers, killer cells were frequently seen to kill again. While this finding unambigiously demonstrated that killer T cells can kill multiple target cells, it brings up the intriguing question of how frequently such recycling occurs and how much it contributes to short-term ^{51}Cr-release assays. Is it significant that in Zagury's experiments described above, less than 50% (17 of 48) of effector cells were actually observed to kill more than once, or was this a result of damage during the handling of such cells? The issues no longer revolve around whether killer T cells can kill several target cells, but how often they do, and whether effector-cell populations are heterogeneous in this respect.

The $64,000 Question

The prime quest of all studies on T-cell-mediated lysis remains the definition of how the killer cell effects target-cell destruction. Of the suggestions offered to account for this event, most attention has been paid to the proposition that target-cell destruction is caused by a soluble mediator released from the lymphocyte in response to an antigen "trigger." This hypothesis, initially proposed by Granger and Kolb (1968), has received support principally for two reasons: (1) it is conceptually attractive, making T-cell-mediated cytolysis dependent on the product of an "activated" lymphoid cell in the same manner as are so many other cellular immune phenomena; (2) there is a body of supportive experimental evidence, most notably the observation that stimulated lymphoid-cell cultures produce a cytotoxic factor, which has been termed *lymphotoxin.* Although there is much to commend the candidature of lymphotoxin as the mediator of T-cell-induced cytolysis, its acceptance has not been universal, for there remain a number of experimental observations that are difficult to explain.

First, kinetic evidence shows that target-cell destruction results from single collisions with an effector lymphocyte (Wilson, 1965; Berke *et al.,* 1969; Henney, 1971). If a soluble mediator were being secreted into the milieu, lysis would eventually be independent of such collision. It is not, even after extensive incubation periods.

Second, when cultures containing mixed target-cell populations are employed, effector cells kill only those cells bearing homologous antigen; there is no lysis of "innocent bystander" cells (Cerottini and Brunner, 1974). Lymphotoxin, on the other hand, is nonspecific in its action. Furthermore, medium obtained from cultures in which large numbers of target cells have been destroyed is not lytic toward other target cells, nor does it enhance the activity of effector-T-cell populations (Henney, unpublished observations).

A series of recent observations on the relationship between mediator production and the cytolytic potential of lymphocytes casts further doubts on the

Table VI. Effect of Antilymphotoxin Serum on Cell-Mediated Cytotoxicity[a]

Hartley-strain guinea pig spleen cells	Ovalbumin added to culture	Rabbit serum (final dilution)	Specific cytolysis (%)	
			Hepatoma target cells	P815 target cells
P-815 immune	None	None	0	36.9±0.4
	None	Anti-LT (1:20)	–	40.6±1.1
	None	Preimmune (1:20)	–	44.9±0.5
Hepatoma-immune	None	None	28.4±0.2	0
(line 10 strain 2)	None	Anti-LT (1:20)	27.8±0.1	–
	None	Preimmune (1:20)	27.9±0.2	–
Ovalbumin-immune	None	None	2.3±3.0	0
	50 μg/ml	None	52.8±8.9	25.8±2.0
	50 μg/ml	Anti-LT (1:40)	22.2±2.4	1.7±0.4
	50 μg/ml	Preimmune (1:40)	54.8±8.7	19.4±1.6
Normal	50 μg/ml	None	9.1±2.2	0
	50 μg/ml	Anti-LT (1:40)	0	0.3±0.7
	50 μg/ml	Preimmune (1:40)	0	0

[a]Hartley strain guinea pigs were immunized intraperitoneally with one of the following: (1) 500 μg ovalbumin in CFA in rear footpad, (2) 3×10^7 P815 cells of the DBA/2 strain, or (3) 3×10^7 line 10 hepatoma cells syngeneic to strain 2 guinea pigs. In each case, spleen cells were harvested 10 days later and used as a source of effector cells. Both ^{51}Cr-hepatoma and ^{51}Cr-P815 cells were used as targets in a 4-hr assay employing a lymphocyte/target cell multiplicity of 100:1. The rabbit antiserum tested was included throughout the culture period. Specific cytolysis was calculated by the method of Brunner et al. (1968), using target cells incubated in the absence of lymphoid cells as control.

role of lymphotoxin in T-cell-mediated lysis. It was found that the cytolytic activity of a lymphoid-cell population could readily be dissociated experimentally from its ability to produce soluble mediators (Henney et al., 1974). Thus, treatment of lymphocytes with a number of drugs (e.g., cholera enterotoxin, colchicine, and vinblastine) ablated the direct lytic activity of these populations, but left unaffected their ability to produce soluble mediators (including lymphotoxin) in the presence of antigen or mitogen (Henney et al., 1974).

A recent observation made in collaboration with Drs. Gately and Mayer provides perhaps the most incisive argument to date against a role for lymphotoxin in T-cell-mediated lysis. A potent rabbit antilymphotoxin antiserum (Gately et al., 1975), which effectively neutralized both antigen- and mitogen-induced guinea pig lymphotoxin, failed to affect the in vitro lytic activity of guinea pig effector cells raised by alloimmunization (Table VI). This negative finding was strengthened by the observation that a lymphotoxin-mediated lytic system (ovalbumin-immune spleen cells cultured with ^{51}Cr targets in the presence of ovalbumin) *was* inhibited by the antiserum (Table VI).

One also finds it difficult to explain why, if lysis is dependent on a soluble mediator, the killer cell itself is not affected during interaction with target cells. The studies described in this review (Kuppers and Henney, 1976) and those of Golstein (1974) clearly establish that killer cells are not resistant to attack.

In sum, while the experimental evidence to date speaks strongly against the involvement of a freely permeating soluble mediator in T-cell-mediated lysis, it is probably premature to totally discount such a possibility. It is conceivable that a mediator is involved, but that it is delivered, and is effective, only over very short distances.

In addition to discussions of soluble mediators in T-cell-mediated lysis, two alternative mechanisms are currently receiving considerable attention: one implicates intercytoplasmic connections between killer and target cells, the other focuses on effector cell membrane enzyme systems.

It has been suggested that intercytoplasmic connections between effector and target cells, which would allow cell—cell communication without reference to the *milieu exterieur,* might be the key to lymphocyte-induced lysis (Sura *et al.,* 1967; Selin *et al.,* 1971). Although these interactions are frequent among homogeneous cell populations, there have been only isolated reports claiming the existence of such connections between lymphocytes and heterologous target-cell types. A number of investigators have been unable to detect any focal membrane changes such as membrane fusion or the junction type of membrane specialization (e.g., Biberfield and Johansson, 1975). It seems inherently unlikely that intercytoplasmic connections are a common event in lymphocyte—target cell interactions, or that they are an important feature of cytolysis. A principal reason for this assertion is the time factor: the lytic event seems to occur much too fast (probably on the order of 30—60 sec; Martz, 1975; MacDonald, 1975) to allow the formation of intercytoplasmic connections between interacting cells.

There are a number of recent observations that raise the possibility that T-cell-medited lysis may occur totally at the level of interacting cell membranes. The most direct information in this regard is a preliminary report that isolated plasma membranes derived from lymph nodes of contact-sensitized (oxazolone-painted) mice can be cytotoxic toward tumor cells *in vitro* (Ferluga and Allison, 1975). Unfortunately, these studies were not controlled for normal lymphocytes, nor were the plasma membranes well characterized. Although the significance of the oxazolone painting for "sensitization" is as yet unclear, these fascinating observations clearly warrant further investigation. It should be added that the cytotoxic activity of isolated membranes is a totally unexpected finding, for there have been repeated demonstrations that viable effector cells are required to effect lysis. In the past, heated, frozen—thawed, sonicated, and

X-irradiated cells have uniformly failed to exhibit lytic activity. Indeed, such preparations fail to inhibit the lytic activity of viable cells.

A further intriguing observation implies that cell-mediated cytotoxicity may be due to a membrane-associated phospholipase (Frye and Friou, 1975). In a non-T-cell-mediated cytotoxic system [the lysis of chicken erythrocytes (CRBC) by mouse spleen cells in the presence of mouse anti-CRBC antibody], Frye and Friou found that lysis was significantly inhibited by phoshatidylcholine and by a known inhibitor of phospholipase A, D,L-2,3 distearoyloxypropyl (dimethyl)-2(hydroxyethyl)-ammonium acetate (Rosenthal's inhibitor). Whether these reagents also interfere with T-cell-mediated lysis remains to be established. Furthermore, Frye and Friou's experiments were uncontrolled for specificity, and one wonders whether other lipids or even hydrophobic peptides could inhibit cytolysis. If phospholipase A is a feature of the killing mechanism, current information suggests that (1) enzyme activation must be associated with antigen–receptor coupling, and (2) the target for lytic attack is the lecithin component of the lipid bilayer, so that membrane damage would be caused by lysolecithin. In this context, it is interesting to note that Henkart and Blumenthal (1975) recently observed altered conductance across a synthetic lipid bilayer in the presence of antibody and lymphoid cells.

It would seem important to establish soon which component of the plasma membrane is the target of the T cell's lytic attack, a subject that is at the center of this laboratory's current research efforts.

ACKNOWLEDGMENTS

The author wishes to thank J. Eric Bubbers, Rudolf C. Kuppers, Marshall Plaut, Richard Thorn, and H. Kirk Ziegler, all of whom were involved in various aspects of these studies.

The original work reported was supported by Grant AI 10280 from the National Institute of Allergy and Infectious Disease, and Contracts NO1-CB-43932 and NO1-CB-43965 from the National Cancer Institute during the tenure of a Research Career Development Award from the National Institute of Allergy and Infectious Disease.

This chapter is communication No. 253 from the O'Neill Memorial Research Laboratories.

REFERENCES

Berke, G., and Fishelson, Z., 1975, Localization of aggregated cell surface antigens of target cells bound to cytotoxic T lymphocytes, *J. Exp. Med.* **142**:1011.

Berke, G., and Gabison, D., 1975, Energy requirements of the binding and lytic steps of T lymphocyte-mediated cytolysis of leukemic cells *in vitro, Eur. J. Immunol.* **5**:671.

Berke, G., Gabison, D., and Feldman, M., 1975, The frequency of effector cells in populations containing cytotoxic T lymphocytes, *Eur. J. Immunol.* **5**:813.

Berke, G., Sullivan, K.A., and Amos, B., 1972, Rejection of ascites tumor allograft. I. Isolation, characterization and *in vitro* reactivity of peritoneal lymphoid effector cells from BALB/c immune mice to EL4 leukosis, *J. Exp. Med.* **135**:1334.

Berke, G., Ax, W., Ginsburg, H., and Feldman, M., 1969, Graft rejection in tissue culture. II. Quantification of the lytic action on mouse fibroblasts by rat lymphocytes sensitized on mouse embryo monolayers, *Immunology* **16**:643.

Bevan, M., and Cohn, M.J., 1975, Cytotoxic effects of antigen and mitogen induced T cells on various targets, *J. Immunol.* **114**:559.

Biberfield, P., and Johansson, A., 1975, Contact areas of cytotoxic lymphocytes and target cells: An electron microscopic study, *Exp. Cell Res.* **94**:79.

Binz, H., and Wigzell, H., 1975, Shared idiotypic determinants on B and T lymphocytes reactive against the same antigenic determinants. III. Physical fractionation of specific immunocompetent T lymphocytes by affinity chromatography using anti-idiotypic antibodies, *J. Exp. Med.* **152**:1231.

Brunner, K.T., and Cerottini, J.-C., 1971, Cytotoxic lymphocytes as effector cells of cell-mediated cytotoxicity, in: *Progress in Immunology,* p. 385 (B. Amos, ed.), Academic Press, New York.

Brunner, K.T., Mauel, J., Cerottini, J.-C., and Chapuis, B., Quantitative assay for the lytic action of immune lymphoid cells on ^{51}Cr-labelled allogeneic target cells *in vitro:* Inhibition by isoantibody and by drugs, *Immunology* **14**:181.

Bubbers, J.E., and Henney, C.S., 1975a, Studies on the synthetic capacity and antigenic expression of glutaraldehyde fixed target cells, *J. Immunol.* **114**:1126.

Bubbers, J.E., and Henney, C.S., 1975b, Studies on the mechanism of lymphocyte-mediated cytolysis. V. The use of cytochalasins A and B to dissociate glucose transport from the lytic event, *J. Immunol.* **115**:145.

Cerottini, J.-C., and Brunner, K.T., 1974, Cell mediated cytotoxicity, allograft rejection and tumor immunity, *Adv. Immunol.* **18**:67.

Cerottini, J.-C., Nordin, A.A., and Brunner, K.T., 1970a, *In vitro* cytotoxic activity of thymus cells sensitized to alloantigens. *Nature (London)* **227**:72.

Cerottini, J.-C., Nordin, A.A., and Brunner, K.T., 1970b, Specific *in vitro* cytotoxicity to thymus derived lymphocytes sensitized to alloantigens, *Nature (London)* **228**:1308.

Cerottini, J.-C., Engers, H.D., MacDonald, H.K., and Brunner, K.T., 1974, Generation of cytotoxic T lymphocytes *in vitro.* II. Effect of repeated exposure to alloantigens on the cytotoxic activity of long-term mixed leucocyte cultures, *J. Exp. Med.* **140**:719.

Crone, M., Koch, C., and Simonsen, M., 1972, The elusive T cell receptor, *Transplant Rev.* **10**:36.

Ferluga, J., and Allison, A.C., 1974, Observations on the mechanism by which T-lymphocytes exert cytotoxic effects, *Nature (London)* **250**:673.

Ferluga, J., and Allison, A.C., 1975, Cytotoxicity of isolated plasma membranes from lymph node cells, *Nature (London)* **255**:708.

Forman, J.C., and Kettman, J., 1976, Specificity of cytotoxic effector cells for hapten-modified targets, *Fed. Proc. Fed. Amer. Soc. Exp. Biol.* **35**:474 (abstract).

Forman, J.C., Mongar, J.L., and Gomperts, B.D., 1973, Calcium ionophores and the movement of calcium ions following the physiological stimulus to a secretory process, *Nature (London)* **245**:249.

Frye, L.D., and Friou, G.J., 1975, Inhibition of mammalian cytotoxic cells by phosphatidylcholine and its analogue, *Nature (London)* **258**:333.

Gately, M., Gately, C., Henney, C.S., and Mayer, M.M., 1975, Studies on lymphokines: The production of antibody of guinea pig lymphotoxin and its use to distinguish lymphotoxin from migration inhibitory factor and mitogenic factor, *J. Immunol.* **115**:817.

George, W.J., Polson, J.B., O'Toole, A.G., and Goldberg, N.D., 1970, Evaluation of guanosine 3'5' cyclic phosphate in rat heart after perfusion with acetylcholine, *Proc. Natl. Acad. Sci. U.S.A.* **66**:398.

Golstein, P., 1974, Sensitivity of cytotoxic T cells to T cell-mediated cytotoxicity, *Nature (London)* **252**:81.

Golstein, P., and Fewtrell, C., 1975, Functional fractionation of human cytotoxic cells using differences in their cation requirements, *Nature (London)* **255**:491.

Golstein, P., and Gomperts, B.D., 1975, Non-T cell-mediated cytolysis requires Mg^{++} but not a Ca^{++}: An argument against a conventional "stimulus-secretion" mechanism for cytolysis, *J. Immunol.* **114**:1264.

Golstein, P., and Smith, E.T., 1976, The lethal hit stage of mouse T and non-T cell-mediated cytolysis: Differences in cation requirements and characterization of an analytical "cation pulse" method, *Eur. J. Immunol.* **6**:31.

Granger, G.A., and Kolb, W.P., 1968, Lymphocyte *in vitro* cytotoxicity: Mechanisms of immune and non-immune small lymphocyte mediated target cell destruction, *J. Immunol.* **101**:111.

Green, H., Barrow, P., and Goldberg, B., 1959a, Effect of antibody and complement on permeability control in ascites tumor cells and erythrocytes, *J. Exp. Med.* **110**:699.

Green, H., Fleischer, R.A., Barrow, P., and Goldberg, B., 1959b, The cytotoxic action of immune gamma globulin and complement on Krebs ascites tumor cells. II. Chemical studies, *J. Exp. Med.* **109**:511.

Hadden, J.W., Hadden, E.M., Haddox, M.K., and Goldberg, N.D., 1972, Guanosine 3'5' cyclic monophosphate: A possible intracellular mediator of mitogenic influences in lymphocytes, *Proc. Natl. Acad. Sci. U.S.A.* **69**:3024.

Henney, C.S., 1971, Quantitation of the cell-mediated immune response. I. The number of cytolytically active mouse lymphoid cells induced by immunization with allogeneic mastocytoma cells, *J. Immunol.* **107**:1558.

Henney, C.S., 1973a, Studies on the mechanism of T cell mediated cytolysis, *Transplant Rev.* **17**:37.

Henney, C.S. 1973b, Studies on the mechanism of lymphocyte-mediated cytolysis. II. The use of various target cell markers to study cytolytic events, *J. Immunol.* **110**:73.

Henney, C.S., 1974a, Estimation of the size of a T cell induced lytic lesion, *Nature (London)* **249**:456.

Henney, C.S., 1974b, Relationships between cytolytic activity of thymus derived lymphocytes and cellular cyclic nucleotide concentrations, in: *Cyclic AMP, Cell Growth and the Immune Response* pp. 195–209 (W. Braun, C.W. Parker, and L.M. Lichtenstein, eds.), Springer-Verlag, New York.

Henney, C.S., 1975, T cell mediated cytolysis: Consideration of the role of a soluble mediator, *J. Reticuloendothel. Soc.* **17**:231.

Henney, C.S., and Bubbers, J.E., 1973a, Antigen-T lymphocyte interactions: Inhibition by cytochalasin B, *J. Immunol.* **111**:85.

Henney, C.S., and Bubbers, J.E., 1973b, Studies on the mechanism of lymphocyte-mediated cytolysis. I. The role of divalent cations in cytolysis by T lymphocytes, *J. Immunol.* **110**:63.

Henney, C.S., and Lichtenstein, L.M., 1971, The role of cyclic AMP in the cytolytic activity of lymphocytes, *J. Immunol.* **107**:610.

Henney, C.S., and Mayer, M.M., 1971, Specific cytolytic activity of lymphocytes: Effect of antibodies against complement components C_2, C_3 and C_5, *Cell. Immunol.* **2**:702.

Henney, C.S., Bourne, H.R., and Lichtenstein, L.M., 1972, The role of cyclic 3'5'-adenosine monophosphate in the cytolytic activity of lymphocytes, *J. Immunol.* **108**:1526.

Henney, C.S., Gaffney, J., and Bloom, B.R., 1974, On the relation of soluble mediators to T cell mediated cytolysis, *J. Exp. Med.* **140**:837.

Henkart, P., and Blumenthal, R., 1975, Interaction of lymphocytes with lipid bilayer membranes: A mode for lymphocyte-mediated lysis of target cells, *Proc. Natl. Acad. Sci. U.S.A.* **72**:2789.

Kamat, R., and Henney, C.S., 1975, Studies on T cell clonal expansion. I. Suppression of killer T cell production *in vivo*, *J. Immunol.* **115**:1592.

Kuppers, R.C., and Henney, C.S., 1976, Evidence for direct linkage between antigen recognition and lytic expression in effector T cells, *J. Exp. Med.* **143**:684.

Lichtenstein, L.M., Gillespie, E., Bourne, H.R., and Henney, C.S., 1972, The effects of a series of prostaglandins on *in vitro* models of the allergic response and cellular immunity, *Prostaglandins* **2**:519.

Lichtenstein, L.M., Henney, C.S., Bourne, H.R., and Greenough, W.B., 1973, The effect of cholera toxin on *in vitro* models of immediate and delayed hypersensitivity: Further evidence for the role of cAMP, *J. Clin. Invest.* **52**:691.

MacDonald, H.R., 1975, Early detection of potentially lethal events in T cell-mediated cytolysis, *Eur. J. Immunol.* **5**:251.

Mage, M.G., and McHugh, L.L., 1975, Specific partial depletion of graft *vs.* host activity by incubation and centrifugation of mouse spleen cells on allogeneic spleen cell monolayers, *J. Immunol.* **115**:911.

Martz, E., 1975, Early steps in specific tumor cell lysis by sensitized mouse T lymphocytes. I. Resolution and characterization, *J. Immunol.* **115**:261.

Martz, E., 1976a, Multiple target cell killing by the cytolytic T lymphocyte and the mechanism of cytotoxicity, *Transplantation* **21**:5.

Martz, E., 1976b, Functional adhesion and the calcium requirement in T lymphocyte-mediated killing, *Fed. Proc. Fed. Amer. Soc. Exp. Biol.* **35**:248 (abstract).

Martz, E., and Benacerraf, B., 1973, An effector cell independent step in target cell lysis by sensitized mouse lymphocytes, *J. Immunol.* **111**:1538.

Martz, E., Burakoff, B., and Benacerraf, B., 1974, Interpretation of the sequential release of small and large molecules from tumor cells by low temperature during cytolysis mediated by immune T cells or complement, *Proc. Natl. Acad. Sci. U.S.A.* **71**:177.

Mauel, J., Rudolf, H., Chapuis, B., and Brunner, K.T., 1970, Studies of allograft immunity in mice. II. Mechanism of target cell inactivation *in vitro* by sensitized lymphocytes, *Immunology* **18**:517.

Moller, E., 1965, Contact-induced cytotoxicity by lymphoid cells containing foreign isoantigens, *Science* **147**:873.

Plaut, M., Lichtenstein, L.M., Gillespie, E., and Henney, C.S., 1973, Studies on the mechanism of lymphocyte mediated cytolysis. IV. Specificity of the histamine receptor on effector T cells, *J. Immunol.* **111**:389.

Plaut, M., Bubbers, J.E., and Henney, C.S., 1976, Studies on the mechanism of lymphocyte-mediated cytolysis. VII. Two stages in the T cell-mediated lytic cycle with distinct cation requirements, *J. Immunol.* **116**:150.

Rasmussen, H., 1970, Cell communication, calcium ion, and cyclic adenosine monophosphate, *Science* **170**:404.

Rosenau, W., 1968, Target cell destruction, *Fed. Proc. Fed. Amer. Soc. Exp. Biol.* **27**:34.

Rubens, R.P., and Henney, C.S., 1977, Studies on the mechanism of lymphocyte-mediated cytolysis. VIII. The use of Con A to delineate a distinctive killer T cell subpopulation. *J. Immunol.* **118**:180.

Rubin, R.P., 1974, *Calcium and the Secretory Process,* Plenum Press, New York.

Selin, D., Wallach, D.F.H., and Fischer, H., 1971, Intercellular communication in cell-mediated cytotoxicity. Fluorescein transfer between H-2^d target cells and *H-2^b* lymphocytes *in vitro, Eur. J. Immunol.* 1:453.

Strom, T.B., Carpenter, C.B., Garovoy, M.R., Austen, K.F., Merrill, J.P., and Kaliner, M., 1973, The modulating influence of cyclic nucleotides upon lymphocyte-mediated cytotoxicity, *J. Exp. Med.* 138:381.

Stulting, R.D., and Berke, G., 1973, Nature of lymphocyte-tumor interaction. A general method for cellular immunoabsorption, *J. Exp. Med.* 137:932.

Sura, S.N., Chernyakhovskaya, Y.U., Kadaghidze, A.G., Fuks, B.B., and Svet-Moldavsky, G.J., 1967, Cytochemical study of interaction between lymphocytes and target cells in tissue culture, *Exp. Cell Res.* 48:656.

Thorn, R.M., 1974, Thesis, University of Pennsylvania.

Thorn, R.M., and Henney, C.S., 1976a, Studies on the mechanism of lymphocyte-mediated cytolysis. VI. A reappraisal of the requirement for protein synthesis during T cell-mediated lysis, *J. Immunol.* 116:146.

Thorn, R.M., and Henney, C.S., 1976b, Enumeration of specific cytotoxic T cells, *Nature (London)* 262:75.

Todd, R., 1975, Functional characterization of membrane components of cytotoxic peritoneal exudate T lymphocytes. II. Trypsin sensitivity of the killer cell receptor, *Transplantation* 20:314.

Wagner, H., and Feldman, M., 1972, Cell-mediated immune response *in vitro.* I. A new *in vitro* system for the generation of cell-mediated cytotoxic activity, *Cell. Immunol.* 3:405.

Wagner, H., and Rollinghoff, M., 1974, T cell-mediated cytotoxicity: Discrimination between antigen recognition, lethal hit and cytolysis phase, *Eur. J. Immunol.* 4:475.

Waterfield, J.D., Waterfield, E., and Moller, G., 1975, Lymphocyte-mediated cytotoxicity against tumor cells. I. Con A activated cytotoxic effector cells exhibit immunological specificity, *Cell. Immunol.* 17:392.

Wedner, H.J., Dankner, R., and Parker, C.W., 1975, Cyclic GMP and lectin-induced lymphocyte activation, *J. Immunol.* 115:1682.

Werkele, H., Lonai, P., and Feldman, M., 1972, Fractionation of antigen-reactive cells on a cellular immunoadsorbent: Factors determining recognition of antigens by T lymphocytes, *Proc. Natl. Acad. Sci. U.S.A.* 69:1620.

Wilson, D.B., 1965, Quantitative studies on the behavior of sensitized lymphocytes *in vitro.* I. Relationship of the degree of destriction of homologous target cells to the number of lymphocytes and to the time of contact in culture and consideration of the effects of isoimmune serum, *J. Exp. Med.* 122:143.

Zagury, D., Bernard, J., Thierness, N., Feldman, M., and Berke, G., 1975, Isolation and characterization of individual functionally reactive cytotoxic T lymphocytes: Conjugation, killing and recycling at the single cell level, *Eur. J. Immunol.* 5:818.

Chapter 8

Mechanism of T-Cell-Mediated Cytolysis:
The Lethal Hit Stage

Pierre Golstein* and Evan T. Smith

Department of Zoology, University College London
London, England

I. INTRODUCTION

The existence of cell-mediated cell-destruction systems in higher organisms (extensively reviewed by Perlmann and Holm, 1969, and Cerottini and Brunner, 1974) raises two basic questions, namely: (1) *Why;* i.e., what is the selective advantage for the reproductive multicellular individual of possessing cytotoxic devices? (2) *How*; i.e., by which mechanism(s) is a cell able to destroy another cell? This chapter deals exclusively with the latter question, delineated as follows:

First, only model cytotoxicity experiments done *in vitro* will be described or discussed, irrespective of whether similar cytotoxic phenomena occur or do not occur *in vivo*. Cell-mediated cytotoxicity will thus be considered here, not from a utilitarian immunologic point of view, but as a problem of cell physiology studied under test-tube conditions.

Second, among the various cell types that are able to exert cytotoxicity *in vitro,* we shall consider mainly thymus-derived lymphocytes (T cells). Non-T-cell-mediated cytotoxicity systems will occasionally be discussed to emphasize the differences observed between some of them and T-cell-mediated cytotoxicity. Cytotoxic T cells can be obtained through sensitization of normal T cells with allogeneic cells. Mouse antiallogeneically sensitized cytotoxic cells

*Present address: Centre d'Immunologie de Marseille-Luminy, 13288 Marseille Cedex 2, France.

were shown to be T cells (Cerottini *et al.*, 1970), with no participation of non-T cells whether sensitization had been *in vivo* (Golstein *et al.*, 1972b; Golstein and Blomgren, 1973) or *in vitro* (Wagner, 1971; Lohmann-Matthes and Fischer, 1972; Andersson *et al.*, 1973). While the experiments presented below were done with *in vitro* sensitized mouse spleen cells, the discussion will also include results obtained with *in vivo* sensitized cells of various origins. It will be assumed that we are in all cases dealing with T cells, and that they all act through the same cytotoxic mechanism irrespective of their origin or mode of sensitization.

Third, T-cell-mediated cytotoxicity may express itself not only as cytolysis, but also as cytostasis. If so, it is not known whether cytolysis and cytostasis represent two different phenomena or different degrees of the same phenomenon, and whether the same cytotoxic T cells are involved in both cases. Only cytolysis, as measured by the percentage of ^{51}Cr released by injured prelabeled target cells, will be considered in this chapter.

Fourth, the T-cell-mediated cytolytic process can be fractionated into three stages, recognition, lethal hit, and target-cell disintegration, as discussed in detail in the next section. Experimental results pertinent to the former and the latter stages will be reviewed only briefly. The main emphasis will be on a study of the mechanism of the intermediate, lethal hit stage.

II. THE THREE STAGES OF T-CELL-MEDIATED CYTOLYSIS

The present subdivision of the mechanism of T-cell-mediated cytolysis into three stages (discussed in Section II.C) results from an overlap of two different two-stage subdivisions (discussed in Sections II.A and II.B).

A. Two-Stage Subdivision into Recognition and Lytic Stages

Amos (1962) suggested that the cytolytic process included a specific recognition stage followed by a lytic stage, the mechanism of which would then be nonspecific. Indeed, evidence in favor of specific surface recognition of the target cell by the cytolytic cell accumulated over the next few years. It was first observed that sensitized lymphocytes tended to be adsorbed in greater number on "relevant" target cells (i.e., on target cells bearing determinants against which the lymphocytes were sensitized) than on nonrelevant ones (Koprowski and Fernandes, 1962; Rosenau, 1963; Wilson, 1965), which, however, did not prove that cells actually involved in cytolysis were preferentially adsorbed. Specific depletion of cytolytic activity after incubation on relevant cell monolayers

(Brondz, 1968; Golstein *et al.*, 1971; Berke and Levey, 1972) followed by elution of adsorbed cytolytic cells from the monolayers (Golstein *et al.*, 1971; Berke and Levey, 1972) gave strong evidence in favor of specific adsorption of cytolytic cells and thus of specific receptors at the surface of these cells. These experiments not only suggested an anatomic substratum for the postulated specific recognition stage, but also provided a technique for the study of this stage (see Section III). They gave no information as to postrecognition lytic events.

B. Two-Stage Subdivision into Effector-Cell-Dependent and -Independent Stages

Destruction of target cells is usually assessed through the release of ^{51}Cr from prelabeled cells over a period of several hours. It was recently realized that the continuous presence of functional effector cells was not necessary for ^{51}Cr release to proceed. Indeed, effector cells can be functionally inactivated only a few minutes after the beginning of a cytotoxicity experiment (while there is still no significant ^{51}Cr release) without suppressing subsequent specific ^{51}Cr release from the target cells. Results of this sort were obtained through effector-cell inactivation with a thermic shock (Miller and Dunkley, 1974; Wagner and Röllinghoff, 1974), with antiserum plus complement (Martz and Benacerraf, 1973), or with addition of EDTA (Mauel *et al.*, 1970; Henney and Bubbers, 1973a; Martz and Benacerraf, 1973; Martz, 1975; MacDonald, 1975), the latter causing, among other effects, the effector–target cell complexes to dissociate (Stulting and Berke, 1973; Martz, 1975). These results allowed the experimental isolation and study of an effector-cell-independent target-cell-disintegration stage. They gave little information as to pre-target-cell-disintegration events.

C. Three-Stage Subdivision into Recognition, Lethal Hit, and Target-Cell-Disintegration Stages

The results described above suggested the existence of an intermediate stage, following recognition, still requiring the presence of functional effector cells, and during which an irreversible lesion of the target cell takes place. We probably owe the first clear conceptual division into three stages to Wagner and Röllinghoff (1974). The existence of the intermediate stage was also implicit in the discussions by Martz (1975) about "programming for lysis." Isolation and characterization of this key stage, the lethal hit stage, was realized using a calcium pulse technique (Golstein and Smith, 1976; see also Section IV.C), thus giving full experimental support to the concept of a three-stage subdivision.

III. RECOGNITION

By definition, we shall call the "recognition stage" of T-cell-mediated cytolysis the sequence of events, within this process, that corresponds to the sequence of events leading to specific adsorption of cytotoxic T cells on a monolayer. We shall consider neither the nature of the T-cell receptor nor the nature of the recognized target-cell structure. We shall restrict ourselves to a short discussion of the mechanism by which these structures combine during the recognition stage.

When studies were made of the parameters governing either specific adsorption of cytotoxic cells onto monolayers (Brondz, 1968; Golstein *et al.*, 1971; Berke and Levey, 1972) or specific "conjugation" of effector and target cells (Berke *et al.*, 1975), four groups of results were obtained.

First, it was found that specific recognition by cytolytic T cells was a temperature-dependent phenomenon, occurring at 37°C, but not, or to a far

Table I. Drug-Induced Inhibition and Reversal of Specific
Adsorption of Cytotoxic T Cells on Fibroblast Monolayers

Drug[a]	Final concentration	Specific adsorption[b,c]	
		Inhibition (%)[d]	Reversal (%)[e]
Azide	4×10^{-2} M	68 (27,123)	−3 (−27,12)
DMSO	4%	86 (75,102)	−3 (−12, 8)
Phenol	10^{-2} M	89 (55,112)	8 (−20,45)
Cytochalasin B	10 μg/ml	100 (50,180)	−21 (−80,19)
Theophylline	10^{-2} M	46 (−21,117)	−9 (−20,−4)

[a]In every experiment, cytotoxic cells were processed as described below, but in the absence of fibroblast monolayers, in order to check drug reversibility under these experimental conditions.

[b]Each figure is the mean of 3 or 4 independently obtained values, the extremes of which are given in parentheses.

[c]Cytotoxic *b* anti-*d* cells were incubated for 2 hr at 37°C on either *b* or *d* glutaraldehyde-fixed fibroblast monolayers. Nonadsorbed cells were washed and tested for their cytotoxicity. The lower cytotoxicity of nonadsorbed cells from *d* monolayers with respect to that of cells from *b* monolayers was expressed as percentage specific adsorption.

[d]Cytotoxic cells were incubated at 37°C in the presence of a given drug for 10 min prior to, and throughout, the adsorption period. The percentage inhibition was obtained by comparing the values of percentage specific adsorption in the presence of a drug with control values in the absence of any drug.

[e]Cytotoxic cells were incubated on monolayers for 2 hr in the absence of drugs, which were then added for a further incubation period of 30 min at 37°C. The percentage reversal was obtained by comparing the values of percentage specific adsorption with delayed addition of a drug with control values in the absence of any drug. Note the absence of high positive figures of percentage reversal.

lesser extent, at 4°C (Golstein *et al.*, 1971; Wekerle *et al.*, 1972; Berke and Gabison, 1975). This is a sharp contrast to the temperature-independence of antigen recognition by B cells (Wigzell, 1970), and is in very good agreement with the temperature-dependence of antigen recognition by other types of T cells (Hämmerling *et al.*, 1975; Benacerraf *et al.*, 1975).

Second, specific recognition by cytolytic T cells required the presence of divalent cations in the extracellular medium, and Mg^{2+} was more efficient than Ca^{2+} in this respect (Stulting and Berke, 1973; Golstein and Smith, 1976; Plaut *et al.*, 1976).

Third, specific recognition could be inhibited (but not reversed) by a range of drugs, namely, azide (Wekerle *et al.*, 1972; Berke and Gabison, 1975; Todd, 1975; Table I), cyanide (Berke and Gabison, 1975), cytochalasin B (Henney and Bubbers, 1973b; Stulting *et al.*, 1973; Table I), dimethylsulfoxyde (DMSO, Table I), dinitrophenol (Wekerle *et al.*, 1972; Berke and Gabison, 1975; Todd, 1975), iodoacetate (Berke and Gabison, 1975), phenol (Table I), and theophylline (Table I).

Fourth, specific adsorption could be achieved using fixed monolayers (Golstein *et al.*, 1972a; Wekerle *et al.*, 1974; Bubbers and Henney, 1975; Stulting *et al.*, 1975), which suggests that monolayers need not be metabolically active during adsorption. Hence, the results described above would not reflect target-cell metabolic requirements for adsorption, but would apply to the cytolytic T cells themselves. A word of caution should be given about the concentration of fixative used in these experiments. With the batch of glutaraldehyde used in our earlier work (Golstein *et al.*, 1972a), monolayers fixed with a 0.25% solution (this being the lowest concentration to confer satisfactory resistance of fixed monolayers to trypsin) supported significant specific adsorption of cytolytic cells. Other groups usually had to resort to much lower concentrations. With another batch of glutaraldehyde, fixation at a concentration of 0.02% conferred to fibroblast monolayers significant resistance to trypsin and to drugs, thus enabling us to perform the specific adsorption experiments described in Table I. Higher concentrations with this batch of glutaraldehyde resulted in lower levels of specific adsorption. Whatever the exact concentration of glutaraldehyde used for fixation of monolayers supporting specific adsorption, the degree of fixation at this concentration was shown through relative resistance of the treated monolayers to trypsinization and drugs, and through their inability to incorporate either nucleotides (Bubbers and Henney, 1975) or amino acids (Bubbers and Henney, 1975; Stulting *et al.*, 1975) into macromolecules.

In summary, the temperature-dependence and the effect of metabolic inhibitors, together with the feasibility of adsorption on fixed monolayers, strongly suggest that specific recognition requires an active metabolic process at the level of the cytolytic T cell itself. Also, divalent cations, preferentially Mg^{2+}, are necessary. It might be that some degree of active cell motility or flattening or both are required for a cytolytic T cell to position itself onto an adsorbing cell. This, however, would not entirely account for the characteristics of specific adsorption mentioned above, since, for instance, (1) our drug inhibition experiments (Table I) involved centrifugation of the cytolytic T cells on the monolayers (Kedar et al., 1974), and (2) antigen recognition also has different temperature requirements for B and T cells in the case of soluble antigens. It may then be that some movement of the receptors at the surface of a cytolytic T cell is necessary for specific adsorption. Receptors could move either in the plane of the membrane to ensure a high local concentration of receptors toward the adsorbing monolayer cell, or they could move perpendicularly to the plane of the membrane in a masked–unmasked pattern. This process may itself be Mg^{2+}-dependent and thus entirely account for the characteristics of specific adsorption. Alternatively, it may be Mg^{2+}-independent (like capping, for instance; Taylor et al., 1971), and specific recognition would then have to include at least another, Mg^{2+}-dependent step. More thorough studies on the role of Mg^{2+} may well provide essential clues as to the mechanism of specific recognition by T cells.

IV. LETHAL HIT

A. Introduction

The lethal hit stage follows recognition and includes events leading to target-cell disintegration. The obvious importance of this key stage of T-cell-mediated cytolysis is not matched by any detailed knowledge as to its mechanism. The lack of a direct experimental approach explains the paucity of data available so far. This in turn generated a wide range of hypotheses, of which two extremes are as follows:

First, toxicity for the target-cell membrane might be through direct contact with the somehow aggressive effector-cell membrane. This type of membrane–membrane mechanism was advocated by, for instance, Ferluga and Allison (1975), who showed that purified membrane fractions from oxazolone-sensitized mouse lymph node cells were able to lyse tumor cells in vitro. Although the relevance of these results to the mechanism of specific T-cell-mediated cytolysis has not yet been established, they certainly are consistent with the possibility of a direct membrane–membrane interaction. A simple version of the latter would be a "membrane–enzyme–membrane" mechanism by which an effector-cell-surface enzyme would attack the target-cell surface anchored through specific recognition, in a direct one-step process.

Second, at the other end of the range of hypotheses, the formation during the recognition stage of an immune complex at the effector-cell surface could trigger this cell to release a substance secondarily toxic to the target cell. Many such stimulus–secretion systems whereby a surface-triggered cell releases some of its products have been described (for reviews, see Rubin, 1970, and Becker and Henson, 1973). A popular version of this model as applied to cell-mediated cytolysis was that the toxic substance ("lymphotoxin") was released in the extracellular fluid and did not display any specificity in its subsequent lytic activity. Direct search for lymphotoxin(s) provided contradictory results (see the references in Golstein, 1974). In any case, the demonstration of the presence of a cytotoxic substance in an effector–target cell mixture supernatant does not demonstrate its relevance to the mechanism of specific T-cell-mediated cytolysis; conversely, its absence does not exclude the possibility of a role for short-lived or short-range-acting extracellular factors.

We think that both one-step membrane–enzyme–membrane and stimulus–secretion–extracellular lymphotoxin models, *in their simplest forms*, are unlikely candidates for explaining the mechanism of the lethal hit stage. They are not consistent, the latter with a requirement for *polarity*, the former with a requirement for *metabolic complexity* (two major characteristics of the lethal hit stage of T-cell-mediated cytolysis, as shown in Sections IV.B and IV.C). They may contribute, however, to the actual, more complex lytic mechanism.

B. Polarity

The effector T cell is not lysed either during or after the lytic process (Häyry *et al.*, 1972; Koren *et al.*, 1973) and, moreover, is able to kill other target cells (Berke *et al.*, 1972; Cerottini and Brunner, 1974). The survival of the cytolytic T cell can be explained in one of two mutually exclusive ways. First, the cytolytic cell may be resistant to the mechanism of lysis. Second, the cytolytic cell may be sensitive to, but protected from, the mechanism of lysis, which would be polarized toward the target cell.

The demonstration that cytolytic cells are in fact sensitive to the mechanism of lysis was achieved as follows (Golstein, 1974): A first batch of sensitized antiallogeneic cells was prepared, e.g., (C57Bl/6×CBA)F_1 hybrid anti-Balb/c (H-2^b×H-2^k anti-H-2^d, b×k anti-d for short), which are cytolytic to d target cells. A second batch of sensitized cells was prepared, e.g., k anti-b, which should destroy cytolytic cells from the first batch if those are sensitive to cytolysis. In practice, b×k anti-d cells and k anti-b cells were coincubated overnight. The lysis or at least the functional inactivation of the former was demonstrated through a very substantial drop in the residual anti-d activity compared with controls. It should be emphasized that in this genetic combination, recognition and subsequent cytolysis in mixtures of the two batches of cytolytic cells can occur in only one direction, thus eliminating the possibility of unwanted blocking or "interkill" phenomena. Also, the effect of k anti-b cells on $b \times k$ anti-d cells was not observed if the former were pretreated with anti-Θ antiserum plus complement (Golstein, 1975). Qualitatively analogous results were obtained by Martz and Benacerraf (1976); quantitative discrepancies may very well be due to the fact that a reciprocal combination of cytolytic cells, allowing interkill, was used by this author. Similar findings were also reported by Wagner et al. (1975).

Thus, the cytolytic cell would appear to be sensitive to lysis by another cytolytic cell. It is not lysed, however, when it destroys a target cell. This strongly suggests that the cytolytic cell must be protected from the lytic mechanism, which has to be polarized toward the target cell. There are admittedly a few, perhaps less likely, alternative explanations to our results, such as resistance of cytolytic cells limited to the short time when they actually kill, or existence of a different mechanism for lysis of tumor target cells and lymphoid cytolytic cells.

As discussed previously (Golstein, 1974), polarity would not be consistent with an "all-lymphotoxin" mechanism for the lethal hit: a lymphotoxin (defined as a nonspecifically cytotoxic substance) released in the extracellular fluid by the effector cell on recognition would destroy in a nonpolarized way the effector cell as well as the target cell. Soluble factors may still be involved, however, e.g., if directly injected by the killing cell into the target cell, or as an extracellular agent completing the sublytic effects of membrane—membrane interactions (see below).

C. Metabolic Complexity:
A Study Using an Analytical Ca^{2+} Pulse Method

The lethal hit stage could be experimentally isolated and manipulated using a Ca^{2+} pulse method (Golstein and Smith, 1976). This method stemmed from systematic studies on the divalent cation requirements of cell-mediated cytolysis.

1. Divalent Cations and Cell-Mediated Cytolysis: The Ca^{2+} Pulse Method

(a) Different Cation Requirements of Different Cell-Mediated Cytotoxicity Systems. In T-cell-mediated systems, it was first found that the inhibitory effect of EDTA added at the beginning of the experiments could be reversed on addition of Ca^{2+} or Mg^{2+}, the former being more effective in this respect, with murine (Mauel et al., 1970; Henney and Bubbers, 1973a) and human (Dickmeiss, 1974) effector cells. More recently, experiments using relatively cation-free media to which either Mg^{2+} or Ca^{2+} was added confirmed the Ca^{2+} requirement of human and murine T-cell-mediated cytolysis (Golstein and Fewtrell, 1975; Golstein and Smith, 1976; Plaut *et al.*, 1976). In non-T-cell-mediated systems, lysis of antibody-coated erythrocytes by murine peritoneal cells and by a subpopulation of human peripheral blood cells was found to be divalent-cation-independent (Scornik and Cosenza, 1974; Golstein and Fewtrell, 1975), whereas their lysis by murine spleen cells at low antiserum concentration and by another subpopulation of human peripheral blood cells required Mg^{2+} (Golstein and Gomperts, 1975; Golstein and Fewtrell, 1975; Golstein and Smith, 1976). On the other hand, Ca^{2+} is required for lysis of antibody-coated tumor cells by human peripheral blood cells (Golstein and Fewtrell, 1975).

(b) Different Cation Requirements of Different Stages Within T-Cell-Mediated Cytolysis. Three series of observations led us to propose (Golstein and Smith, 1976) that each of the three stages of T-cell-mediated cytolysis has its peculiar cation requirements. First, Mg^{2+} is sufficient at the recognition stage (Stulting and Berke, 1973; Golstein and Smith, 1976; Plaut *et al.*, 1976). Second, neither Ca^{2+} nor Mg^{2+} is necessary at the target-cell-disintegration stage, since the latter can take place in the presence of EDTA (Mauel *et al.*, 1970; Henney and Bubbers, 1973a; Martz and Benacerraf, 1973; Martz, 1975; Mac-Donald, 1975). Third, there is an absolute requirement for Ca^{2+} in this system (see references in the preceding section), which must therefore apply to lethal hit stage events. To summarize, Mg^{2+} is sufficient at the recognition stage, Ca^{2+} is necessary at the lethal hit stage, and neither Ca^{2+} nor Mg^{2+} is required at the target-cell-disintegration stage.

(c) The Ca^{2+} Pulse Method. Since the Ca^{2+} requirements were restricted to the lethal hit stage, the following method could be set up as an experimental handle to investigate this stage (Golstein and Smith, 1976): Briefly, cytolytic T cells and ^{51}Cr-labeled target cells were mixed in the presence of Mg^{2+} in wells of microplates, which were immediately centrifuged. Recognition could take place, but not lethal hit because of the absence of Ca^{2+}. Ca^{2+} was then added to support lethal hit stage events, which were stopped a few minutes later by the addition of EDTA. ^{51}Cr release occurred during the subsequent incubation period. The successive addition of Mg^{2+}, Ca^{2+}, and finally EDTA provided a convenient, very simple way of isolating and studying the lethal hit stage (Fig. 1). With the indicated time schedule, the Ca^{2+} pulse (i.e., the interval of time between addition of Ca^{2+} and addition of EDTA) was contaminated by a minimum amount of recognition or target-cell-disintegration events (Golstein and Smith, 1976). The Ca^{2+} pulse includes some, but not necessarily all, lethal hit stage events. In the presence of Mg^{2+} alone, the cytolytic process would go through recognition and putative Ca^{2+}-independent lethal hit stage events before falling short of the first Ca^{2+}-requiring event. Following addition of Ca^{2+}, the addition of EDTA could interfere not only with the lethal hit through removal of Ca^{2+}, but also with effector-target-cell adherence through removal of Ca^{2+} *and*

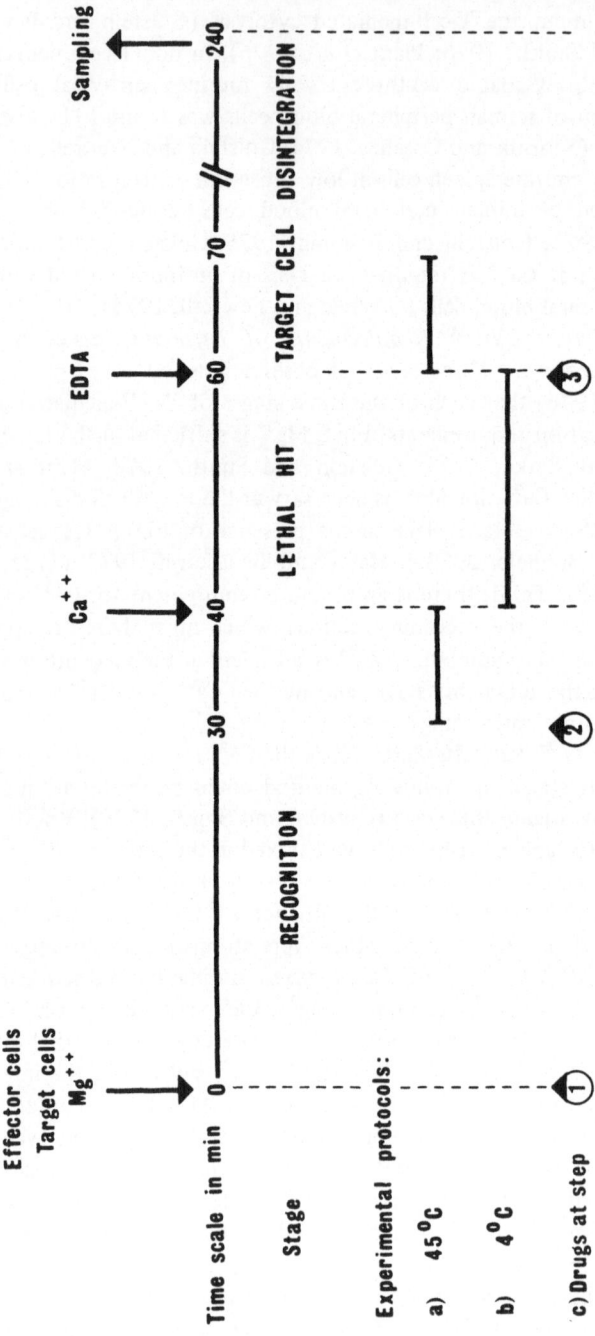

Fig. 1. The Ca^{2+} pulse method and its use with thermic shocks, temperature shifts, and drugs. On a common backbone of sequential addition of Mg^{2+}, Ca^{2+}, and EDTA, experiments involving thermic shocks (protocol a), temperature shifts (protocol b), and addition of drugs (protocol c) gave the results shown in Tables II, III, and IV, respectively.

Mg^{2+}. However, our unpublished experiments of addition of first Mg^{2+}, then Ca^{2+}, then EGTA in the presence of an excess of Mg^{2+}, and finally EDTA suggested that the lethal hit could be stopped by mere removal of Ca^{2+}, the dissociation of effector-target-cell complexes being unnecessary. Strictly speaking, the Ca^{2+} pulse method enables us to isolate, not necessarily the lethal hit stage as a whole, but a process within it stretching from its first to its last Ca^{2+}-dependent event.

For the experiments described below, the medium was a modified Eagle's medium specially prepared without $CaCl_2$ and $MgCl_2$, with 1% heat-inactivated fetal calf serum, 0.25 mM EGTA, and 0.50 mM Mg^{2+}, thus ensuring the presence of an excess of Mg^{2+} with no free Ca^{2+} until added. After *in vitro* sensitization as described previously (Golstein, 1974; Golstein and Smith, 1976), k anti-d and reciprocally sensitized control d anti-k effector cells were tested for their cytotoxicity against P815, d target cells as follows: Each V-shaped well of LS-MVC-96 Linbro microplates received a mixture of 5×10^3 ^{51}Cr-labeled P815 cells and 10^5 effector cells, in the presence of an excess of Mg^{2+}. After centrifugation of the microplates ($280g$, 2 min) and incubation for 40 min at $37°C$, Ca^{2+} was added to a final concentration of 0.50 mM, incubation proceeded for 20 min at $37°C$, and EDTA was added to a final concentration of 1 mM. The final volume was 200 μl per well. The sequential addition of 50-μl aliquots did not macroscopically disturb the cell pellet at the bottom of each well. After a further period of incubation of 3 hr, the plates were centrifuged again, the radioactivity of a 100-μl aliquot from each well was compared with the radioactivity of 5×10^3 target cells, and cytolysis was expressed as the percentage of ^{51}Cr released from the target cells in triplicate wells. Results are tabulated either as percentage ^{51}Cr release, as specific ^{51}Cr release (the difference between the percentage of ^{51}Cr released from d target cells alone and from d target cells in the presence of k anti-d or d anti-k effector cells; the latter was not significantly different from the ^{51}Cr released from d target cells alone), or as percentage inhibition (specific ^{51}Cr release in the absence of a drug minus specific release in its presence, expressed as a percentage of the former). On this experimental backbone, temperature shifts were made or drugs were added as described in Fig. 1.

2. Requirement for Functional Effector Cells

Within mixtures of effector and target cells, the effector cells can be selectively inactivated without any apparent damage to the target cells, through the use of a controlled thermic shock (Miller and Dunkley, 1974; Wagner and Röllinghoff, 1974). We incubated mixtures of effector and target cells at $45°C$ for 10 min, either just before or just after the Ca^{2+} pulse. Table II shows that such a treatment given before the Ca^{2+} pulse suppressed cytolysis, which demonstrates the necessity for active effector cells during the Ca^{2+} pulse. When given

Table II. Impact on T-Cell-Mediated
Cytolysis of a Thermic Shock Applied
Before or After the Ca^{2+} Pulse[a]

Experiment No.	Thermic shock[b]	Specific ^{51}Cr release (%)	Inhibition (%)
1	None	20	–
	Prepulse	2	90
	Postpulse	22	–10
2	None	16	–
	Prepulse	1	94
	Postpulse	14	12
3	None	39	–
	Prepulse	7	82
	Postpulse	35	10

[a]Cytotoxicity tests were performed as described in the text, except that plastic tubes (ref. 2003, Falcon) were used instead of microplates to allow for 45°C incubations in a water bath.
[b]Triplicate tubes incubated at 45°C for 10 min as indicated in Fig. 1, protocol a, either before or after the Ca^{2+} pulse.

after the Ca^{2+} pulse, it did not suppress cytolysis, which confirms that effector cells are not required any more at the target-cell-disintegration stage.

3. Temperature-Dependence

Cytolysis was suppressed if the Ca^{2+} pulse was performed at 4°C instead of 37°C (Table III). This demonstrates the temperature-dependence of at least one of the events occurring during the lethal hit stage. It should be kept in mind that not only this stage, but also recognition (Golstein et al., 1971; Wekerle et al., 1972; Berke and Gabison, 1975) and target-cell disintegration (Martz et al., 1974; Ferluga and Allison, 1974), are temperature-dependent.

4. Inhibition by Drugs

The purpose of investigating the inhibitory effect of drugs on the lethal hit stage was threefold. First, inhibition by several very different drugs would suggest for the lethal hit a complex mechanism, rather than a one-step simple enzymatic effect. Second, sequencing of drug-sensitive steps may provide a way of subdividing the lethal hit stage. Third, some drugs may affect the lethal hit stage of T-cell-mediated cytolysis and other cytolytic or model systems differently, suggesting that there are differences among these effector mechanisms.

(a) Reversible Inhibition by Azide, DMSO, Phenol, Cytochalasin B, and

Theophylline. Preliminary experiments helped to select the drugs listed in Table IV, most of which were previously shown to affect cytolysis either as a whole or at the recognition stage, while no definitive information was available as to their effect on the lethal hit stage (Wekerle *et al.*, 1972; Wolberg *et al.*, 1973; Kemp and Berke, 1973; Cerottini and Brunner, 1972; Plaut *et al.*, 1973; Henney and Bubbers, 1973b; Stulting *et al.*, 1973; Henney *et al.*, 1972; Strom *et al.*, 1972; Ferluga *et al.*, 1972; Berke and Gabison, 1975; Todd, 1975). Dose–inhibition experiments were performed with each drug to select concentrations giving maximum inhibition of cytolysis without being toxic to target cells. Also, it was found necessary to add drugs 10 min before the addition of Ca^{2+} and not just before it (results not shown). Each drug was tested at each step in at least four independent experiments, and Table IV summarizes the results expressed as average percentage of inhibition. Only dextran inhibited to some extent when added at the target-cell-disintegration stage, which is consistent with previous results suggesting a physical effect of this agent (Henney, 1974; Ferluga and Allison, 1974). That all other drugs tested did not inhibit target-cell disintegration argues against the necessity for complex target-cell metabolic events at this stage.

In the protocol described in Fig. 1, a drug can be demonstrated to inhibit the lethal hit stage if (1) it blocks when added before the Ca^{2+} pulse; and (2) it does not block when added after the Ca^{2+} pulse, since it would then be impossible to show blocking at an earlier stage; and (3) it does not reverse specific recognition, since this would modify the significance of a block when

Table III. Impact of Cold on T-Cell-Mediated Cytolysis During the Ca^{2+} Pulse

Experiment No.	Temperature during Ca^{2+} pulse[a]	Specific ^{51}Cr release (%)	Inhibition (%)
1	37°C	33	–
	4°C	4	88
	Control[b]	25	24
2	37°C	33	–
	4°C	3	91
	Control[b]	24	27
3	37°C	28	–
	4°C	1	96
	Control[b]	16	23

[a]Microplates incubated either at 37°C or at 4°C during the Ca^{2+} pulse, as indicated in Fig. 1, protocol b.
[b]Control groups were incubated for 20 min at 4°C just before the Ca^{2+} pulse. Similar results (not shown) were obtained in two other experiments with controls incubated for 20 min at 4°C just after the Ca^{2+} pulse.

Table IV. Inhibition of T-Cell-Mediated Cytolysis by Drugs
Added at Various Steps of the Lytic Process

Inhibitor[a]	Concentration[b]	Averaged[c] inhibition (%) when inhibitor added at step:		
		(1)	(2)	(3)
Azide	4×10^{-2} M	103 (78,117)	83 (71,109)	−4 (−30,13)
Iodoacetate	$5-10 \times 10^{-5}$ M	86 (67,103)	58 (27, 88)	−11 (−47,10)
DMSO	4%	101 (89,113)	71 (64, 80)	4 (−20,20)
Phenol	10^{-2} M	105 (96,113)	94 (72,136)	−5 (−17,12)
Cytochalasin B	10 µg/ml	99 (86,113)	69 (43, 83)	−6 (−21,13)
Colchicine	$3-10 \times 10^{-5}$ M	50 (33, 60)	39 (6, 71)	−7 (−16,12)
Theophylline	10^{-2} M	94 (79,106)	89 (73,106)	−11 (−32,14)
Dextran T 40	4%	76 (67, 83)	47 (19, 71)	40 (39,42)

[a]Sodium azide, iodoacetic acid, and colchicine (BDH Chemicals); dimethylsulfoxide (DMSO, Fisons Analytical); cytochalasin B (Calbiochem); theophylline (Sigma Chemicals); dextran T 40 (mol. wt. 40,000, Pharmacia).
[b]Figures refer to final concentrations in wells after the Ca^{2+} pulse.
[c]Each inhibitor was tested in at least 4 independent experiments at the steps shown in Fig. 1, protocol c. Thus, each figure represents the mean of at least 4 independently obtained values of percentage inhibition, the extremes of which are given in brackets.

the drug is added before the Ca^{2+} pulse. Condition (1) was fulfilled by all drugs listed in Table IV. Condition (2) eliminates dextran. Condition (3) was investigated by checking the ability of these drugs to detach effector cells specifically adsorbed onto fibroblast monolayers. In practice, this type of experiment can be done with reversible inhibitors only. Unpublished experiments showed that all drugs listed had reversible effects, except for colchicine, which was therefore eliminated, and iodoacetate, which will be further discussed in Section IV.C.4(b). The five remaining drugs, although blocking the specific adsorption of cytolytic cells, did not reverse it (see Table I), thereby fulfilling condition (3). It is very unlikely that the effect of drugs added just before the Ca^{2+} pulse (Table IV) is due to inhibition of new recognition events occurring during the Ca^{2+} pulse, since the observed levels of inhibition are much more than the percentage of new recognition events contaminating the Ca^{2+} pulse (Golstein and Smith, 1976). Thus, we believe that azide, DMSO, phenol, cytochalasin B, and theophylline all block the lethal hit stage of T-cell-mediated cytolysis.

It should be noted that all these drugs inhibit both recognition and lethal hit (Tables I and IV). Thus, they all have at least two sites of impact on the cytolytic process as a whole.

It was further reasoned that if events within the lethal hit followed a linear metabolic pathway, it may be possible to establish a sequence of drug-induced metabolic blocks. This can be tested by adding two drugs sequentially within the Ca^{2+} pulse, as described in Fig. 2, protocol a. Suppose two reversible inhibitors x

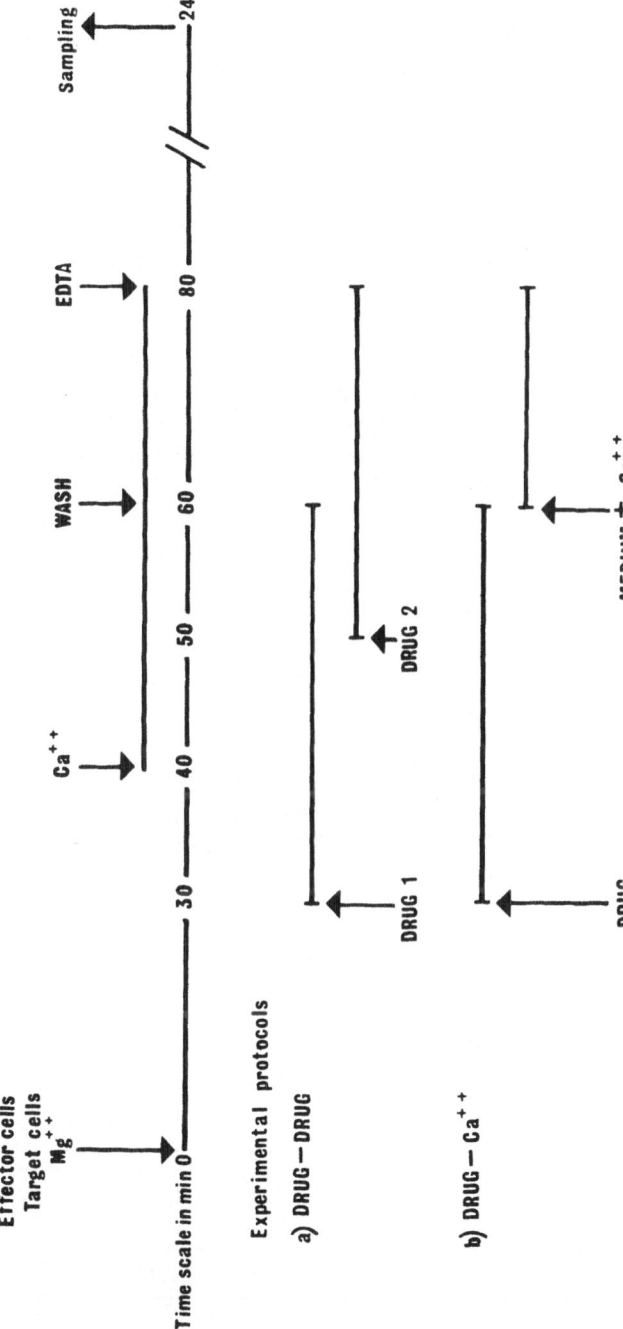

Fig. 2. The Ca²⁺ pulse method and its application to "sequencing" experiments. Protocol a consisted of addition of two drugs in succession (with an overlap that was necessary to ensure full inhibition by the second drug before removing the first one). The successive addition of a drug and medium with or without Ca²⁺ (protocol b) gave the results shown in Table X. The cell pellets were "washed" as follows: The plates were centrifuged, supernatants were carefully removed using a hypodermic needle fitted to a suction device, 0.1 ml of the appropriate solution was added to each well, and the process was repeated once.

and y, with x blocking a step situated before the step blocked by y, in a linear metabolic pathway. Drug x followed by drug y should give maximum inhibition, while drug y followed by drug x should give little inhibition. We repeatedly tested every paired combination of five drugs. In no case did we find any convincing evidence for a situation similar to the one described above, i.e., any indication of a sequence for the steps blocked by a given pair of drugs (results not shown). This may still mean that the lethal hit stage follows a linear metabolic pathway, but with multiple targets for each drug overlapping with those of other drugs. Alternatively, all drugs may act on the same event within the lethal hit stage, either through convergent pathways or directly (although the latter possibility seems unlikely; see below).

Indeed, most of these drugs are known to have multiple effects, and caution should be exercised before ascribing their action to a given metabolic step or to the alteration of a particular structure. It seems possible, however, to draw some conclusions from our results as to the complexity of the lethal hit mechanism. Known major effects of azide, phenol and DMSO, cytochalasin B, and theophylline are, respectively, blocking of electron transport, cell membrane disorganization, impairment of microfilament function, and increase of intracellular cAMP. Even if these drugs blocked the lethal hit through an effect other than their major ones, it seems unlikely that they would *directly* interfere with the same metabolic event. We should thus tentatively conclude that the clear-cut impact of these drugs on the lethal hit stage argues against a one-step mechanism, in favor of metabolic complexity.

(b) Irreversible Inhibition by Iodoacetate. In a model stimulus–secretion system, namely, the immunologic release of chemical mediators from lung fragments, there is an inhibitory effect of iodoacetate (an SH reagent, which blocks in particular the enzyme 3-phosphoglyceraldehyde dehydrogenase, thus inhibiting the glycolytic pathway). Indeed, the effect of iodoacetate could be

Table V. Effect on T-Cell-Mediated Cytolysis of Iodoacetate Added at Various Intervals Before the Ca²⁺ Pulse[a]

Cytotoxic cells	Iodoacetate added at the following times before addition of Ca^{2+}.					No iodoacetate added
	40 min	15 min	10 min	5 min	0	
k anti d	31	31	33	39	62	63
d anti k	28	24	25	24	25	25

[a]Cytolysis is expressed as percentage ^{51}Cr released from d target cells, at an effector/target cell ratio of 20:1, with or without iodoacetate (BDH Chemicals) at a final concentration of 10^{-4} M.

Table VI. Absence of Pyruvate Bypass at Varying Concentrations of Iodoacetate-Induced Inhibition of T-Cell-Mediated Cytolysis[a]

	Iodoacetate (M):	0	10^{-4}	10^{-4}	10^{-4}	10^{-4}	10^{-4}
Cytotoxic cells	Pyruvate (M):	0	0	5×10^{-3}	10×10^{-3}	20×10^{-3}	40×10^{-3}
k and d		41	22	27	28	27	30
d and k		17	21	23	21	22	23

[a] Ten minutes before the Ca^{2+} pulse, addition of 10^{-4} M iodoacetate and pyruvate (Sigma) at various concentrations. The experimental conditions were otherwise as in Table V.

bypassed by adding pyruvate, which strongly suggested a role for the glycolytic pathway in mediator release (Orange et al., 1971). We investigated the effect of iodoacetate and pyruvate in the present system.

Iodoacetate at a final concentration of 10^{-4} M was added to an ongoing cytotoxicity test at various intervals before the addition of Ca^{2+}. Almost complete inhibition was observed when 10 min elapsed between addition of drug and addition of Ca^{2+} (Table V; note that the concentration of iodoacetate that almost completely inactivated cytolytic T cells within 10 min was not obviously detrimental to the tumor target cells as judged by ^{51}Cr release over a period of time of several hours). Since iodoacetate can block, but not reverse, the specific recognition stage (Berke and Gabison, 1975) and does not inhibit the target-cell-disintegration stage (see Table IV), its effect when added just before the Ca^{2+} pulse must be at the lethal hit stage.

We then tested whether inhibition by iodoacetate could be prevented by adding pyruvate. We found that iodoacetate still blocked even in the presence of comparatively high concentrations of pyruvate, 400 times that of iodoacetate (Table VI). Cytolytic cells were irreversibly blocked by preincubating them, before the cytotoxicity test, with iodoacetate either with or without pyruvate; the results were the same whether pyruvate was present or not during the subsequent cytotoxicity test. They were also the same when using two different sources of iodoacetate (BDH and Fisons) and two different sources of pyruvate (BDH and Sigma), making it unlikely that our reagents were somehow inappropriate (results not shown).

Thus, iodoacetate irreversibly blocks the lethal hit stage of T-cell-mediated cytolysis. The present results are in contrast with those obtained in two other systems. First, the same concentrations of iodoacetate did not inhibit hemolysis by a macrophage-cell line (Walker and Demus, 1975). Second, the iodoacetate-induced block of a model stimulus–secretion system could be bypassed by pyruvate (Orange et al., 1971). That this is not the case here suggests that the iodoacetate-inhibited process within the lethal hit stage is not, or not only, glycolysis.

5. Role of Ca^{2+}

Extracellular Ca^{2+} is necessary to the lethal hit stage of T-cell-mediated cytolysis, which to our knowledge may be the only hard fact as yet about the role of Ca^{2+} in this phenomenon. When we tried to investigate it further (because of possible analogies with stimulus–secretion systems, and because Ca^{2+} might provide a means of studying the mechanism of the lethal hit), we came across a series of unexpectedly negative results.

First, preliminary unpublished experiments with M. H. Freedman gave no evidence of a ^{45}Ca uptake by effector cells significantly higher in the presence than in the absence of the relevant target cells. Similar techniques were sufficient to demonstrate Ca^{2+} influx in antigen-stimulated mast cells (Foreman et al., 1973); they may admittedly be of too low sensitivity in the present situation, and it may very well be that positive results will be obtained using improved techniques.

Second, when we looked for indirect evidence for a role of Ca^{2+} intake in subsequent cytotoxicity, we could not obtain it. We tried to induce cytotoxicity of d anti-k cells for d target cells, by "forcing" Ca^{2+} intake with a Ca^{2+} ionophore, A 23187. Use of the latter produced nonimmune mast-cell degranulation (Foreman et al., 1973). Table VII shows that the addition of the ionophore, in a Ca^{2+}-containing medium, did not induce d anti-k cells to lyse d target cells nonspecifically. It was then thought that not only Ca^{2+} entry, but also close contact between effector and target cells, might be necessary for cytotoxicity to occur. Under normal circumstances (e.g., k anti-d effector cells confronting d target cells), specific recognition would then provide both the trigger leading to Ca^{2+} entry and the close contact necessary for subsequent kill. We tested the effect on cytotoxicity of combinations of the Ca^{2+} ionophore A 23187 and an

Table VII. Effect of a Ca^{2+} Ionophore on T-Cell-Mediated Cytolysis[a]

Cytotoxic cells:	k anti-d			d anti-k			
Ratios:	50:1	10:1	2:1	50:1	10:1	2:1	None
Ionophore A23817							
10^{-6} M	66	55	36	27	27	27	26
10^{-7} M	70	62	47	27	26	25	29
None	71	63	45	28	29	27	28

[a]Cytotoxicity, expressed as percentage ^{51}Cr release, at various ratios of effector to d target cells, in the presence of various concentrations of ionophore (note that 10^{-6} M was probably toxic to effector cells; at 10^{-5} M, not shown, there was a definite toxicity toward target cells). There was no induction of nonspecific cytotoxicity by d anti-k cells.

Table VIII. Effect of a Ca^{2+} Ionophore Plus an *Axinella* Extract on T-Cell-Mediated Cytolysis[a]

Axinella[b]:	6μg/ml			0.6 μg/ml			None		
Ionophore A 23187:	10^{-5} M	10^{-6} M	None	10^{-5} M	10^{-6} M	None	10^{-5} M	10^{-6} M	None
Cytotoxic cells									
k anti-*d*	45	55	46	52	64	60	58	70	69
d anti-*k*	30[c]	23	21	32	24	21	31	25	21

[a]Cytolysis is expressed as percentage ^{51}Cr released from *d* target cells, at an effector/target cell ratio of 20:1.
[b]An extract of *Axinella polyploides,* kindly provided by Dr. M. Crumpton via Dr. Janossy. This preparation had demonstrable agglutinating ability at a concentration of 3 μg/ml.
[c]Note the toxicity of ionophore 10^{-5} M for target cells and probably also effector cells. There was no demonstrable induction of nonspecific cytotoxicity by *d* anti-*k* cells.

Table IX. Reversal of Drug-Induced Block in the Presence or in the Absence of Ca^{2+}

	Specific ^{51}Cr release with the following drugs in the prewash stage:					
Postwash addition of[a]:	Azide	DMSO	Phenol	Cytochalasin B	Theophylline	None
Drug + Ca^{2+}	1	12	7	7	7	25
Medium alone	5	12	6	9	7	18
Medium + Ca^{2+}	12	19	21	24	24	19

[a]Following protocol b in Fig. 2, drugs were added to mixtures of effector and target cells, then removed by washing and replaced either with the same drug or with medium with or without Ca^{2+}. Cytotoxicity was at about the same level whether drug or medium without Ca^{2+} was added. Reversal occurred only with Ca^{2+}-containing medium. This experiment was done three times with similar results.

extract from *Axinella polyploides* (Asherson *et al.,* 1973). The latter alone induced agglutination but no nonspecific cytolysis under our experimental conditions. Neither did the addition of the Ca^{2+} ionophore induce cytotoxicity of *d* anti-*k* cells toward *d* target cells (Table VIII). Thus, within the limits of this experiment, Ca^{2+} intake, even in the presence of an agglutinating agent, does not seem to be sufficient for induction of cytolysis.

Third, we could not dissociate drug-induced metabolic blocks from Ca^{2+}-requiring steps. Henney and Bubbers (1973a) previously attempted to sequence cytochalasin B- and EDTA-sensitive events, however, for the cytolytic process as a whole. Within the lethal hit stage, if the Ca^{2+}-requiring step(s) occur(s) before the step(s) sensitive to a given drug, reversal of the inhibition caused by this drug should take place in the absence as well as in the presence of Ca^{2+}. This was tested for each drug as described in Fig. 2, protocol b. The results (Table IX) show that the reversal of inhibition observed when the drug was replaced with Ca^{2+}-containing medium did not in fact occur in the absence of Ca^{2+}. It may be that one or more of the drugs we investigated block a hypothetical Ca^{2+} uptake by effector cells. However, all our experiments involving drugs gave the same results when performed in the absence or in the presence of the Ca^{2+} ionophore A 23187 (unpublished results). Alternatively, the results shown in Table IX could mean that Ca^{2+} is required at and/or after each drug-sensitive step. In any case, we could not show that Ca^{2+} was not necessary after the drug-sensitive steps.

Thus, while we know that Ca^{2+} is necessary to the lethal hit stage of T-cell-mediated cytolysis, we do not know exactly at which step(s) it is necessary, and we have no evidence as yet, either direct or indirect, as to the necessity, let alone any determining effect, of Ca^{2+} intake by effector cells in this system. This is in sharp contrast to the results obtained in a model stimulus–secretion system, mast-cell degranulation, in which ionophore-induced Ca^{2+} entry is sufficient to trigger degranulation events (Foreman *et al.,* 1973).

D. Discussion

1. The Lethal Hit Is Probably Not an Exclusive One-Step Membrane–Membrane Phenomenon

The metabolic complexity of the lethal hit makes it unlikely that this stage is restricted to membrane interactions, at least in their simplest forms, such as a direct one-step deleterious effect of an effector-cell membrane on the target-cell membrane. This does not exclude the possibility of membrane–membrane phenomena as part of a more complex process.

2. The Lethal Hit Is Probably Not an Exclusive Stimulus–Secretion Phenomenon

On the one hand, the lethal hit stage presents similarities to stimulus–secretion systems. An immune complex is formed at the effector-cell membrane and could provide the stimulus. There is a requirement for extracellular Ca^{2+}, and the process is temperature-dependent and can be blocked with several metabolic inhibitors.

On the other hand, several characteristics of the lethal hit make it unlikely that this is a pure stimulus–secretion phenomenon. First of all, there is a requirement for polarity. There is also an inhibition with iodoacetate that cannot be reversed with pyruvate. There is neither direct nor indirect evidence as yet for Ca^{2+} intake by the effector cells. However, this does not exclude the possibility of some stimulus–secretion pathways contributing to the lethal hit as part of a more complex process.

3. So What Is the Lethal Hit?

It is satisfying (although only moderately so) to know what the lethal hit may not be. As to what it actually is, we know only that any candidate mechanism should account for both *polarity* and *metabolic complexity*. Examples of possible mechanisms are given below, in a necessarily schematic way.

(a) Mechanisms Involving Soluble Cytolytic Molecules. These would have in common the release of soluble cytolytic molecules, through some type of stimulus–secretion process, from a shielded (vesicular?) location in the effector-cell cytoplasm. On release, the cytolytic molecules may be directly injected into the target cell (but there is no unambiguous evidence in favor of transfer of material from effector to target cell). Alternatively, inactive cytolytic molecules may be released in the extracellular fluid. They would become activated only secondarily by fixation onto the receptor–surface antigen complex, and would then lyse the target cell in a polarized way. We tested this hypothesis as follows: After incubation for 30 min in the presence of Mg^{2+}, allowing for recognition, mixtures of effector and target cells were blocked with azide before the lethal hit stage. Putative cytolytic molecules were then provided by adding supernatants from nonblocked mixtures of effector and target cells in the presence of Ca^{2+}. Table X shows that no cytolysis was generated when supernatants from nonblocked cells were added to azide-blocked complexes of effector and target cells. It could be argued that azide may interfere with the cytolytic effect. However, we did the same type of experiment, with the same results, using cell complexes blocked not by azide but by Ca^{2+} deprivation and supernatants treated with EGTA to selectively remove Ca^{2+} (unpublished results). Thus, we obtained no evidence in favor of this "hybrid" (soluble cytolytic molecules plus immune complex) mechanism for the lethal hit.

(b) Mechanisms Involving Membrane-Bound Cytolytic Molecules. Such molecules would become *actively* positioned on the effector-cell membrane at the zone of contact with the target cell, directed toward the latter, which they would then lyse. Membrane-bound esterases would be obvious candidates, since at least some cell-mediated cytolytic systems can be blocked with organophosphorus inhibitors (Ferluga *et al.,* 1972) or phosphatidylcholine (Frye and Friou,

Table X. Inability of Supernatants to Bypass an Azide-Induced Inhibition of the Lethal Hit[a]

		Ca²⁺: −	+	+	+	+
		Azide: −	−	+	+	+
	Cytotoxic cells				Sup.[b] k anti-d	Sup.[b] d anti-k
Expt. 1	k anti-d	23	68	21	19	28
	d anti-k	21	23	22	21	23
Expt. 2	k anti-d	26	65	26	28	26
	d anti-k	26	26	23	24	24

[a]Mixtures of effector and target cells, at a ratio of 150:1, were incubated in the presence of Mg^{2+} for 30 min, then for a further 15 min in the presence of azide. *Supernatants* from other similar cell mixtures (however, not treated with azide, and incubated for 30 min with Mg^{2+}, then for 15 min in the presence of Ca^{2+}) were added at a final concentration of 1:2, as well as Ca^{2+} in some of the experimental groups. Note that the addition of supernatants from ongoing cytolytic reactions did not bypass azide-induced inhibition. Values indicate per cent of ^{51}Cr released.
[b]Supernatants from mixtures of d target cells and effector cells.

1975). Such enzymes might also be targets for the blocking effect of iodoacetate [see Section IV.C.4(b)], and might account for the cytolytic activity of cell membranes (Ferluga and Allison, 1975).

Location of the cytolytic molecules may be on the inner side of membranes of cytoplasmic vesicles. On recognition, these vesicles would migrate by a metabolically active process toward the cell membrane. Cell membrane and vesicle membrane would fuse, and continuity would be established in such a way that the former inner side of the membrane vesicle would now face the extracellular space, or rather the target cell membrane, which it could lyse.

Alternatively, the cytolytic molecules may be already located at the effector-cell membrane, though in an inactive form. Activation would occur on binding of these molecules to the receptors complexed to target-cell antigens. Binding would (1) require metabolism-dependent movements of the inactive cytolytic molecules at the membrane, (2) be a or the Ca^{2+}-dependent phenomenon, and (3) account for the polarity of the subsequent lytic activity. Among several interesting features, this model does not imply any stimulus—secretion mechanism, or any Ca^{2+} intake.

V. TARGET-CELL DISINTEGRATION

Consecutively to the irreversible lesion inflicted by the effector cell during the lethal hit stage, the target cell undergoes a disintegration process, which has the following main characteristics:

First, it does not require the presence of functional effector cells, as reviewed in previous sections. Indeed, microcinematographic studies showed that the effector cell may leave the target cell before the occurrence of any obvious morphological alteration of the latter (Ax *et al.*, 1968; Koren *et al.*, 1973).

Second, there is an efflux from the target cell of components, first of small, later of larger, molecular weight (Henney, 1973; Martz *et al.*, 1974; Ferluga and Allison, 1974). Efflux of ^{51}Cr-labeled material, but not of ^{86}Rb, could be blocked with solutions of dextrans of given molecular sizes (Henney, 1974; Ferluga and Allison, 1974).

Third, there is a temperature-dependence of both ^{86}Rb and ^{51}Cr release (Martz *et al.*, 1974; Ferluga and Allison, 1974), which was attributed to the sealing at low temperature of target-cell-membrane primary lesions rather than to the involvement of an enzymic reaction in or on the target cell during disintegration, although the latter does not seem to have been completely excluded as yet.

Fourth, none of a range of drugs that inhibit the first two stages of lysis inhibits this one, under conditions allowing blocking by dextran (see Table IV).

These observations are consistent with the possibilities that (1) target-cell disintegration does not require any active target-cell metabolism, and that (2), moreover, within the target-cell-disintegration stage, the events following an initial leak of small molecules induced by the lethal hit may be of purely osmotic nature.

VI. SUMMARY AND CONCLUSIONS

The mechanism of T-cell-mediated cytolysis could be divided into three stages: specific recognition, lethal hit, and target-cell disintegration. We briefly discussed the mechanism of the former and latter stages. We examined in detail the physiology of the lethal hit stage, using in particular a recently developed analytical Ca^{2+} pulse method, and established some of the constraints to which the mechanism of the lethal hit has to comply. This allowed us to exclude some candidate mechanisms, while contributing to a characterization of the actual one.

Main characteristics of the lethal hit stage were found to be, on the one hand, polarity, and, on the other hand, requirement for Ca^{2+}; temperature-dependence; and sensitivity to azide, DMSO, phenol, cytochalasin B, theophylline, and iodoacetate, which seem to reflect a degree of metabolic complexity. The requirement for both polarity and metabolic complexity makes it very unlikely that *simple* membrane–membrane or stimulus–secretion systems are exclusively responsible for the lethal hit. Examples of possible alternative mechanisms are given.

It should be stressed that what is true for one type of cell-mediated cytolysis is not necessarily true for others as well. Indeed, the strict Mg^{2+} requirements of the lethal hit stage of non-T-cell-mediated hemolysis stands in sharp contrast to the strict Ca^{2+} requirement of the lethal hit stage of T-cell-mediated cytolysis (Golstein and Smith, 1976). This observation may be one of the first indications of different mechanisms operating in various types of cell-mediated cytotoxicity systems at the lethal hit stage. Further systematic comparative studies may be of considerable interest.

A better understanding of the lethal hit process may be reached by exploiting further the Ca^{2+} pulse method in conjunction with specific probes. It is not necessary to underline the potential importance of an elucidation of the mechanisms of cell-mediated cytolysis from the point of view of both fundamental and applied research.

ACKNOWLEDGMENTS

The authors are grateful to Miss Lynda Strong for excellent technical assistance.

This work was supported by the Imperial Cancer Research Fund, the British Medical Research Council and the Institut National de la Santé et de la Recherche Médicale.

VII. REFERENCES

Amos, D.B., 1962, The use of simplified systems as an aid to the interpretation of mechanisms of graft rejection, *Prog. Allergy* 6:468.

Andersson, L.C., Nordling, S., and Häyry, P., 1973, Allograft immunity *in vitro*. VI. Autonomy of T lymphocytes in target cell destruction, *Scand. J. Immunol.* **2**:107.

Asherson, G.L., Ferluga, J., and Janossy, G., 1973, Non-specific cytotoxicity by T cells activated with plant mitogens *in vitro* and the requirement for plant agents during the killing reaction, *Clin. Exp. Immunol.* **15**:573.

Ax, W., Malchow, H., Zeiss, I., and Fischer, H., 1968, The behavior of lymphocytes in the process of target cell destruction *in vitro, Exp. Cell Res.* **53**:108.

Becker, E.L., and Henson, P.M., 1973, *In vitro* studies of immunologically induced secretion of mediators from cells and related phenomena, *Adv. Immunol.* **17**:93.

Benacerraf, B., Unanue, E.R., Dorff, M.E., and Kennedy, L.J., 1975, Binding of the terpolymer of L-glutamic acid, L-alanine, L-tyrosine by mouse thymic lymphocytes: Inhibition by anti-*H-2* alloantisera, in: *Membrane Receptors of Lymphocytes,* pp. 127–130 (M. Seligmann, J.L. Preud'homme, and F. M. Kourilsky, eds.), North-Holland Publishing Co., Amsterdam.

Berke, G., and Gabison, D., 1975, Energy requirements of the binding and lytic steps of T lymphocyte mediated cytolysis of leukaemic cells *in vitro. Eur. J. Immunol.* **5**:671.

Berke, G., and Levey, R.H., 1972, Cellular immunoadsorbents in transplantation immunity. Specific *in vitro* deletion and recovery of mouse lymphoid cells sensitized against allogeneic tumours, *J. Exp. Med.* **135**:972.

Berke, G., Sullivan, K.A., and Amos, D.B., 1972, Tumor immunity *in vitro:* Destruction of a mouse ascites tumor through a cycling pathway, *Science* **177**:433.

Berke, G., Gabison, D., and Feldman, M., 1975, The frequency of effector cells in populations containing cytotoxic T lymphocytes, *Eur. J. Immunol.* **5**:813.

Brondz, B.D., 1968, Complex specificity of immune lymphocytes in allogeneic cell cultures, *Folia Biol.* **14**:115.

Bubbers, J.E., and Henney, C.J., 1975, Studies on the synthetic capacity and antigenic expression of glutaraldehyde-fixed target cells, *J. Immunol.* **114**:1126.

Cerottini, J.-C., and Brunner, K.T., 1972, Reversible inhibition of lymphocyte-mediated cytotoxicity by Cytochalasin B, *Nature (London) New Biol.* **237**:272.

Cerottini, J.-C., and Brunner, K.T., 1974, Cell mediated cytotoxicity, allograft rejection and tumour immunity, *Adv. Immunol.* **18**:67.

Cerottini, J.-C., Nordin, A.A., and Brunner, K.T., 1970, Specific *in vitro* cytotoxicity of thymus-derived lymphocytes sensitised to alloantigens, *Nature (London)* **228**:1308.

Dickmeiss, E., 1974, Comparative study of antibody-dependent and direct lymphocyte-mediated cytotoxicity *in vitro* after alloimmunisation in the human. II. Chemical inhibitors, *Scand. J. Immunol.* **3**:817.

Ferluga, J., and Allison, A.C., 1974, Observations on the mechanism by which T lymphocytes exert cytotoxic effects, *Nature (London)* **250**:673.

Ferluga, J., and Allison, A.C., 1975, Cytotoxicity of isolated plasma membranes from lymph node cells, *Nature (London)* **255**:708.

Ferluga, J., Asherson, G.L., and Becker, E.L., 1972, The effect of organophosphorus inhibitors, *p*-nitrophenol and cytochalasin B on cytotoxic killing of tumor cells by immune spleen cells, and the effect of shaking, *Immunology* **23**:577.

Foreman, J.C., Mongar, J. L., and Gomperts, B.D., 1973, Calcium ionophores and movement of calcium ions following the physiological stimulus to a secretory process, *Nature (London)* **245**:249.

Frye, L.D., and Friou, G.J., 1975, Inhibition of mammalian cytotoxic cells by phosphatidyl-choline and its analogue, *Nature (London)* **258**:333.

Golstein, P., 1974, Sensitivity of cytotoxic T cells to T cell mediated cytotoxicity, *Nature (London)* **252**:81.

Golstein, P., 1975, Cell mediated cytolysis. Foetal liver cells as non-T effector cells, *in vitro* educated spleen cells as T effector cells, Proceedings of the XIth International Cancer Congress, *Excerpta Med. Int. Congr. Ser.* pp. 280–284.

Golstein, P., and Blomgren, H., 1973, Further evidence for autonomy of T cells mediating specific *in vitro* cytotoxicity: Efficiency of very small amounts of highly purified T cells, *Cell. Immunol.* 9:127.

Golstein, P., and Fewtrell, C., 1975, Functional fractionation of human cytotoxic cells using differences in their cation requirements, *Nature (London)* 255:491.

Golstein, P., and Gomperts, B.D., 1975, Non-T cell mediated cytolysis of antibody-coated sheep red blood cells requires Mg^{++} but not Ca^{++}: An argument against a conventional "stimulus secretion" mechanism for cytolysis, *J. Immunol.* 114:1264.

Golstein, P., and Smith, E.T., 1976, The lethal hit stage of mouse T and non-T cell mediated cytolysis: Differences in cation requirements and characterisation of an analytical "cation pulse" method, *Eur. J. Immunol.* 6:31.

Golstein, P., Svedmyr, E.A.J., and Wigzell, H., 1971, Cells mediating specific *in vitro* cytotoxicity. I. Detection of receptor-bearing lymphocytes, *J. Exp. Med.* 134:1385.

Golstein, P., Svedmyr, E.A.J., and Blomgren, H., 1972a, Specific adsorption of cytotoxic thymus-processed lymphocytes (T cells) on glutaraldehyde-fixed fibroblast monolayers, *Eur. J. Immunol.* 2:380.

Golstein, P., Wigzell, H., Blomgren, H., and Svedmyr, E.A.J., 1972b, Cells mediating specific *in vitro* cytotoxicity. II. Probable autonomy of thymus-processed lymphocytes (T cells) for the killing of allogeneic target cells, *J. Exp. Med.* 135:890.

Hämmerling, G.J., Lonai, P., and McDevitt, H.O., 1975, Specificity and temperature requirements for T cell interaction with an antigen, in: *Membrane Receptors of Lymphocytes*, pp. 121–126 (M. Seligmann, J.L. Preud'homme, and F.M. Kourilsky, eds.), North-Holland Publishing Co., Amsterdam.

Häyry, P., Andersson, L.C., Nordling, S., and Virolainen, M., 1972, Allograft response *in vitro, Transplant. Rev.* 12:91.

Henney, C.S., 1973, Studies on the mechanism of lymphocyte-mediated cytolysis. II. The use of various target cell markers to study cytolytic events, *J. Immunol.* 110:73.

Henney, C.S., 1974, Estimation of the size of a T cell-induced lytic lesion, *Nature (London)* 249:456.

Henney, C.S., and Bubbers, J.E., 1973a, Studies on the mechanism of lymphocyte-mediated cytolysis. I. The role of divalent cations in cytolysis by T lymphocytes, *J. Immunol.* 110:63.

Henney, C.S., and Bubbers, J.E., 1973b, Antigen–T lymphocyte interactions: Inhibition by cytochalasin B, *J. Immunol.* 111:85.

Henney, C.S., Bourne, H.R., and Lichtenstein, L.M., 1972, The role of cyclic $3',5'$-adenosine monophosphate in the specific cytolytic activity of lymphocytes, *J. Immunol.* 108:1526.

Kedar, E., Ortiz de Landazuri, M., Bonavida, B., and Fahey, J.L., 1974, Cellular immunoadsorbents. An improved technique for specific depletions of cytotoxic (T) lymphoid cells, *J. Immunol. Methods* 5:97.

Kemp, A.S., and Berke, G., 1973, Inhibition of lymphocyte-mediated cytolysis by the local anaesthetics benzyl and salicyl alcohol, *Eur. J. Immunol.* 3:674.

Koprowski, H., and Fernandes, M.V., 1962, Autosensitization reaction *in vitro*. Contactual agglutination of sensitized lymph node cells in brain tissue culture accompanied by destruction of glial elements, *J. Exp. Med.* 116:467.

Koren, H.S., Ax, W., and Freund-Moelbert, E., 1973, Morphological observations on the contact-induced lysis of target cells, *Eur. J. Immunol.* 3:32.

Lohmann-Matthes, M.-L., and Fischer, H., 1972, Specific cytotoxicity of a mouse thymocyte population sensitised *in vitro* against *H-2* alloantigens, *Eur. J. Immunol.* 2:290.

MacDonald, H.R., 1975, Early detection of potentially lethal events in T cell-mediated cytolysis, *Eur. J. Immunol.* 5:251.

Martz, E., 1975, Early steps in specific tumor cell lysis by sensitized mouse T lymphocytes. I. Resolution and characterization, *J. Immunol.* 115:261.

Martz, E., and Benacerraf, B., 1976, Multiple target cell killing by the cytolytic T lymphocyte and the mechanism of cytotoxicity, *Transplantation* 21:5.

Martz, E., and Benacerraf, B., 1973, An effector cell-independent step in target cell lysis by sensitized mouse lymphocytes, *J. Immunol.* 111:1538.

Martz, E., Burakoff, S.J., and Benacerraf, B., 1974, Interruption of the sequential release of small and large molecules from tumor cells by low temperature during cytolysis mediated by immune T cells or complement, *Proc. Natl. Acad. Sci. U.S.A.* 71:177.

Mauel, J., Rudolf, H., Chapuis, B., and Brunner, K.T., 1970, Studies of allograft immunity in mice. II. Mechanism of target cell inactivation *in vitro* by sensitized lymphocytes, *Immunology* 18:517.

Miller, R.G., and Dunkley, M., 1974, Quantitative analysis of the ^{51}Cr release cytotoxicity assay for cytotoxic lymphocytes, *Cell. Immunol.* 14:284.

Orange, R.P., Kaliner, M.A., and Austen, K.F., 1971, The immunological release of histamine and slow-reacting substance of anaphylaxis from human lung. III. Biochemical control mechanisms involved in the immunologic release of the chemical mediators, in: *Biochemistry of the Acute Allergic Reactions,* pp. 189–204 (K.F. Austen and E.L. Becker, eds.), Blackwell Scientific Publications, Oxford.

Perlmann, P., and Holm, G., 1969, Cytotoxic effects of lymphoid cells *in vitro, Adv. Immunol.* 11:117.

Plaut, M., Lichtenstein, L.M., and Henney, C.S., 1973, Studies on the mechanism of lymphocyte-mediated cytolysis. III. The role of microfilaments and microtubules, *J. Immunol.* 110:771.

Plaut, M., Bubbers, J.E., and Henney, C.S., 1976, Studies on the mechanism of lymphocyte-mediated cytolysis. VII. Two stages in the T cell mediated lytic cycle with distinct cation requirements, *J. Immunol.* 116:150.

Rosenau, W., 1963, Interaction of lymphoid cells with target cells in tissue culture, in: *Cell-Bound Antibodies,* p. 75 (B. Amos and H. Koprowski, eds.), The Wistar Institute Press, Philadelphia.

Rubin, R.P., 1970, The role of calcium in the release of neurotransmitter substances and hormones, *Pharmacol. Rev.* 22:389.

Scornik, J.C., and Cosenza, H., 1974, Antibody-dependent cell-mediated cytotoxicity. III. Two functionally different effector cells, *J. Immunol.* 113:1527.

Strom, T.B., Deisseroth, A., Morganroth, J., Carpenter, C.B., and Merrill, J.P., 1972, Alteration of the cytotoxic action of sensitized lymphocytes by cholinergic agents and activators of adenylate cyclase, *Proc. Natl. Acad. Sci. U.S.A.* 69:2995.

Stulting, R.D., and Berke, G., 1973, Nature of lymphocyte–tumor interaction. A general method for cellular immunoadsorption, *J. Exp. Med.* 137:932.

Stulting, R.D., Berke, G., and Hiemstra, K., 1973, Evaluation of the effects of cytochalasin B on lymphocyte-mediated cytolysis, *Transplantation* 16:684.

Stulting, R.D., Todd, R.F., III., and Amos, D.B., 1975, Lymphocyte-mediated cytolysis of allogeneic tumour cells *in vitro.* II. Binding of cytotoxic lymphocytes to formaldehyde-fixed target cells, *Cell. Immunol.* 20:54.

Taylor, R.B., Duffus, W.P.H., Raff, M.C., and de Petris, S., 1971, Redistribution and pinocytosis of lymphocyte surface immunoglobulin molecules induced by antiimmunoglobulin antibody, *Nature (London) New Biol.* **233**:225.

Todd, R.F., 1975, Inhibition of binding between cytotoxic (T) lymphocytes and tumor target cells by inhibitors of energy metabolism, *Transplantation* **20**:350.

Wagner, H., 1971, Cell-mediated immune response *in vitro:* Independent differentiation of thymocytes into cytotoxic lymphocytes, *Eur. J. Immunol.* **1**:498.

Wagner, H., and Röllinghoff, M., 1974, T cell-mediated cytotoxicity: Discrimination between antigen recognition, lethal hit and cytolysis phase, *Eur. J. Immunol.* **4**:745.

Wagner, H., Trostmann, H., Pfizenmaier, K., and Röllinghoff, M., 1975, The cytotoxic activity of mouse T lymphocytes against allogeneic cytotoxic T cells, *Z. Immunitaetsforsch.* **150**:81.

Walker W.S., and Demus, A., 1975, Antibody-dependent cytolysis of chicken erythrocytes by an *in vitro*-established line of mouse peritoneal macrophages, *J. Immunol.* **114**:765.

Wekerle, H., Lonai, P., and Feldman, M., 1972, Fractionation of antigen reactive cells on a cellular immunoadsorbent: Factors determining recognition of antigens by T lymphocytes, *Proc. Natl. Acad. Sci. U.S.A.* **69**:1620.

Wekerle, H., Kölsch, E., and Feldman, M., 1974, T cell recognition of cell-surface antigens. II. Antigen recognition is necessary yet not sufficient for triggering T cell-mediated immunity, *Eur. J. Immunol.* **4**:246.

Wigzell, H., 1970, Specific fractionation of immunocompetent cells, *Transplant. Rev.* **5**:76.

Wilson, D.B., 1965, Quantitative studies on the behavior of sensitized lymphocytes *in vitro.* I. Relationship of the degree of destruction of homologous target cells to the number of lymphocytes and to the time of contact in culture and consideration of the effects of isoimmune serum, *J. Exp. Med.* **122**:143.

Wolberg, G., Hiemstra, K., Burge, J.J., and Singler, R.C., 1973, Reversible inhibition of lymphocyte-mediated cytolysis by dimethyl sulfoxide (DMSO), *J. Immunol.* **111**:1435.

Chapter 9

Mechanism of Specific Tumor-Cell Lysis by Alloimmune T Lymphocytes: Resolution and Characterization of Discrete Steps in the Cellular Interaction

Eric Martz

Department of Pathology
Harvard Medical School
Boston, Massachusetts

I. INTRODUCTION

A. Overview

A cytolytic thymus-derived lymphocyte (CTL)* is a specialized cell the recognized function of which is immune killing. CTLs are generated by a process of antigen-induced clonal selection, proliferation, and differentiation. Each CTL apparently recognizes a single *H-2* alloantigen. CTL targets are eukaryotic tissue cells bearing specific membrane-associated antigen, such as virus-infected autologous cells, grafted cells of genetically different origin, tumor cells, or autologous cells made more immunogenic by chemical modification. CTLs are believed to play a uniquely important role in physiological immune tissue destruction (for

---

*Abbreviations used in this chapter: (ADCC) antibody-dependent cell-mediated cytotoxicity; (cAMP) cyclic adenosine monophosphate; (CCB) cytochalasin B; (CMF) "calcium-and-magnesium-free" medium; (CTL) cytolytic thymus-derived lymphocyte; (DCM) dextran-containing medium; (EDTA) ethylenediaminetetraacetate, a divalent ion chelator; (EGTA) ethylene glycol-*bis* (β-amino-ethyl-ether) *N,N'*-tetraacetic acid, a calcium-specific chelator; (KCIL) killer-cell-independent lysis; (TSL) T-lymphocyte-mediated specific lysis.

which serum immunoglobulins are usually insufficient), probably utilizing mono-nuclear phagocytes as an amplifying mechanism.

CTLs inflict irreversible damage on specific antigen-bearing target cells within minutes after contact. However, the CTLs themselves remain unharmed, capable of repeated killing encounters. Adjacent bystander cells lacking specific antigen are also spared. These properties make the as yet totally obscure mechanism by which CTLs effect damage to target cells a fascinating problem in cell biology, as well as one of practical importance in immunology.

In this chapter, we will review recent studies, primarily those from our own laboratory, concerning the mechanism of killing by CTLs. The generation of CTLs, the nature of the antigen-specific receptor molecules employed by CTLs, and the nature of the target antigens recognized by CTLs are outside the scope of this review. Our main contribution has been to provide a technique that resolves the CTL–target cell interaction into three component steps. This technique provides virtually complete interruption between steps, which has permitted quantitative characterization of each step. Moreover, it provides a general method for elucidating the sites of drug action on T-lymphocyte-mediated specific lysis (TSL), which we have recently begun to exploit.

B. Nature of CTLs

Several independent methods have shown that the cytolytic activity in murine splenic or peritoneal cells following intraperitoneal tumor allograft rejection resides very largely or exclusively in thymus-derived lymphocytes (Cerottini and Brunner, 1974; Martz, 1975b). These CTLs can kill target cells *in vitro* alone and unaided by other cell types, including adherent or phagocytic cells, B lymphocytes, null lymphocytes, or other subpopulations of T lymphocytes (Brunner and Cerottini, 1971; Golstein *et al.*, 1972a; Golstein and Blomgren, 1973; Cantor and Boyse, 1975).

C. Nature of Target Cells

CTLs can kill syngeneic, allogeneic, or xenogeneic mammalian tissue cells, including macrophages (Brondz *et al.*, 1975), fibroblasts (Brunner *et al.*, 1967; Berke *et al.*, 1969), lymphocytes (Brunner *et al.*, 1967; Strom *et al.*, 1973c; Bevan and Cohn, 1975), adherent tumor-cell monolayers (Wilson, 1965), and nonadherent tumor cells (Brunner *et al.*, 1966; Canty and Wunderlich, 1970). CTLs are apparently unable to lyse erythrocytes or pathogenic microorganisms. The reason for the former is a mystery, since erythrocytes have surface *H-2* antigens and are readily lysed by other means, but an explanation for the latter can be surmised from recent studies indicating that the CTL receptor is limited to recognizing allogeneic or modified syngeneic major histocompatibility complex antigens (Bevan, 1975; Doherty and Zinkernagel, 1975; Shearer *et al.*, 1975; Burakoff *et al.*, 1976). Thus, CTL progenitors are probably "blind" to any cell so phylogenetically unrelated to vertebrates as to lack a cross-reacting major histocompatibility system.

D. Mechanism of Killing by CTLs

The mechanism by which CTLs damage target cells is unknown. Some insight, however, comes from several observations. First, the CTL is unharmed during the lytic interaction, and each single CTL cell can kill multiple target cells sequentially (Zagury *et al.*, 1975; Sanderson, 1976b; Martz and Benacerraf, 1976). This raises the possibility that CTLs might be resistant to their own toxin. It appears that CTLs can be inactivated by other CTLs (Golstein, 1974; Kuppers and Henney, 1976, 1977) but the possibility of a limited resistance to their own lethal hit has not been ruled out (Martz and Benacerraf, 1976).

Second, bystander cells lacking appropriate antigen, when mixed among CTLs killing specific target cells, remain unharmed (Cerottini and Brunner, 1974; Martz, 1975b). This implies that a nonspecific, stable toxin is not released by CTLs during killing (cf. Henney, 1975). This is corroborated by the failure to detect toxic activity in supernatants (Cohen and Feldman, 1971; Häyry *et al.*, 1972) or disrupted CTL preparations (Berke *et al.*, 1972a; Martz and Benacerraf, 1973b; Martz, unpublished observations). The latter findings also speak against the involvement of a specific toxin.

One striking and interesting exception to the selectivity with which CTLs attack specific antigen-bearing target cells occurs in the presence of plant lectins. When used at agglutinating concentrations during the 4-hr assay, these agents cause CTLs to kill target cells nonspecifically, as most clearly shown by Bevan and Cohn (1975). It is not clear whether simple agglutinin-induced proximity of a susceptible target-cell membrane is sufficient to trigger TSL, or whether the agglutinins must also trigger the specific CTL receptors in a nonspecific way (see Section VIII.B.2).

Third, irreversible damage is done to the target cell within a few minutes after contact (see Section V.A.). Thus, any hypothesis for the mechanism of TSL must be compatible with the speed of CTL action.

Finally, studies of the effects of drugs on TSL (see Table IV) yield some insight. Protein synthesis is not required by the CTL during killing, nor apparently is any protein depleted during killing (Thorn and Henney, 1976). It seems unlikely that any complex metabolic activity is required in the target cell for it to be lysed, since cells treated with sufficient glutaraldehyde to abolish incorporation of leucine, uridine, and thymidine are lysed efficiently by CTLs (Bubbers and Henney, 1975b).

Inhibitors of TSL include agents affecting cytoskeletal functions (cytochalasin B, colchicine), inhibitors of energy metabolism, local anesthetics, and cyclic AMP (see Table IV). Removal of divalent ions inhibits TSL, and calcium seems to play a special role in supporting CTL-administered damage (see Sections IV.C and V.E.). Since each of these agents has a broad range of effects, it is difficult to draw any mechanistic conclusions. However, elucidation of the step in the process of TSL at which each inhibitor acts may help (see Section VII).

Two known mediators of cytolysis, complement (Cerottini and Brunner, 1974) and lymphotoxin (Henney *et al.*, 1974; Gately *et al.*, 1976), seem unlikely to play a crucial role in TSL, although neither can be positively ruled out from present data.

Antibodies have often been used (without complement) to probe CTL–target cell interactions through attempts to block crucial membrane components. It has long been known that antibodies specific for target cell antigens can block TSL (see Table IV). Attempts to block TSL with antisera directed to components of the CTL membrane, however, have met with little success. In particular, antisera to immunoglobulins, CTL *H-2* specificities and Thy 1 do not block TSL (see Table IV). Kimura (1974) reported the production of an antiidiotype-like antiserum capable of blocking TSL, but this has neither been followed up nor confirmed. Thus, little information about molecules on the CTL membrane involved in TSL has resulted from this approach.

E. Importance of CTLs *in Vivo*

TSL was selected for our studies of an immune cell-mediated effector mechanism because this mechanism alone, among the several kinds of immune cytolysis that have been identified *in vitro,* is virtually certain to play a central and crucial role in graft rejection *in vivo.*

Specific allograft rejection can be induced by intravenous injection of virtually pure activated T lymphocytes into neonatally thymectomized (Sprent and Miller, 1972) or thymectomized, irradiated, and bone-marrow reconstituted mice (Rouse and Wagner, 1972). Activated B lymphocytes were insufficient (Freedman *et al.*, 1972), and macrophage function seemed unnecessary in some (Freedman *et al.*, 1972) but not all situations (Rouse and Wagner, 1972). Although the T cell populations used in these studies were rich in CTL activity, the role of the non-CTL-activated T cells probably included in these populations (Cantor and Boyse, 1975) has not been examined.

The selectivity of damage during allograft rejection supports a major role for CTLs, as distinct from macrophages, in graft rejection. Syngeneic bystander tissue is spared in graft rejection, even when imbedded in a matrix of rejected tissue (Klein and Klein, 1972; Mintz and Silvers, 1970). In contrast, bystander tissue is damaged when activated macrophages accumulate in delayed hypersensitivity reactions (Zbar et al., 1970; Bernstein et al., 1971; Wisniewski and Bloom, 1975).

II. TECHNICAL CONSIDERATIONS IN THE ASSAY OF TSL

Details of all procedures used in obtaining the data discussed in this review are given in previous and forthcoming publications from our laboratory. The purpose of this section is to explain in general terms the rationale behind the selection of certain procedures and methods.

A. Assay Container

For optimal TSL, we use 12X75 mm round-bottomed test tubes, and the cell mixture is centrifuged before incubation is begun to establish maximal intercellular contact. Plastic tubes (Falcon, Inc., Oxnard, California) are preferred because the cells slide down the uniformly rounded inside bottom to form circular pellets; glass tubes have irregular, lumpy inside bottoms, resulting in a lack of uniformity in pellet configurations, although we have no evidence that this increases variation in the results.

When the number of target cells per tube is less than approximately 1×10^4, TSL becomes less efficient (at constant sensitized/target cell ratios). The reason is believed to be that there is inadequate intercellular contact on the relatively large round bottom of the tube, since the same number of cells (e.g., 2×10^3 target cells) is killed optimally in a "V" well (Linbro Scientific Co., New Haven, Connecticut, IS-MVC-96).

Canty and Wunderlich (1970) introduced the use of petri dishes for assaying TSL. As they showed, however, insufficient intercellular contact occurs for efficient TSL unless the dishes are rocked. In several comparisons using sensitized peritoneal cells (sensitized/target cell ratio 10:1) or spleen cells (ratio 50:1) with 3×10^4 P815 cells per culture, we have always observed substantially more efficient TSL in precentrifuged stationary tubes than in rocked dishes (Martz, unpublished observations). Similar results were reported by Wagner and Röllinghoff (1974).

B. Nature and Limitations of Radiochromium Release

1. Estimation of Target-Cell Lysis by Release of Radiochromium

Taken literally, the term *lysis* means solubilization. We define lysis operationally as specific radiochromium release. While the latter does not signify total solubilization of the cell, it does indicate loss of plasma-membrane integrity sufficient to release cytoplasmic constituents of up to 3,000 daltons, and probably all soluble cytoplasmic macromolecules (see Section II.B.3).

Several factors complicate the estimation from radiochromium release of the percentage of the target-cell population lysed at any point in time. First, the most appropriate correction for spontaneous release is not known (see Section II.B.2). Second, less than 100% of the cell-associated radiochromium is solubilized immediately after T-cell-mediated lysis, usually about 65% for tumor cells (Martz and Benacerraf, 1973b; Burakoff *et al.*, 1975). Worse, this percentage depends on the way in which lysis is brought about. Detergent or distilled water lysis probably solubilizes most, freeze–thaw less, T-lymphocyte-mediated lysis still less, and antibody and complement least (Burakoff *et al.*, 1975). The nature of the culture medium is important: more isotope is soluble in EDTA-containing media (Martz and Benacerraf, 1973b), less in media at high pH (Stulting and Berke, 1973b) or with certain polyvalent cations, e.g., barium (Berke and Amos, 1973). Finally, once lysis has released the immediately soluble isotope, insoluble isotope is slowly solubilized with continued incubation at 37°C, probably by enzymatic degradation of associated particulates (Martz and Benacerraf, 1973b). There is some evidence that the percentage of isotope that is soluble varies even with incubation time after labeling, and with culture conditions (Martz and Benacerraf, 1973b).

Thus, only large differences in specific release (> 20%) can confidently be interpreted as differences in percent target-cell lysis. Smaller differences, *even though statistically significant,* may result from any of the artifacts mentioned above, and in many cases may not reflect differences in lysis.

2. Correction for Spontaneous Release

Unfortunately, target cells labeled with radiochromium slowly release the isotope in the absence of any immunologic damage. Hence, isotope released in the presence of immunologic effector cells (*e*) must be corrected for this so-called "spontaneous" release (*c*). The simplest correction, *e–c*, is often used, but underestimates the percentage of the target-cell population specifically lysed if spontaneous release is largely due to slow leakage from viable cells, rather than to spontaneous cell death (Martz, 1976a). When spontaneous release results from slow leakage from living cells, the best correction to estimate specific lysis is

$(e-c)/(1-c)$ (for an example, see Martz, 1976a). For this reason, we have used the latter computation, although the choice is arbitrary, since the mechanism of spontaneous release of radiochromium is not known (Stulting and Berke, 1973a). With either correction, misunderstandings can be avoided if two rules are followed: (1) always state the value of spontaneous release; (2) when spontaneous release exceeds about 35%, either correction becomes dubious, and it is best simply to give e and c.

3. Cytostructural Significance of Specific Radiochromium Release

Functionally, induced release of radiochromium signifies an advanced and irreversible state of deterioration. Presumably, gross discontinuities in the plasma membrane must occur to release radiochromium. Evidence supporting these beliefs is of three kinds. First, release of electrolytes or certain small metabolites always precedes the release of radiochromium. This has been shown for complement-mediated damage (Burakoff et al., 1975; cf. Green et al., 1959), as well as for TSL (Henney, 1973a; Martz et al., 1974; Martz, 1976a; Sanderson, 1976a). Second, specific radiochromium release correlates well with other measures of cell death, such as loss of cloning ability and trypan blue uptake (Wigzell, 1965; Brunner et al., 1966; Sullivan et al., 1972; Burakoff and Martz, unpublished observations; see also Section V.D.). Third, Sanderson (1976a) recently showed that specific release of [^{14}C]leucine-labeled material occurs at the same rate as ^{51}Cr during TSL, and that the former, unlike the latter, is released in a form excluded from Sephadex G25 (i.e., greater than 5000 daltons). Thus, soluble cytoplasmic proteins are probably released simultaneously with ^{51}Cr during TSL.

Recently, we estimated, by Sephadex chromatography, the molecular size of radiochromium-labeled moieties released from P815 cells (Martz, 1976b). The isotope is associated with a slightly heterogeneous peak in the size range of 2000–4000 daltons, irrespective of whether release is spontaneous, or is induced by freezing and thawing, antibody and complement, or TSL. These findings are in accord with recent reports by Kurth and Medley (1975) and Sanderson (1976a), but differ from the results of Henney (1973a), who reported a much larger size. Despite attempts to use identical conditions, we were unable to repeat the latter finding. Once chromate enters the cell, it is probably reduced immediately to Cr^{3+}, which has been shown to bind irreversibly to proteins (reviewed by Martz, 1976b). The chemical nature of the radiochromium-associated soluble cell constituents is not known.

4. Alternatives to Radiochromium

Despite the problems with estimation of lysis from radiochromium release, it is still frequently the best choice. ^{86}Rb, a potassium analogue, is a very sensitive indicator of early membrane damage, but tumor cells spontaneously release 50% in less than an hour (Henney, 1973a; Martz, 1976a). Isotopically labeled 2-deoxyglucose (Martz, unpublished observations) and 2-amino-iso-butyric acid (a nonmetabolizable amino acid; Burakoff *et al.,* 1975) have spontaneous release rates little better than [86]Rb. Nicotinamide, however, is spontaneously released at a tolerable rate, 50% in 7 hr (Martz *et al.,* 1974). It is released during TSL sooner than [51]Cr (Martz *et al.,* 1974; Sanderson, 1976a) and apparently in chemically unaltered form (Martz, 1976b). It provides a more sensitive indicator than radiochromium in titrations with antisera and complement (Kurth and Medley, 1975). Its main disadvantage is that an over-night incubation is required to get sufficient amounts into target cells.

A number of other molecules, both small and large, have rates of sponta-neous release comparable to that of ^{51}Cr, and are specifically released at the same rate as ^{51}Cr during TSL (Sanderson, 1976a). Whether any of these avoid some of the problems associated with ^{51}Cr, without introducing new ones, has not been worked out.

Thus, in many cases, radiochromium release is preferable. Its attractive features include rapid labeling, low spontaneous release, indication of irreversible damage, simplicity, speed, precision, and automation. It is subject to many artifacts, however, and the data must be intelligently evaluated.

III. RESOLUTION OF TSL INTO STEPS

We recently introduced a technique, the *detachment-and-dispersion* method, which resolves three discrete steps in TSL. This method provides, for the first time, rapid and virtually complete interruption of the lytic interaction following each of the first two steps. Before discussing our findings with this method, we shall first review findings obtained with other methods concerning steps in TSL.

A. Other Methods of Resolution

1. Specific Adhesion of CTLs to Antigenic Cell Monolayers

Brondz (1968) first showed that CTL activity is specifically depleted in the nonadherent cell population recovered following incubation of the lymphocytes on antigenically appropriate macrophage monolayers. Golstein *et al.* (1971) and Berke and Levey (1972) extended this approach by recovering specifically enriched CTL activity in the population of lymphoid cells adhering to fibroblast monolayers bearing antigens to which the CTL were sensitized. This result indicated that CTLs were binding to antigenic target cells by virtue of specific receptors, and this binding has been considered to represent the first step in the CTL–target cell interaction. Ratios of CTL activity in adherent/nonadherent lymphoid populations have subsequently been used to study the mechanism of CTL–target cell adhesion (see Sections IV and VII and Table IV). The main limitation of this approach has been that considerable nonspecific adhesion of lymphocytes to the monolayer keeps the enrichment ratios rather low. Hence, the technique is more qualitative than quantitative, and has not been adapted to give the precisely timed kinetic analyses possible with the dispersion technique. Moreover, unlike dispersion, this approach measures the recognition phase of TSL indirectly, since the adhesions are not measured by virtue of their direct progression to lysis. Thus, results obtained with monolayer adhesion need not always reflect the character of those particular adhesions that actually progress to lysis.

2. Interruption by Cessation of Rocking

Certain investigators, following Canty and Wunderlich (1970), have assayed TSL in rocked petri dishes (see Section II.A). In this assay configuration, rocking is necessary to obtain efficient TSL, since otherwise the cells are too widely dispersed in the dish to establish frequent contacts. Berke and Sullivan (1973) showed that after 30 min of rocking (at which time little specific lysis had occurred), continued rocking was unnecessary for continued target cell lysis. Moreover, this was true even when EDTA was added after 30 min of rocking. Stulting and Berke (1973) had found that EDTA could detach CTL adhering to specific target-cell monolayers. Therefore, they suggested that following 30 min of interaction with CTLs, target cells entered an intermediate state in which lysis was not complete, but could subsequently progress to completion even though the effector cells were detached by EDTA, i.e., in the absence of continued effector-cell participation. This interpretation, that there exists a prolonged killer-cell-independent stage of lysis, has subsequently been confirmed by three independent methods (Martz and Benacerraf, 1973b; Wagner and Röllinghoff, 1974; Martz, 1975a).

Other "stop-rock" experiments showed that (1) killer-cell-independent lysis was stopped at low temperatures (Berke and Sullivan, 1973), and (2) the initial CTL–target cell interaction (presumably including adhesion) is less temperature-sensitive than are subsequent events required for killing (Berke et al., 1972b). These points have also been confirmed by independent methods (Martz and Benacerraf, 1975; Wagner and Röllinghoff, 1974; Martz, 1975a).

The stop-rock method does not provide complete interruption of TSL following killer-cell-dependent events, since some specific lysis is seen in dishes never rocked (Canty and Wunderlich, 1970; Berke *et al.*, 1972b; Berke and Sullivan, 1973). Nevertheless, it was the first approach that indicated that TSL consists of a short, killer-dependent interaction followed by a long, killer-independent phase of lytic radiochromium release, and it has permitted substantial characterization of each phase (see also Table I).

3. Inactivation of CTLs by Antiserum and Complement

Ongoing TSL can be interrupted by the addition of anti-*H-2* serum, prepared so as to react with the CTLs but not the target cells, together with complement (Martz and Benacerraf, 1973b). Under proper conditions, this inactivates the CTLs within 30 min. This method provided the first unequivocal resolution of TSL into killer-cell-dependent and -independent phases. After CTLs and target cells were incubated together for 1 hr (at which time specific lysis was 10%), addition of anti-killer antiserum plus complement failed to stop subsequent radiochromium release from the majority of the target-cell population during the next few hours. Since controls demonstrated that the CTLs were totally inactivated, the target-cell lysis was described as *killer-cell-independent* (Martz and Benacerraf, 1973b; Martz *et al.*, 1974). This finding was recently confirmed by Sanderson and Taylor (1975). The term *killer-cell-independent lysis* (KCIL) has been used to mean that lysis proceeds in the absence of participation by intact killer cells; it is not meant to exclude the possibility of continued participation by subcellular fragments or products of the CTLs that may remain attached to or inside the target cell.

This method permitted the characterization of the temperature-dependence and irreversibility of KCIL (Martz and Benacerraf, 1973b, 1975; Martz *et al.*, 1974) and the observation that KCIL is accelerated when Ca^{2+} and Mg^{2+} are removed with EDTA (Martz *et al.*, 1974). Precise timing of the killer-dependent phase was not possible, however, due to the relatively slow nature of inactivation of CTLs by antiserum and complement.

4. Resolution by a Sequence of Pharmacologically Inhibited Steps

If two drugs inhibit TSL reversibly by acting at different steps in the lytic interaction, this can be detected by "inhibitor-sequencing" experiments.

For the sake of discussion, let us suppose that inhibitor *1* blocks an earlier step in the lytic interaction, and inhibitor *2* blocks a later step, both steps, however, preceding radiochromium release. Cultures initiated in the presence of inhibitor *1*, and then washed in medium containing inhibitor *2*, will proceed to the later step, where they will remain blocked; no lysis will ensue. When the inhibitors are applied in the reverse order, however, lysis should ensue: cultures initially blocked at the later step will have already completed the earlier step when inhibitor 2 is replaced with inhibitor 1.

Experiments of this type were first reported by Henney and Bubbers (1973a). Their results suggested that EDTA inhibited a step later than cytochalasin B or prostaglandin E. The levels of lysis observed were small, however, and the EDTA–cytochalasin result could not be repeated (Cerottini et al., 1974). Subsequent work by Plaut et al. (1976) has clarified this situation. In the original studies by Henney and Bubbers (1973a), insufficient EDTA was used to chelate all Mg^{2+}. As will be discussed below, Mg^{2+} is sufficient for physical adhesion to occur between CTLs and target cells, but not for efficient target-cell lysis. Adhesion is prevented when EDTA is present in excess (see Section IV.C), which explains the results of the study by Cerottini et al. (1974). As will also be discussed below, there is good evidence that cytochalasin B blocks the initial adhesive recognition step. It is therefore apparently true that removal of Ca^{2+} (leaving Mg^{2+}) inhibits a later step in TSL than does cytochalasin B. The situation with prostaglandin E is not yet so clearly resolved, since there is conflicting evidence on the effects of cyclic nucleotides on the adhesion step (see Section VII).

Henney (1973b) elsewhere reported additional sequence data for colchicine. Putting all their data together, the conclusions are that cytochalasin B, prostaglandin E, and colchicine all act at an earlier step than does EDTA (at concentrations leaving some free Mg^{2+}). Additionally, their data are consistent with the possibilities that the first three drugs all act on the same step, or that cytochalasin B may act at an earlier step than prostaglandin E, which may act at the same or an earlier step than colchicine.

Inhibitor-sequencing experiments seem a very promising approach to resolution of steps in TSL, and more effort of this type will, it is to be hoped, yield additional insights in the future.

5. Inactivation of CTLs at 45°C

Following the demonstration by Miller and Dunkley (1974) that CTLs can be inactivated by a 10-min exposure to 45°C, Wagner and Röllinghoff (1974) exploited this to interrupt ongoing TSL. Since target cells are spared by this treatment, this constituted the second method for unequivocal resolution of the killer-dependent from the killer-independent phases of TSL. More important, in this way they provided the first demonstration that the killer-cell-dependent administration of the lethal hit can take place in a few minutes. (Exact timing is complicated by uncertainty about the events taking place during the 10-min inactivation.) They also confirmed the temperature-dependence of killer-independent lysis by this independent method.

6. Manipulation of Divalent Cations

It has long been known that divalent cations are required for TSL (Mauel *et al.*, 1970), and the observations that lysis continues after addition of EDTA to an ongoing interaction (Mauel *et al.*, 1970) were first viewed as evidence for the existence of a phase of KCIL by Berke and Sullivan (1973). Recently, this phenomenon has been precisely timed. Under conditions in which EDTA largely prevents TSL when added at initiation of the cultures, MacDonald (1975) showed that addition of EDTA as little as 30 sec after initiation allows substantial lysis during the following 90 min. This procotol clearly detects a very rapid event(s), which MacDonald termed *damage*. Mere addition of EDTA, however, does not detach all adhesions, and permits continued damage to occur (Martz, 1975b; see also Section V.E.). Hence, the earliest event detected by this protocol is almost certainly adhesion, not damage.

The distinct roles of Ca^{2+} and Mg^{2+} in TSL are discussed in Sections IV.C and V.E. It is concluded there that Mg^{2+} alone is sufficient for the formation of a physical adhesion between CTLs and target cells, but that Ca^{2+} is necessary for that adhesion optimally to progress to killing. Resolution of TSL can thus be accomplished solely through manipulation of divalent cations as follows. Cultures are initiated in Mg^{2+} without Ca^{2+}, which permits the first step (adhesive recognition), but retards the second step, damage. Addition of Ca^{2+} accelerates damage. Finally, damage can be interrupted by utilizing EDTA, permitting observation of isolated KCIL.

This rationale has recently begun to be exploited by Golstein and Smith (1976; see also Chapter 8) and by Plaut *et al.* (1976). One problem with this method is that the recognition event occurring in the absence of calcium may be unphysiological (see Section IV.C.5). Another problem is that TSL is by no means stopped, although it is slowed substantially, by media containing Mg^{2+} (see Section V.E). Finally, mere addition of EDTA does not completely stop ongoing TSL (Martz, 1975b; see also Section V.E). These problems are largely avoided by the detachment-and-dispersion technique.

B. Resolution by Detachment and Dispersion

Recently, we have developed an approach that resolves three steps in TSL (Martz, 1975a). The interruption after each of the first two steps is virtually complete and very fast. This has permitted characterization of each step with greater quantitation and more precise timing than have any of the methods described above. The first step, adhesion, is detected by specific lysis following dispersion of cell clusters (without detachment) under conditions preventing further adhesions from forming. The second step, programming for lysis, is detected by specific lysis following detachment of CTLs from targets and subsequent dispersion. The third step, KCIL, is observed after allowing sufficient time for CTLs to program target cells for lysis, and then utilizing detachment and dispersion (see Fig. 1 and Table I).

1. Dispersion

The rationale behind dispersion is the following: Much evidence suggested that intercellular contact is required for CTL-mediated lysis, and that an early step in CTL–target cell interaction is the formation of an adhesion between the membranes of the two cells (see Section III.A.1). We reasoned that if CTL–target cell mixtures were sufficiently widely dispersed, no intercellular contacts would occur; thus, no adhesions could form and no lysis could ensue. If some target cells were permitted to adhere to CTLs prior to cell dispersion, however, the resulting cell clusters might remain intact, permitting completion of the lytic interaction subsequent to dispersion (see Fig. 1). Thus, the specific lysis following dispersion would equal the percentage of the target cells that had adhered to CTLs prior to dispersion.

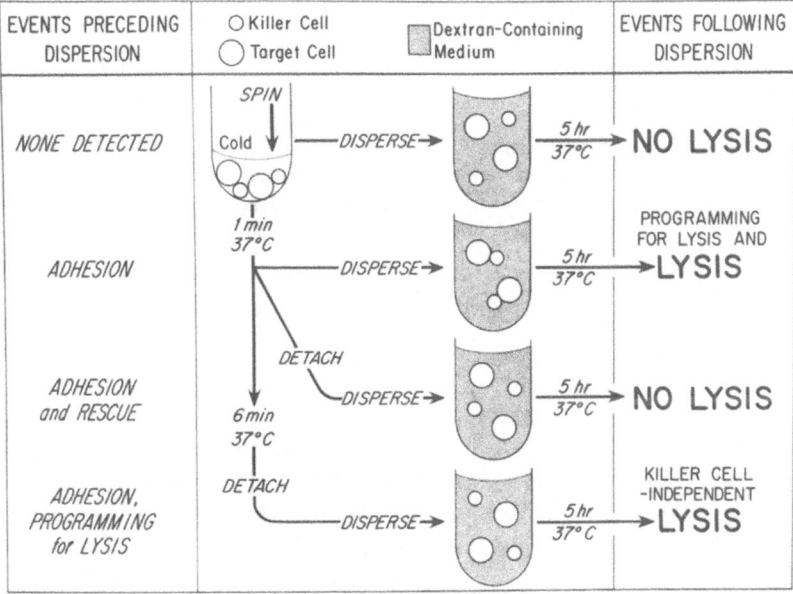

Fig. 1. Schematic diagram showing method for resolution and quantitation of three steps (adhesion, programming for lysis, and killer-cell-independent lysis) in specific T-lymphocyte-mediated cytolysis.

Table I. Definitions and Characteristics of Three Steps in T-Lymphocyte-Mediated Specific Lysis[a]

	Adhesion	Programming for lysis	Killer-cell-independent lysis
Operational definition of initiation	Undefined. Presumably triggered by receptor–antigen interaction following intercellular membrane contact.	Undefined. Could begin anytime after contact is established.	When detachment or inactivation of the CTL fails to prevent lysis.
Operational definition of completion	When dispersion fails to prevent lysis.	When detachment and dispersion fail to prevent lysis.	When radiochromium is released.
Time required for half-maximum	1 min	5 min	100 min
Q_{10} (22–37°C)	2.7	7.4	1.6
Q_{10} (37–40°C)	1.0	5.7	>1
Divalent-cation requirements	Mg^{2+} sufficient; Ca^{2+} ineffective; Ca^{2+} and Mg^{2+} synergize.	Ca^{2+} accelerates about 3.6×.	None required; EDTA accelerates.
Effects on target-cell-membrane integrity	None detected.	[86]Rb lost concomitantly.	Small metabolites lost more rapidly than radiochromium.
Loss of target-cloning ability	No. Rescued by detachment and dispersion.	Probably sooner, but not later than programming for lysis.	

[a]For supporting data and references, see appropriate sections of the text.

The stop-rock experiments of Berke *et al.* (1972b) and Berke and Sullivan (1973; see also Section III.A.2) have a similar rationale, and adhesions that form during rocking are undoubtedly detected by lysis after rocking is stopped. This method has not provided total separation between adhesion and subsequent events, however, since interruption by cessation of rocking is incomplete: some specific lysis is seen in dishes never rocked (Canty and Wunderlich, 1970; Berke *et al.*, 1972b; Berke and Sullivan, 1973).

During the development of our dispersion method, Sanderson and Taylor (1975) independently tried interrupting CTL-mediated lysis by dispersion based on slow rolling to keep cells in suspension, and recognized the possibility that their data might reflect formation of stable adhesions.

In the development of our own approach, the first problem was to find a practical, rapid, and economical method of dispersion that could totally prevent cell interaction and subsequent target lysis in CTL–target cell mixtures. Initially, we tried spreading the cells out in large plastic petri dishes, but found that some specific lysis always occurred despite extreme precautions to avoid agitation of the plates during incubation (however, cf. Berke *et al.*, 1975). Next, we considered suspending the cells in a large volume of medium that was made sufficiently viscous and dense to prevent significant settling out of the cells. To thicken the medium, we wanted an inert polymer. Dextran seemed appropriate, and a preparation with an average molecular weight of 500,000 was used to minimize any possible osmotic interference with lysis (Henney, 1974; Ferluga and Allison, 1974; Burakoff *et al.*, 1975). Specific lysis was prevented for at least 7 hr when 3×10^4 P815 cells and 40 sensitized cells per P815 cell were suspended in 2 ml culture medium containing 10% dextran (Martz, 1975a).

Our belief that the dextran-containing medium (DCM) prevented CTL-mediated killing by maintaining distance between cells, rather than by a pharmacological or osmotic effect, was supported by the following evidence: Smaller volumes of DCM permitted some specific lysis. Also, after 2 hr of incubation of cell suspensions in DCM, rapid specific lysis could be initiated by centrifuging the cells into a pellet to establish intercellular contact.

Mixtures of CTLs and target cells were centrifuged at 4°C to establish intercellular contact, and the cell pellets were incubated up to several hours on ice. Following dispersion by suspension in DCM and incubation for several hours at 37°C, no specific lysis occurred (Martz, 1975a). This showed that any interactions that may have occurred in the cold were too fragile to withstand the dispersion procedure (see Fig. 1, top line). This finding was of practical value, since mixed cell pellets can be stored on ice for considerable periods of time without the occurrence of detectable interactions between CTLs and target cells.

2. Quantitation of Adhesion by Radiochromium Release

Culture tubes containing mixed cell pellets, prepared at 0–4°C, were incubated for various times at 37°C, and the cells were then dispersed and incubation continued for 6 hr to allow all lytic interactions to reach completion. After only 1 min at 37°C, half the target-cell population lysed following dispersion (see Figs. 1 and 2; Martz, 1975a). The event responsible for this could have been either (1) adhesion of CTL cells to half the target cells (with or without damage to the target cell), or (2) if no stable adhesion is formed, contact-induced damage to the half of the target cells had become irreversible in 1 minute. The second possibility seems unlikely, since the target cells can be rescued (see Section III.B.5). The first hypothesis requires that cells of the sensitized population be observed adhering to 50% or more of the target cells. As discussed in Section III.B.3, this has been confirmed, microscopically.

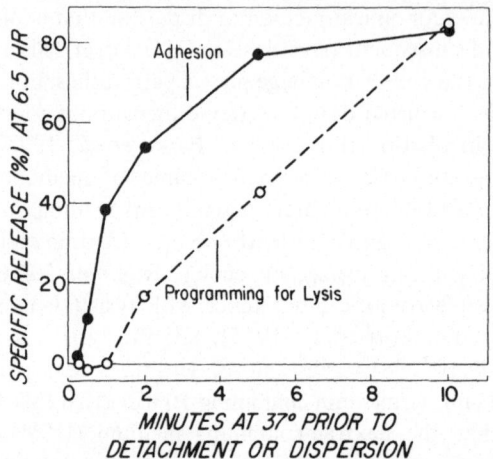

Fig. 2. Typical kinetics of adhesion and programming for lysis at 37°C. Centrifuged cell pellets containing 1×10^4 radiochromium-labeled P815 cells and 20 sensitized cells (nonadherent C57BL/6 peritoneal cells 9 days after intraperitoneal allografting with 2×10^7 P815 cells) per P815 target cell were made in 12×75 mm plastic test tubes at 0–4°C in 0.05 ml culture medium. The tubes were then placed in a 37°C water bath for the times indicated on the abcissa. To measure adhesion (●——●), interaction was interrupted by dispersion (addition of 2 ml culture medium containing 10% dextran and resuspension by vortexing). To measure programming for lysis (○————○), interaction was interrupted by detachment with EDTA (see Section III.B.4), followed immediately by dispersion. (Divalent cations in the dextran-containing medium used for dispersion remain in excess after neutralizing the EDTA.) In both cases, dispersed cultures were then incubated at 37°C for 6.5 hr to permit all lytic interactions to complete radiochromium release. Spontaneous radiochromium release was measured in identically treated control cultures from which sensitized cells were omitted, and was 24–27%.

We conclude that the specific radiochromium release that follows dispersion by suspension in DCM provides a sensitive and quantitative assay for the percentage of target cells adhering to CTLs (see Table I). This assay is capable of precise timing, enabling one to follow the kinetics of adhesion formation (see Figs. 1 and 3). The adhesions detected are remarkably stable (resist vigorous vortexing), and hence variability in the vigor of mixing used during dispersion produces little if any variation in the results (Martz, 1975a). Lysis following dispersion in DCM reaches a plateau level in 4–5 hr (unpublished data); hence, we routinely sample cultures for radiochromium release after incubation at 37°C for 5 hr (or, in some earlier experiments, 6 hr) following dispersion.

3. Morphological Corroboration of Adhesion

Size was used to distinguish sensitized lymphocytes (about 6 μm diameter) from P815 tumor cells (about 12 μm diameter) in early studies of CTL-mediated killing (Brunner *et al.,* 1966). In this way, we were able to estimate the percentage of target cells adhering to sensitized cells by observation with low-power bright-field microscopy (Martz, 1975a; cf. Berke *et al.*, 1975). This percentage was never less than, and usually exceeded, the percentage of target cells adhering to CTLs estimated by specific radiochromium release following dispersion and suspension in DCM.

4. Induced Detachment

EDTA, a nontoxic chelating agent that removes free calcium and magnesium from the culture medium, has long been used to induce detachment of cells from each other and from culture substrata. Stulting and Berke (1973b) showed that CTL adhering to antigenic cell monolayers could be detached with EDTA.

We explored this approach, and, after testing a number of variables, we selected a protocol that induces detachment of all CTLs adhering to target cells (Martz, 1975a). This protocol consists of exposing the cell clusters to 10 mM EDTA for 10 min at 37°C, followed by vigorous vortex shearing for 10 sec to complete detachment of the weakened adhesions. Morphological cluster counts demonstrated that at any time after adhesions had formed, this procedure left less than 5% of the target-cell population adhering to sensitized cells (Martz, 1975a).

The effect of EDTA on adhesions was found to be time- and temperature-dependent (Martz, 1975a). Vigorous vortex shearing alone detached few adhesions (Martz, 1975a). Although adhesions did not form at 0°C, once formed at higher temperatures, they did not detach at 0°C (Martz, 1975a).

5. Rescue After Adhesion

As described above, target cells to which CTLs have adhered go on to lyse following dispersion of the cell mixture (see Figs. 1 and 2). If the CTL are detached quickly enough, however, the target cells are "rescued," since they then fail to lyse following dispersion (see Fig. 1). Rescue at 37°C requires detachment within a few minutes (see Fig. 2). Thus, formation of a stable adhesion is not *per se* sufficient to cause the lysis of a target cell (cf. Sanderson, 1976b).

6. Programming for Lysis

When detachment is delayed by more than a few minutes at 37°C, it no longer rescues the target cells (see Figs. 1 and 2). After 7 min at 37°C, half the target-cell population is committed to lyse following detachment and dispersion (Martz, 1975a) (see Fig. 2). This rapid action of the CTL on the target cell that commits it to KCIL was termed *programming for lysis* (Martz, 1975a; see also Section VIII.B.4).

Detachment followed by dispersion provides a sensitive, quantitative assay for the percentage of the target-cell population that has been programmed to lyse at any point in time* (see Table I). Note that the 2 ml DCM used for dispersion contains sufficient calcium and magnesium to remain in excess after neutralizing the EDTA used for detachment. Hence, the cells are exposed to divalent cation depletion for only 10 min. Nevertheless, this may accelerate KCIL, since following dispersion in DCM, lysis plateaus by 3 hr. We routinely sample at 5 hr, since sampling earlier than 5 hr may not allow cultures that were not treated with EDTA to reach plateau levels of lysis.

7. Killer-Cell-Independent Lysis

In order to study KCIL, it is desirable to inactivate or detach the CTLs from target cells (which have already been programmed to lyse) by a method that does little damage to the target cells. Among the three methods now known, inactivation of CTLs by alloantiserum and complement is probably the one that interferes least with the subsequent kinetics of KCIL (Martz and Benacerraf, 1973b). When cells are prepared in this way, KCIL is accelerated in the continuous presence of EDTA (Martz *et al.*, 1974). However, EDTA does not induce lysis in target cells that may have sustained otherwise sublytic levels of damage (Martz, 1975b). Detachment of CTLs with EDTA requires exposure of the target cells to EDTA for only 10 min, but this may accelerate subsequent lysis. Hence, this method may not be ideal for kinetic studies of "undisturbed" KCIL. Moreover, the DCM used for subsequent dispersion may slow KCIL by a diffusion-limiting effect (see Section VI.C), even though high-molecular-weight dextran is used to minimize osmotic protection. Finally, heating to 45°C to inactivate CTLs, even though only 10 min is required, may also accelerate KCIL (Miller and Dunkley, 1974; Wagner and Röllinghoff, 1974).

---

*One minor technical problem connected with this assay is the possibility that programming for lysis may sometimes continue after the addition of EDTA, i.e., during the 10-min incubation at 37°C prior to vigorous vortexing, which constitutes the detachment procedure. This does not always occur, since, following substantial adhesion at 15°C, detachment and dispersion sometimes yield zero specific radiochromium release (e.g., Fig. 1 and Table 1 in Martz, 1975a). On other occasions, however, small but significant levels of programming for lysis are observed following incubation at 15°C (e.g., Figs. 3 and 4 in Martz, 1975a; Table 1 in Martz, 1975b). In these latter instances, it is unclear whether the programming for lysis occurred at 15°C prior to addition of EDTA, or at 37° during detachment. In any case, it has been unequivocally demonstrated that over periods of hours, substantial levels of programming for lysis can occur at 37°C after the addition of EDTA to ongoing interactions (Martz, 1975b). It is possible that the detachment procedure can be modified to overcome this problem. In the meantime, however, this minor uncertainty should be borne in mind (see Section V.A).

IV. CHARACTERISTICS OF ADHESION

A. Rapidity

Adhesion of CTLs to target cells is extremely rapid, often having been detected in 15 sec (Martz, 1975a). In 13 experiments, half-maximum adhesion occurred in 0.25–1.9 min (mean 0.79 min; Martz, 1975a). These times were measured with sensitized target cell ratios of more than 10, and cells had been pressed into contact by centrifugation at $4°C$ prior to placing tubes in the $37°C$ water bath. High ratios are not essential, however. In a recent experiment utilizing a sensitized (non adherent peritoneal)/target cell ratio of 1.5:1, 31% of the target-cell population (2×10^5 cells/tube) adhered to CTL in 2 min at $37°C$. Adhesion within minutes has also been noted by Berke et al. (1975).

The percentage of target cells adhering to CTLs does not readily plateau (except when it reaches 100% at high ratios). Adhesion slows with time, but continues to increase. For example, in the experiment mentioned above (sensitized/target cell ratio 1.5:1), between 2 min and 20 min, adhesion increased from 31 to 50%. Since this was measured at $37°C$, CTLs might have programmed some target cells to lyse, spontaneously detach, and moved on to adhere to additional target cells. The adhesion assay (dispersion without detachment) does not distinguish target cells adhering to CTLs from those no longer adhering to CTL, but programmed to lyse during earlier adhesive events.

However, even at $15°C$ (where programming for lysis does not occur; see Section IV.B), adhesion does not reach a clear plateau. For example, in one experiment at $15°C$ utilizing sensitized spleen/target cell ratio of 13:1, adhesion was 20% by 7 min, 37% by 30 min, but continued to increase to 48% by 90 min, and 63% by 225 min. It seems that the CTL population makes some adhesions very rapidly, but continues slowly to gather more and more target cells into stable adhesive clusters for a prolonged time. Insufficient experiments have been done at low ratios at $15°C$ to estimate the maximum number of target cells that can adhere to one sensitized cell.

B. Temperature-Dependence

Adhesion is substantially less temperature-dependent than programming for lysis. The quantitative comparison possible with the dispersion assay (Table I) confirms and extends the earlier qualitative finding of Berke et al. (1972b). Adhesion is more temperature-dependent than KCIL (Table I). It is quite possible that the temperature-dependence of the formation of adhesions sufficiently stable to withstand dispersion reflects the properties of secondary membrane "zipping-up" movements, rather than the putative primary receptor–antigen interaction. Qualitatively, however, the failure of CTLs to adhere to target cells at $0°C$ (Golstein *et al.*, 1971; Stulting and Berke, 1973b; Martz, 1975a; Berke *et al.*, 1975) is in accord with the failure of unsensitized T-lymphocytes to bind antigen in the cold (Hämmerling and McDevitt, 1974; Kennedy *et al.*, 1975; Basten *et al.*, 1975).

Recently, Cerottini and Brunner (1977) have shown that the temperature-dependence of adhesion is markedly less for CTLs produced in a secondary immune response than for CTLs produced in a primary response *in vitro*.

C. Role of Divalent Cations in Adhesion

1. Previous Evidence

Stulting and Berke (1973b) first showed that Mg^{2+} promotes adhesion of CTLs to specific antigenic cell monolayers more effectively than Ca^{2+}. This has recently been confirmed by Golstein and Smith (1976) and Plaut *et al.* (1976). Other evidence suggests that while EDTA interferes with the initiation of TSL (Martz, 1975b; Plaut *et al.*, 1976), Mg^{2+} without Ca^{2+} is sufficient to permit initiation, but retards completion of TSL (Plaut *et al.*, 1976). This is consistent with the concept that Mg^{2+} is sufficient for the initial adhesive recognition event, but that Ca^{2+} is necessary for completion of TSL.

2. Importance of EGTA

The most definitive evidence showing that Mg^{2+} is sufficient for adhesion comes from the use of EGTA (see Section IV.C.3), a ligand that chelates calcium much more strongly than magnesium (Portzehl *et al.*, 1964). EGTA is very effective at chelating Ca^{2+} in the presence of excess Mg^{2+} (i.e., where the total Mg^{2+} concentration exceeds the total EGTA concentration). EDTA also binds Ca^{2+} more strongly than Mg^{2+}, but the difference in binding strength is much less, so EDTA does not reduce the free Ca^{2+} concentration substantially when the total Mg^{2+} concentration exceeds the EDTA concentration (for an example, see Section IV.C.3). Unfortunately, no ligand exists that can chelate Mg^{2+} in the presence of excess free Ca^{2+}.

3. Sufficiency of Magnesium for Adhesion

We have recently studied the role of divalent cations in the adhesion of CTLs to tumor target cells using specific radiochromium release following dispersion in DCM to quantitate adhesion. The results of these studies will be reported elsewhere in detail (Martz, manuscript in preparation), but the main conclusions will be summarized here. In these studies, sensitized cells and radiochromium-labeled P815 target cells were "precleaned" separately by incubating for 30 min at 37°C in a *calcium-and-magnesium-free* culture medium (CMF) to which 0.1 mM EDTA had been added. Following precleaning, the cells were rinsed in CMF to remove EDTA, and resuspended in media with various divalent cation compositions. The cells were allowed to equilibrate with these final test media for 20 min at 37°C. Finally, aliquots of the CTL and P815 suspensions were mixed and centrifuged in the cold. The mixed cell pellets were then warmed to 37°C for short times to allow adhesion formation. Cells were then immediately dispersed in DCM (containing Ca^{2+} 1.3 mM, Mg^{2+} 1.8 mM), and radiochromium release was measured after 5 hr at 37°C. Since inhibition of TSL by EDTA is completely reversible on addition of Ca^{2+} and Mg^{2+}, CTLs that adhered to target cells in the controlled cation environment will complete TSL on dispersion in DCM.

An example of data obtained by this method is given in Fig. 3, and the overall findings are summarized in Table II.

Tests for the sufficiency of Mg^{2+} in supporting CTL–target cell adhesion were made in culture medium to which no calcium or magnesium was inten-

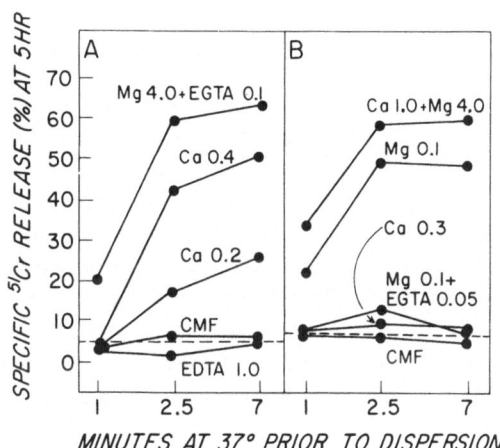

Fig. 3. Role of divalent cations in adhesion. Adhesion was measured as described in Sections III.B.2 and IV.C.3. Concentrations of cations and ligands added are given in millimolar. Basic test media were CMF (A) and Chelex-treated CMF (B). [Other, but unimportant, differences between A and B were as follows: Precleaning was in CMF containing 1 mM EDTA (A) or CMF containing 0.1 mM EDTA (B). Carryover of EDTA used for precleaning into test media was less than 0.01 mM (A) and less than 0.001 mM (B). Equilibration time (prior to testing adhesion) was 10 min (A) and 20 min (B).] Sensitized/ target cell ratios were 15:1. The horizontal dashed lines show the levels of specific release observed in controls, which were not allowed to adhere at 37°C prior to dispersion in dextran; these small but significant levels of lysis represent failure of the DCM completely to prevent new CTL–target interactions following dispersion. Hence, the *dashed lines signify zero adhesion* prior to dispersion. Spontaneous radiochromium release in cultures from which sensitized cells were omitted did not exceed 26%, and was usually 12–22%.

tionally added (except calcium pantothenate), and including 1% fetal calf serum dialyzed against divalent-cation-free saline. Such media are conventionally described as "calcium-and-magnesium-free." Contamination by divalent cations, originating largely from contamination of the reagent grade sodium chloride, is at least 1×10^{-5} M. [No direct measurements were made, but Golstein and Smith (1976) found 4.6×10^{-5} M in similar media by absorption spectrometry.] Our tests were made in the presence of 1×10^{-4} M EGTA. In the presence of excess Mg^{2+}, this is expected to reduce free Ca^{2+} at pH 7.3 to not greater than 7×10^{-8} M (Portzehl et al., 1964; assuming worst-case conditions of total calcium = 5×10^{-5} M, total magnesium = 4×10^{-3} M). (EDTA, if substituted for EGTA under these conditions, would bind only 66% of the calcium, leaving free Ca^{2+} = 1.7×10^{-5}M.) Under these conditions, magnesium was sufficient for adhesion (see Fig. 3A and Table II). While these results are consistent with earlier reports (Stulting and Berke, 1973b; Golstein and Smith, 1976; Plaut et al., 1976), the use of EGTA makes the present results more compelling by several orders of magnitude (in view of the striking synergism with traces of calcium, see Section IV.C.5).

4. Ineffectiveness of Calcium in Supporting Adhesion

When added to CMF, calcium appeared able to support adhesion nearly as well as magnesium (see Fig. 3A and Table II). To explore this situation further, the CMF was stirred overnight at $6°C$ with a chelating cation-exchange resin (Chelex-100, BioRad Labs, Richmond, California) in the sodium form (Martz, manuscript in preparation) in the hope of reducing contamination by divalent cations. When tested in this Chelex-treated medium (after removal of the resin), precleaned cells were unable to adhere in the presence of free Ca^{2+} in the range 2×10^{-5} M through 2×10^{-3} M (e.g., Fig. 3B). Thus, we concluded that calcium alone is unable to support the formation of adhesions between CTLs and P815 target cells. While other studies have suggested that calcium is less effective than magnesium in supporting adhesion (Stulting and Berke, 1973b; Golstein and Smith, 1976; Plaut et al., 1976), this is the first demonstration that in the absence of synergistic levels of other ions, calcium is virtually ineffective.

5. Synergism of Calcium and Magnesium in Supporting Adhesion

The observation that addition of calcium induced adhesion in CMF, but not in Chelex-treated CMF, raised the possibility of synergy between calcium and, presumably, magnesium. Another observation consistent with this possibility was the striking effect of omitting EGTA on the ability of magnesium to promote adhesion in either CMF or Chelex-treated CMF: 1/6 as much Mg^{2+} was adequate for half-maximum adhesion in the absence of EGTA (cf. Fig. 3B and Table II).

Synergy was easily confirmed by direct testing. For example, in one experiment using Chelex-treated CMF, Mg^{2+}, 2×10^{-5} M, gave 8% of maximum adhesion (maximum adhesion occurring in Mg^{2+}, 4×10^{-3} M, with or without Ca^{2+}, 1×10^{-3} M), and Ca^{2+}, 5×10^{-5} M, gave no adhesion. Hence the nonsynergistic adhesion expected in the presence of both would be 8%; the adhesion observed was 60% of maximal, demonstrating superadditive effectiveness. Less striking but clear-cut synergy was also seen in CMF.

Earlier studies have noted synergy in the whole process of TSL (see Section V.E), but have reported a lack of synergy in adhesion using the monolayer adsorption technique (Stulting and Berke, 1973b; Plaut et al., 1976). This underscores the considerably greater sensitivity and quantitation possible with the present dispersion method of studying adhesion.

6. Results with Other Cations

When tested in CMF, manganous ions (Mn^{2+}) were slightly more effective than magnesium in supporting adhesion. Preliminary results suggest that strontium (Sr^{2+}) is ineffective.

Table II. Divalent Cation Concentration Requirements in T-Lymphocyte-Mediated Specific Lysis[a]

Test medium	Variable cation	Adhesion step (isolated by dispersion)		TSL (without interruption)	
		Half-maximum	Optimum	Half-maximum	Optimum
CMF	Ca	0.2	0.4	0.2	0.4–1.0
	Mg	0.04	0.2–10	N.D.[b]	N.D.
Chelex-treated CMF	Ca	Ineffective	Ineffective	N.D.	N.D.
	Mg	0.05	0.2–?	N.D.	N.D.
EGTA	Mg	0.3	1–5	None	(suboptimal peak: 1–10)
Optimum Mg	Ca	<0.00007	<0.00007 to 10	N.D.	~0.05 to >2
Ca ⩾ 0.05	Mg	<0.02	<0.1 to >2	0.03	0.1 to >2

[a] All concentrations are given in millimolar. For further explanation, see Sections IV.C and V.E.
[b] N.D.: Not determined.

V. CHARACTERISTICS OF PROGRAMMING FOR LYSIS

A. Rapidity

The time required for completion of programming for lysis is surprisingly short, when compared with the time required to complete lysis as measured by radiochromium release. In an early series of five experiments (average sensitized/target cell ratio 9:1), the average time required for half-maximum programming for lysis was 7.3 min (Martz, 1975a). In three recent experiments utilizing a cell ratio of 10:1, the time required for half-maximum programming for lysis ranged from 3.0 to 4.5 min. In two experiments with cell ratios of 1.5:1 and 3:1, the half-maximum times were about 9 min. Thus, while the absolute rate of programming for lysis varies somewhat from one series of experiments to another, it usually requires less than 10 min for the majority of the target-cell population to become programmed to lyse (using nonadherent peritoneal effector cells at a sensitized/target cell ratio of about 10:1).

To measure the percentage of the target-cell population that has been programmed to lyse at an exact moment in time, the interruption of programming for lysis must be instantaneous. Inactivation of effector cells by antiserum and complement (Martz, unpublished observations) or by 45°C (Wagner and Röllinghoff, 1974) both permit considerable programming for lysis during the inactivation process, and hence are unsatisfactory for exact timing. Addition of EDTA followed by gentle vortex mixing (the first step in our detachment procedure) may also fall short of complete, instantaneous interruption, at least in certain circumstances (Martz, 1975b; see also Section III.B.6). It is a substantial improvement over either of the previous methods, however, since this method, unlike the other two, completely prevents lysis when applied to CTL–target cell mixtures kept at 0°C prior to beginning the interruption procedure. Moreover, comparison of the kinetics of programming for lysis with loss of cloning ability (see Section V.D) and with specific release of ^{86}Rb (see Section V.C) reinforces the conclusion that the timing observed with this method is not substantially in error.

B. Temperature-Dependence

Programming for lysis is the most temperature-sensitive of the three steps in TSL (see Table I) (Martz, 1975a and manuscript in preparation). Since programming for lysis is much more rapid than KCIL, the latter is the rate-limiting step in TSL above approximately 22°C; below this temperature, programming for lysis becomes rate-limiting. At 15°C, adhesion can occur without significant programming for lysis. This is useful in distinguishing the effects of various treatments on the two steps in TSL (see Section VII).

C. Concomitant Electrolyte Permeability Increase

[86]Rb (a potassium analogue) was shown by Henney (1973a) to be specifically released much more rapidly than radiochromium from target cells undergoing TSL. The utility of ^{86}Rb is frequently restricted, however, by its very rapid rate of spontaneous release. For this reason, we sought a comparably small molecule with a lower rate of spontaneous release, and found that nicotinamide worked well (Martz et al., 1974). Although nicotinamide is specifically released much sooner than radiochromium from P815 cells undergoing TSL, it is specifically released a bit more slowly than is [86]Rb (Martz, 1976a). Thus, among the various isotopic indicators of target-cell damage heretofore described, ^{86}Rb provides the earliest signal, both in TSL and in complement-mediated lysis (Burakoff et al., 1975).

For this reason, we compared the rate of specific release of ^{86}Rb with that of programming for lysis (as defined in Section III.B.6). The former was measured at each point in time simply by cooling, centrifuging, and decanting the culture supernatant for isotopic counting. The latter was measured by specific release of ^{51}Cr during a 5-hr incubation following detachment and dispersion. The amount of ^{86}Rb specifically released at each point in time equaled the percentage of target cells programmed to lyse (Martz, 1976a).

This observation raises the possibility that the first, and perhaps the only, direct damage inflicted on the target cell by the CTL is a membrane lesion permeable to electrolytes and possibly small molecules. Moreover, it corroborates, by an independent and gentler method, our conclusion that the CTL effects crucial and irreversible changes in the target cell within minutes after contact.

D. Loss of Cloning Ability vs. Programming for Lysis

The P815 mastocytoma cell multiplies readily in vitro and can be cloned in soft agar. Loss of cloning ability was an early assay for T-lymphocyte-mediated killing (Brunner et al., 1966), and was used to help establish the validity of radiochromium release as an indicator of cell death (Brunner et al., 1968). Recently, we have returned to cloning studies in order to further characterize the steps now defined in TSL. Our preliminary findings indicate that (1) P815 cells that have adhered briefly to CTLs at 37°C can be rescued from loss of cloning ability by detachment and dispersion, (2) P815 cells that have adhered to CTLs for prolonged periods of time at 15°C can similarly be rescued, and (3) loss of cloning ability occurs not later, but possibly earlier, than the time programming for lysis is completed. Thus, the main conclusions we have drawn about adhesion and programming for lysis assayed by radiochromium release can tentatively be extended to apply equally to the loss of cloning ability of the target cell.

E. Role of Divalent Cations in Programming for Lysis

1. Magnesium

It does not seem feasible to test the role of magnesium in programming for lysis, since programming for lysis cannot occur in the absence of adhesion, and since the latter requires magnesium. Dose–response studies have provided no evidence that magnesium plays a role in programming for lysis distinct from its role in the prerequisite adhesion, since the concentration of magnesium required for TSL does not exceed that required for adhesion (see Table II). The synergy of magnesium with calcium that can be seen in TSL (see Section V.E.2) probably reflects the synergy of these ions in adhesion (Section IV.C.5).

2. Calcium

Mauel et al. (1970) first observed that calcium was more effective than magnesium in reversing inhibition of TSL by EDTA, and this has subsequently been confirmed by many workers (e.g., Henney and Bubbers, 1973a). This, together with the evidence that magnesium is sufficient for adhesion (Section IV.C.3) and that KCIL requires no divalent cations (Martz and Benacerraf, 1973b; Martz et al., 1974), suggests that calcium is specifically required in the programming for lysis step (Golstein and Smith, 1976 and Chapter 8; Plaut et al., 1976). Direct examination of the effect of calcium on programming for lysis, utilizing detachment and dispersion, has not yet been undertaken. At present, therefore, our evidence about the role of calcium comes from studies of the process of TSL as a whole.

Recent reports have tended to convey the impression that the "requirement" for calcium in TSL is absolute (Golstein and Fewtrell, 1975; Golstein and Smith, 1976 and Chapter 8; Plaut et al., 1976). Complete inhibition of TSL by removal of calcium (or both calcium and magnesium) is best seen with short periods of observation or effector cells of low activity. With longer periods of observation and high sensitized/target cell ratios, however, TSL can proceed in the absence of free calcium, and even in the absence of both calcium and magnesium (see below).

We have recently studied TSL in media of defined cation content following separate preincubation of sensitized and target cells in EDTA for 30 min at 37°C. We shall refer below to such cells as *precleaned*.

Even when cells are precleaned and assayed in high concentrations of EDTA (10 mM), significant TSL is observed. Centrifugation at the initiation of incubation can greatly augment the amount of specific lysis occurring in excess EDTA; for example, 50% specific release in 4 hr is possible (Martz, 1975b). This effect of centrifugation in divalent-cation-free media has recently been confirmed by Plaut *et al.* (1976). The limited evidence available (Borle, 1968) suggests that intracellular calcium and magnesium concentrations are not much depleted by extracellular EDTA. Therefore, even with excess EDTA in the bulk medium, tightly packed cells may be able to produce local accumulations of divalent cations sufficient for TSL using intracellular stores. Thus, the question of whether either ion is absolutely required for TSL is difficult to resolve by the straightforward approach, and remains unanswered.

An estimate of the effectiveness of divalent cation chelation at inhibiting TSL can be made by comparing the rates of uninterrupted TSL in the presence of physiological levels of magnesium together with EGTA (which chelates calcium but not magnesium), in EDTA, and in controls. We have completed a series of eight such experiments utilizing precleaned cells (Martz, manuscript in preparation). Rates were based on the times required for half-maximum specific lysis. In control cultures with both Ca^{2+} and Mg^{2+}, at sensitized/target cell ratios of 5–20:1, half-times ranged from 0.6 to 2.5 hr in individual experiments. The ratios of half-times in EGTA + Mg to positive control half-times ranged from 1.9 to 6.1, with a mean of 3.6. Thus, the removal of free Ca^{2+}, leaving free Mg^{2+} at normal levels (1–2 mM), inhibited TSL by 3.6-fold. (Since KCIL is the rate-limiting step in uninterrupted TSL, programming for lysis is probably slowed considerably more than 3.6-fold under these conditions.) Operationally speaking, therefore, while extracellular calcium accelerates TSL severalfold, it is not absolutely required.

Inhibition by EDTA was sufficiently great that half-times could only be estimated by extrapolation. In this way, results from five experiments with cell ratios of 15:1 or 20:1 showed a minimum inhibition of about sevenfold; in three experiments with cell ratios of 5–10:1, inhibition exceeded twentyfold.

It has been reported (Golstein and Smith, 1976; Plaut *et al.*, 1976) that Ca^{2+} and Mg^{2+} have a superadditive effect in promoting TSL. Our results (Martz, manuscript in preparation) confirm this: with Ca^{2+} in the range of 30 to 100 μM, and Mg^{2+} at 100 μM or more, the extent of killing observed in the presence of both ions exceeded that expected from the sum of the TSL observed with each ion separately by three- to sevenfold in a series of four experiments. This synergy could well reflect nothing more than the synergy of Ca^{2+} and Mg^{2+} in the adhesion step (see Section IV.C.5).

If calcium has some specific role in programming for lysis, then TSL as a whole might require more calcium under certain conditions than does adhesion. This appears not to be the case (see Table II). With 2 mM Mg^{2+}, the concentration of Ca^{2+} required for a half-maximum rate of TSL is 20 μM; with the low levels of Mg^{2+} that contaminate so-called "magnesium-free" medium, half-maximum TSL requires 200 μM Ca^{2+} (Martz, manuscript in preparation). Neither value differs significantly from the concentrations required under similar conditions for half-maximum adhesion (see Section IV.C and Table II). The interpretation of these results is further discussed in Section VIII.

VI. CHARACTERISTICS OF KCIL

A. Timing and Temperature-Dependence

As explained in Section III.B.7, inactivation of CTLs by alloantisera and complement is presently thought to be the gentlest way to prepare target cells (previously programmed to lyse) for kinetic studies of KCIL. Using this method, data from six experiments (using sensitized spleen effector cells, which had been stored frozen, at cell ratios 18–32:1) gave an average time for half-maximum radiochromium release of 1.7 hr, and plateau lysis was achieved by 5–6 hr (Martz and Benacerraf, 1975). The effect of cell ratio and other methods of observing KCIL on the rate of KCIL has been systematically investigated.

KCIL is the least temperature-sensitive step in TSL (see Table II), but it can be nearly arrested at 0°C, which is useful for stopping lysis during sampling procedures. The significance of the effect of temperature is unclear (see Section VI.C).

As mentioned above, KCIL does not require divalent cations, and is accelerated in their absence (Martz et al., 1974). Other agents besides EDTA that accelerate KCIL are high temperature (Miller and Dunkley, 1974; Wagner and Röllinghoff, 1974) and lidocaine (Shain and Martz, 1976).

In contrast to the acceleration of the lytic phase of TSL by EDTA, the lytic phase of complement-induced lysis can be blocked by EDTA, even after specific release of ^{86}Rb has occurred (Burakoff et al., 1975). It is not clear whether this reflects differences in methodologies or underlying mechanisms.

B. Irreversibility

Although KCIL can be slowed or stopped at low temperatures, no recovery or repair takes place, since lysis reaches control levels on rewarming to 37°C (Martz and Benacerraf, 1975).

C. Role of Colloid Osmotic Lysis in KCIL

If the primary damage inflicted by CTLs is an electrolyte-permeable membrane lesion, this alone might be sufficient to induce lysis secondarily as a result of colloid osmotic swelling. This has been proposed as the mechanism of complement-mediated lysis (Green et al., 1959; Seeman, 1974; Lauf, 1975). In the latter case, lysis can be prevented, even following damage sufficient to cause loss of ^{42}K or ^{86}Rb, by high concentrations of extracellular macromolecules (Green et al., 1959; Burakoff et al., 1975). Since these macromolecules could balance the colloid osmotic pressure due to intracellular protein, this inhibition has been regarded as due to colloid osmotic protection. Consequently, estimates of the size of the primary complement-induced permeability lesion have been based on the minimum molecular weight of extracellular solutes conferring protection (Green and Goldberg, 1960; Sears et al., 1964).

However, these studies failed to consider an alternative interpretation of the protection by extracellular macromolecular solutes, namely, a barrier to escape by diffusion of intracellular solutes used to monitor lysis (Davies et al., 1968; Seeman, 1972). This latter possibility, which is consistent with all the data, would make estimation of the size of the membrane lesion impossible by the method described above.

Two studies have shown that TSL can be inhibited by extracellular macromolecules following specific release of ^{86}Rb (Henney, 1974; Ferluga and Allison, 1974). Here, too, the data are consistent with either an osmotic or a diffusion-limiting protective mechanism, although the molar concentrations employed favor the latter. These studies therefore do not provide proof of a colloid osmotic mechanism in TSL, nor do they provide reliable estimates of the size of the T-cell-induced lytic lesion.

Despite these difficulties in demonstrating colloid osmotic phenomena, colloid osmotic lysis remains a highly plausible component in TSL.

When we first observed the temperature sensitivity of KCIL, we thought it implied a metabolic process, rather than a purely physical process like colloid osmotic lysis (Martz and Benacerraf, 1974). Subsequently, however, we showed that the supposedly colloid osmotic phase of complement-induced lysis of P815 tumor cells is equally temperature-sensitive (Burakoff et al., 1975). It is possible that minimally damaged tumor cells simply gel at 0°C and trap most intracytoplasmic constituents. In any case, this finding removes any need to postulate requirements above and beyond colloid osmotic lysis during the KCIL phase of TSL.

VII. SITES OF ACTION OF DRUGS INHIBITING TSL

A. Previous Information

Some information about the mechanism of TSL can be surmised from the types of drugs that inhibit or stimulate it (see Section I.D). Considerable effort has been devoted to studies of the effects of drugs, enzymes, and antibodies on TSL, and we have attempted to summarize present knowledge in Table IV. Knowledge of exactly where each drug acts, in the sequence of steps comprising TSL, would increase our understanding of the mechanism of TSL.

Inhibition of specific adhesion of CTLs to antigenic cell monolayers has been shown using EDTA, inhibitors of energy metabolism (azide and dinitrophenol), cytochalasins A and B, and antibody to target *H-2* specificities (for details and references, see Table IV). Inhibition by drugs affecting energy metabolism has recently been confirmed using counts of CTL–target cell clusters (Table IV). Detachment of CTLs adhering to monolayers has been achieved with EDTA, protease, pH 5.5, and partially with antiserum to target *H-2* specificities (Table IV).

Thus, in addition to depending on unimpeded exposure of the relevant target-cell antigens, CTL–target cell adhesion requires divalent cations (see Section IV.C), an energy source, and cytoplasmic microfilament function. Except for cytochalasin A in the latter case, all inhibitors are reversible, and hence these requirements may pertain to the CTL, the target cell, or both. However, the ability of CTL specifically to adhere to and lyse target cells pretreated with sufficient glutaraldehyde to abolish protein synthesis (Bubbers and Henney, 1975b) suggests that the metabolic requirements pertain exclusively to the CTL.

Heretofore, it has not been possible to isolate the programming for lysis step for inhibitor studies. Some conclusions can be drawn, however, from previous work. As has already been discussed (Section V.E), calcium is more important in programming for lysis than in adhesion, and thus Mg–EGTA (or Mg–EDTA) is a specific inhibitor of programming for lysis. Similar activity has also been suggested for two partial inhibitors of TSL, cAMP and colchicine, since little or no interference with adhesion by these agents was detected in one study (Henney and Bubbers, 1973b). However, this merits additional study (see Section VII.C.3).

Inhibition of KCIL has not been observed, except with high concentrations of dextran (Table IV).

B. A General Method for Investigating Sites of Drug Action

We have described how two rapid, early steps in TSL, adhesion and programming for lysis, can be resolved utilizing detachment and dispersion, and quantitated utilizing radiochromium release (Section III). Using this technique, we demonstrated that adhesion, but not programming for lysis, takes place at 15°C. Together, these observations provide the basis for a general method for investigating sites of drug action, which is outlined in Table III.

1. Testing Drugs on Adhesion Formation

To test whether a drug inhibits adhesion formation, mixed cell pellets are prepared in medium with or without drug and incubated for short intervals (0.5–5 min) at 37°C. To assess the percentage of target cells that have adhered to CTLs at each point in time, the cell pellet is dispersed in DCM, and radiochromium release is measured 5 hr later. Provided that the drug is fully reversible (that CTL activity returns after the drug is diluted to ineffective concentrations), CTLs adhering to target cells will complete TSL following dispersion. Dispersion usually dilutes the drug to subinhibitory concentrations, but if it does not, rinsing at 0°C can be carried out prior to dispersion. Thus, inhibition of radiochromium release in this protocol quantitates inhibition of adhesion formation. Separate pretreatment of CTLs and target cells with the drug is possible when the drug is slow-acting. Results can be corroborated by cluster counting (see Section III.B.3), but this is less precise, less quantitative, slower, and more tedious. Cluster counting is the best method, however, for irreversible inhibitors.

2. Testing Drugs for Detachment of Adhesions

If adhesions are allowed to form at 15°C prior to drug addition, reversible drugs can be tested for their ability to detach these adhesions by utilizing dispersion and radiochromium release. Corroboration by cluster counting is feasible (and was used to establish the detaching ability of EDTA; see Section III.B.4). When testing for detachment at 37°C (after drug addition), some programming for lysis may occur prior to drug-induced detachment. This should be measured in controls (by EDTA-induced detachment and dispersion) and discounted from the final radiochromium release, since it might otherwise be misinterpreted as failure of the drug to complete detachment.

3. Testing Drugs on Programming for Lysis

In order to test the effect of a drug on programming for lysis, adhesions are formed at 15°C prior to addition of the drug. After addition of the drug, the temperature is raised to 37°C for short intervals (2–20 min) to permit programming for lysis. The extent of programming for lysis at each time is ascertained by detachment, dispersion, and measurement of radiochromium release 5 hr later.

Table III. A General Method for Determining Sites of Drug Action Utilizing Radiochromium Release Following Detachment or Dispersion or Both

Test	Adhesion[a]	Programming for lysis[a]	KCIL[a]	Comments and Requirements
Adhesion	************* Pellet 37°C → *************	Dispersed and diluted 37°C →	(No change)	•Cells can be preequilibrated with drug. •Drug must be reversible. •Corroboration by microscopic cluster counts.
Programming for lysis	Pellet 15°C →	************* Pellet 37°C → *************	Detach → Dispersed and diluted 37°C	•Drug must be fast-acting. •Drug must be reversible. •Drug must not detach preformed adhesions.
KCIL	Pellet 37°C →	(no change) →	******************** Detach → Dispersed 37°C ********************	•Drug need not be reversible. •Drug must be stable.

[a]Asterisks indicate the presence of drug.

Using this protocol, inhibition of radiochromium release can reflect two possibilities. First, it can reflect direct inhibition of programming for lysis. Second, it can reflect a drug-induced alteration of the structure of the preformed CTL–target cell adhesion, rendering it incompatible with programming for lysis. Drug-induced detachment of the preformed adhesions is a special case of this second possibility, and one that must be controlled for. Even in the absence of drug-induced detachment, however, the second possibility is conceivable.

If the drug fails to affect radiochromium release in this test, this failure may also reflect either of two possibilities. First, failure may result if the drug has no direct effect on programming for lysis (and does not render the preformed adhesions incompatible with programming for lysis). Second, failure may result if the drug fails to take effect quickly enough to interfere with programming for lysis, which is largely completed within 10 min. If necessary, independent tests of the speed with which the drug inhibits TSL can be made to control for this latter possibility.

Tests for drug-induced detachment of adhesions and for direct inhibition of programming for lysis thus complement each other as mutual controls, and it is best to do both in a single experiment. The detachment test requires that the drug be reversible. If the programming for lysis test is run with an irreversible inhibitor, detachment controls can be done by cluster counting.

In conclusion, inhibition (in the absence of detachment) is consistent with direct inhibition of programming for lysis, but cannot be distinguished from drug-induced alteration of the preformed adhesions rendering them incompatible with programming for lysis. Lack of inhibition with a sufficiently fast-acting drug is good evidence against a direct effect of the drug on programming for lysis.

4. Testing Drugs on KCIL

The simplest test for inhibition of KCIL is addition of the drug to an ongoing culture after sufficient time has elapsed for completion of substantial programming for lysis (about 10 min). In this way, inhibition of KCIL by dextrans was shown (see Table IV). Since the dextrans also interfere with adhesion formation, it was necessary to control for this by monitoring specific release of ^{86}Rb. No other agent has been found to inhibit KCIL by this method (see Table IV).

C. Recent Results with Selected Drugs

1. Cytochalasin B

Using the method outlined in Table III, we have recently been able to confirm previous reports that cytochalasin B (CCB), 10 μg/ml, almost completely prevents adhesion formation (Shain and Martz, 1976). Moreover, we have found that CCB has little or no ability to detach preformed adhesions or to inhibit programming for lysis (Shain and Martz, 1976). Although the unlikely possibility of a slow-acting effect on programming for lysis cannot be excluded, we were able to show that CCB blocks adhesion formation within less than 1 min after addition. As suggested by previous reports (see Table IV), CCB had no effect on KCIL. Thus, CCB seems to inhibit TSL solely through prevention of adhesion formation.

Our conclusion that CCB does not inhibit programming for lysis might appear to be in conflict with the recent work by Golstein and Smith (Chapter 8) utilizing the calcium pulse technique, in which they conclude that CCB inhibits the lethal hit. Actually, there is no direct conflict.

First, the inhibition by CCB observed by Golstein and Smith could have resulted from several possibilities other than a direct action of CCB on the lethal hit. For example, CCB may detach adhesions preformed in magnesium *without calcium* (even though adhesions formed in the presence of both calcium and magnesium are largely resistant to detachment by CCB, as shown by Golstein and Smith as well as in our own laboratory).

If, however, we accept the conclusion of Golstein and Smith, the interpretation would be that CCB inhibits a *calcium-dependent* step or steps. On the other hand, our results show that CCB fails to inhibit a *temperature-dependent* step or steps. The two sets of results are consistent, provided we assume that the CCB-sensitive, calcium-dependent step(s) precedes the CCB-insensitive, temperature-dependent step(s).

2. Local Anesthetics

Kemp and Berke (1973b) showed that local anesthetics reversibly inhibit TSL, but do not inhibit KCIL. We studied lidocaine in detail (Shain and Martz, 1976). We found control of pH to be crucial, since lidocaine (a tertiary amine) at 5 mM did not inhibit TSL at pH 6.7, inhibited TSL strongly and reversibly at pH 7.3, and inhibited irreversibly at pH 7.8.

Lidocaine apparently inhibits via the CTLs, since preincubation of the CTLs, but not the target cells, markedly increased inhibition. At pH 7.3, lidocaine, 5 mM, partially inhibited adhesion formation and detached preformed adhesions rapidly. This latter effect prevented us from obtaining evidence on possible direct effects of lidocaine on programming for lysis. However, such effects are clearly not necessary to explain the inhibitory effects of lidocaine on TSL. Lidocaine accelerates KCIL.

Preliminary evidence has been obtained (Martz, work in progress) with two local anesthetic alcohols and with dimethyl sulfoxide (DMSO). DMSO was shown reversibly to inhibit TSL by Wolberg *et al.* (1973), who also found that it did not inhibit KCIL. We have found that DMSO (6%) strongly inhibits adhesion formation (cf. Golstein and Smith, Chapter 8) and detaches preformed adhesions in minutes. Methanol and benzyl alcohol also inhibit adhesion formation.

In general, therefore, the evidence to date indicates that local anesthetics inhibit TSL by interfering with adhesion.

3. Colchicine, Cyclic Nucleotides, and Trypan Blue

We have found trypan blue (0.05%) to be a reversible inhibitor of TSL, and to be a partial inhibitor of adhesion formation. Preliminary evidence with two partial inhibitors of TSL, colchicine (1×10^{-4} M, irreversible) and dibutyryl cyclic AMP (2mM, slowly reversible) suggests that they, too, interfere with adhesion formation. In accord with the latter observation. Golstein and Smith (Chapter 8) have recently reported that theophylline inhibits adhesion formation.

VIII. CONCLUDING REMARKS

A. Stages in TSL

We have described a new method for resolving the cellular interaction in TSL into three discrete stages: adhesion, programming for lysis, and KCIL. The resulting concept of TSL is represented schematically in Fig. 4, and our present knowledge about each stage is summarized in Table I.

Our results show that there exists a mechanism for programming for lysis above and beyond the mere formation of an adhesive attachment between the CTL and target-cell membranes. This is clear since the formation of adhesions with sufficient mechanical strength to withstand dispersion in DCM (our operational definition for adhesion) requires less time and is less temperature-dependent than programming for lysis. Moreover, unlike programming for lysis, adhesion formation is not affected by the extracellular free calcium ion concentration (provided magnesium ions are at physiological levels, i.e., in the vicinity of 2 mM).

There is no evidence contrary to the present belief that KCIL, once initiated by damage to the target-cell membrane (probably occurring during programming for lysis), is an inevitable and irreversible process, probably driven by colloid osmotic influx of water and loss of essential small metabolites.

The time ranges indicated in Fig. 4 for the completion of each stage are our guess of the minimum and maximum at the level of the individual target cell. However, no systematic study of the effect of sensitized/target cell ratio on these times has been undertaken. We do not know whether programming for

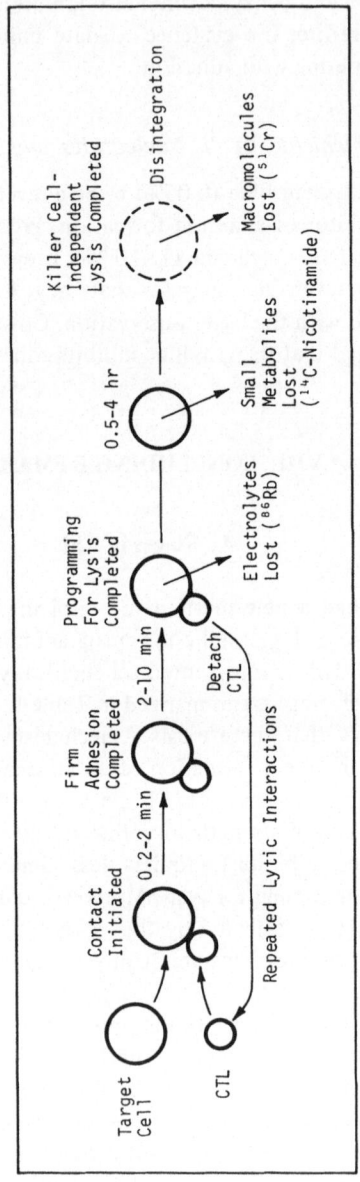

Fig. 4. Schematic representation of T-lymphocyte-mediated specific lysis (TSL). For details about each stage, see Table II.

lysis is quicker when two CTL cells have adhered to a single target cell, or whether additional damage can be done after programming for lysis is completed, or whether such additional damage would shorten KCIL.

Since KCIL plateaus by 4–5 hr, the utility of longer incubation times for assaying weak CTL activity probably depends on the ability of each CTL to move about, establishing a succession of lytic contacts with multiple target cells. Also, some previously triggered CTL-progenitor cells may complete their differentiation into CTL during longer incubation times (Kamat and Henney, 1975).

Caution should be exercised in generalizing the present findings obtained with the detachment-and-dispersion method, since only the C57BL/6 anti-P815 mastocytoma system has been studied in detail. In particular, the killing of target cells other than ascites tumor cells might differ in certain respects.

At the moment, adhesion seems to be the best-characterized stage in TSL. It requires an energy supply, divalent cations, and microfilament function. The significance of inhibition of adhesion by local anesthetics is not clear, since these drugs affect a wide range of cellular functions.

The detachment-and-dispersion method we have introduced for resolving stages in TSL (see Table III) promises to be useful in evaluating the sites of action of the various drugs affecting TSL.

B. Mechanism of Damage

The mechanism by which damage is done to the target cell remains totally obscure. Electrolyte permeability changes observed during programming for lysis suggest that the target cell membrane may be the primary object of attack (Section V.C). Microfilament function is apparently not required during programming for lysis, since addition of cytochalasin B following adhesion fails to prevent damage (Section VII.C.1).

We shall conclude by briefly discussing several questions that help to define the issues remaining unresolved.

1. Is Antigen Recognition Necessary To Initiate Adhesion?

CTLs do not appear to adhere indiscriminately to potential target cells (a possibility that would surely diminish their effectiveness). This is shown by the antigenic specificity observed in the adhesion of CTL to cell monolayers (Brondz, 1968; Golstein et al., 1971; Berke and Levey, 1972), as well as in CTL–target cell adhesion assayed by microscopic counts of cell clusters (Martz, 1975a; Berke et al., 1975). Thus, the receptors function in at least one step: the initiation of adhesion formation.

2. Are the Antigen-Specific Receptors Linked to the Damaging Mechanism?

It is possible that the role of the antigen-specific receptors on the CTL membrane is limited to initiating the adhesion process (the "one-function-receptor" hypothesis); that is, they might not be directly involved in initiating the damage. This is equivalent to saying that simple contact with a CTL membrane is lethal in itself, an idea consistent with the observation that agglutinating concentrations of plant lectins initiate nonspecific killing (Bevan and Cohn, 1975). (Unfortunately, the latter observation is equally consistent with the two-function-receptor hypothesis if one is willing to assume that the lectins studied also interact with the receptors so as to mimic the binding of antigen.)

Some evidence against the one-function-receptor hypothesis has recently been provided by Kuppers and Henney (1976). They studied the interaction of two CTL populations, one sensitized to recognize the second, but the second sensitized to a third party having little or no cross-reaction with the antigens of the first CTL population. They cocultured the two CTL populations, and later measured residual CTL activity (against appropriate tumor target cells) of both types as an index of possible mutual damage. The CTL inactivation, like the receptor—antigen interaction, was largely unidirectional. This suggests that when one CTL specifically recognizes and initiates an adhesion with a second CTL, the latter is damaged (cf. Golstein, 1974; Martz and Benacerraf, 1976). When the second CTL lacks specific receptors for the first, however, it appears unable to damage the first, despite the formation of an adhesion supporting damage in the opposite direction. This suggests that simple contact with a CTL is not lethal in itself, and that the receptors must participate in order to initiate damage (the two-function-receptor hypothesis).

3. Does the Damaging Mechanism Require Activation?

It is possible that the damaging mechanism is completely activated and deployed prior to contact with the target cell. This could be compatible with either the one- or the two-function-receptor hypothesis. In the former case, for example, the damage might be mediated by an enzyme (active and exposed prior to target-cell contact) covalently linked to the receptor. Concentration of the receptor-attached enzyme at the region of adhesion (by receptor—antigen interactions) could be necessary for a lethal level of damage.

Alternatively, the target-damaging mechanism might require triggering, activation, or deployment induced either by adhesive-contact (in the one-function-receptor hypothesis) or by receptor-antigen interaction (in the two-function-receptor hypothesis). Secretion of a toxin would fit this model, provided the secretion does not occur in the absence of contact with an appropriate target cell. There is presently no evidence bearing on the question of whether the damaging mechanism requires activation.

4. Does Programming for Lysis Equal Damage?

The term "programming for lysis" was selected to avoid the implication that patent damage had been inflicted on the target cell at the moment the target cell was first irreversibly committed to KCIL (Martz, 1975a). Actual damage need not have been effected at that time, provided CTL detachment or inactivation leaves on or in the target cell a CTL product capable of inflicting damage later.

Alternatively, primary damage may be stopped by CTL detachment or inactivation. In this case, programming for lysis constitutes irreversible damage. The increased permeability to electrolytes that we have shown in the target-cell membrane during programming for lysis may reflect such irreversible damage.

5. Is Damage Produced Physically or Chemically?

The damage could be done by a physical method, such as a direct interaction of the CTL membrane with the target-cell membrane, possibly making unconventional use of mechanisms otherwise employed in secretory exocytosis. This would explain the similarities in the pharmacology of TSL and secretory phenomena (Henney, 1973b) without requiring the secretion of any chemical mediator in TSL.

On the other hand, a chemical mediator or toxin synthesized by the CTL may produce the damage. If so, consumption of a specialized protein in the process seems unlikely (Thorn and Henney, 1976). Lymphotoxin seems an unlikely candidate for a crucial role in TSL (Gately et al., 1976; Henney et al., 1974), although it has not been totally ruled out.

6. Are There Inhibitors Acting Solely on Programming for Lysis?

To elucidate the mechanism of programming for lysis, it would be most helpful to identify one or more inhibitors (or stimulators) that act solely on that step. Only one treatment is now known to inhibit programming for lysis without diminishing the rate or extent of adhesion formation: removal of Ca^{2+} in the presence of ample Mg^{2+} (most effectively achieved with the ligand EGTA; see Section VI.E). However, Ca^{2+} cannot be said to serve programming for lysis uniquely, since we have shown that it synergizes with low levels of Mg^{2+} in adhesion formation (Section V.C).

This latter observation raises the possibility that the adhesion that forms in Mg^{2+} without Ca^{2+} is unphysiological—a physically firm adhesion, abnormal in structure and incompatible with programming for lysis. Thus, the role of calcium in TSL might be limited to its demonstrated role in adhesion. This is consistent with our observation that the concentration of calcium required for optimal TSL never exceeds the concentration required for optimal adhesion. In short, it is no longer necessary to postulate a role for Ca^{2+} in any subsequent (e.g., hypothetical secretory) events, although such a role cannot be excluded.

Irrespective of whether Ca^{2+} is directly involved in both adhesion formation and programming for lysis, or only in the former, one distinct possibility for the site(s) of action of Ca^{2+} in TSL is the cyclic nucleotide system, including direct effects on both cAMP and cGMP (Strom *et al.,* 1976b).

In any case, at present, no inhibitor of TSL has been shown to act directly on programming for lysis *without interfering with adhesion.* Certainly, a number of inhibitors deserve closer scrutiny in this regard. However, two of the most interesting candidates (colchicine and cAMP) appear to interfere with adhesion in preliminary results in our laboratory (see Section VII.C.3).

To put it the other way around, every inhibitor of TSL examined to date interferes with adhesion (see Table IV), which suggests two possibilities: First, the processes of adhesion and of programming for lysis might have similar underlying mechanisms. Then most agents inhibiting one would do likewise for the other. Second, programming for lysis might be a much simpler process than is adhesion formation. Then any given inhibitor would be more likely to act on the latter.

It is to be hoped that future scrutiny of the pharmacology of each step in TSL, as well as other approaches, will provide definitive answers to some of these questions, and lead to an explanation of this fascinating but enigmatic mechanism.

EXPLANATION FOR TABLE IV: EFFECTS OF DRUGS, ENZYMES, ANTISERA, AND OTHER CHEMICAL AGENTS ON T-LYMPHOCYTE-MEDIATED CYTOLYSIS

This table is restricted to results in the murine allogeneic system, and to studies in which the cytolysis studied was demonstrably T-lymphocyte-mediated. Results with rat TSL from the laboratory of Strom and co-workers are also included. All cytolytic data included are based on short-term radiochromium release studies (4–6 hr incubations), with the exception of some early work by Brondz and co-workers. The author has endeavored to make this list complete, and would appreciate readers calling omissions to his attention.

Concentrations given in units of mg, μg, or ng refer to amounts per milliliter. (2) Numbers in brackets denote references; see the *Key to References* on pp. 352–353.

Abbreviations Used in Table IV.

(+) Complete or nearly complete inhibition (>80%) during the initial phase of specific lysis, i.e., when specific release in drug-free control cultures is usually less than 60%; this designation does not preclude transient (*Tr*) or prolonged (++) inhibition;

(++) prolonged complete or nearly complete inhibition (>80%) persisting beyond the time when drug-free control cultures have reached maximal specific lysis;

(*AC*) tested by inactivation of effector cells by *A*ntiserum and *C*omplement (Section III.A.3);

(*Ad*) tested by *Ad*dition of drug to ongoing interactions (Section VII.B.4);

(*AH*) *A*nti*H*istamine;

(*Au*) *Au*gmentation;

(*CC*) tested by microscopic *C*luster *C*ounting (Section III.B.3);

(*CI*) *C*omplement *I*nhibitor;

(*CN*) agent affecting levels of intracellular *C*yclic *N*ucleotides, i.e., cAMP and cGMP;

(*DD*) tested by *D*etachment and *D*ispersion (Section VII.B.3);

(*Di*) tested by *Di*spersion (Section VII.B.1,2);

(*ED*) tested by addition of *ED*TA (Section III.A.6);

(*En*) inhibitor of *En*ergy metabolism, i.e., oxidative phosphorylation or glycolysis;

(*Es*) inhibitor of serine *Es*terases;

(*FMK*) tested by adhesion of CTLs to aldehyde-*F*ixed cell *M*onolayers (see *MK*);

(*In*) *In*hibition;

(*LA*) *L*ocal *A*nesthetic;

(*MA*) tested by adhesion of sensitized cells to cell *M*onolayers, quantitated by percentage of total cells *A*dhering (Section III.A.1);

(*MK*) tested by adhesion of CTLs to cell *M*onolayers, quantitated by *K*illing activity of adherent and nonadherent lymphocyte populations (Section III.A.1);

(*No*) *No* effect or no substantial effect;

(*Pa*) *Pa*rtial; when referring to inhibition, this means that complete inhibition is not approached, even initially;

(*Ra*) *Ra*pidly;

(*Sl*) *Sl*owly;

(*SR*) tested by *S*top-*R*ock analysis (Section III.A.2);

(*Tr*) *Tr*ansient inhibition; i.e., complete inhibition is approached initially, but later the rate of specific lysis is comparable to the initial rate in drug-free control cultures.

Table IV. Effects of Drugs, Enzymes, Antisera, and Other Chemical Agents on T-Lymphocyte-Mediated Cytolysis

| Agent category | | | | |
Agent, concentration, and effect	Is effect reversible?	Effect on adhesion formation?	Detaches preformed adhesions?	Effect on KCIL?
CN Acetylcholine $10^{-14} - 10^{-9}$ M *Au* [67] Acetylsalicylic acid 1 mg *In,* *Pa* [51] Actinomycin D 3.5 µg *No*				

(Cont'd)

Table IV (Cont'd)

Agent category ↓ Agent, concentration, and effect	Is effect reversible?	Effect on adhesion formation?	Detaches preformed adhesions?	Effect on KCIL?
[9,10,57] 10 μg *In*, *Pa* [15,73]	*Sl* [15]			
CN Adenosine (*In* potentiated by adenosine deaminase inhibitor [88]): ≥ 10^{-5} M *In,Pa* [88]	*Ra* [88]			
Adenosine deaminase inhibitor (potentiates *In* by adenosine [88]): 7.9×10^{-6} M *No* [88]				
5'-Adenosine monophosphate 10^{-3} M *In,Pa* [41]				
Amino-nucleoside-purimycin 50 μg *No* [9,10]				
Antigen, subcellular, from targets, see *H-2*				
En Antimycin A 10^{-6} M *In,*+ [73] 10^{-4} M *In,Pa* [51]				
CI Antisera to C2,C3,C5 *No* [40]				
Antisera to CTL *H-2 No* or slight *Au* [10,15,16, 22,57]				
Antisera to CTL receptor *In,*+ [47]				
Antisera to immunoglobulins *No* [10,17,20,23,				

Table IV (Cont'd)

Agent category	Agent, concentration, and effect	Is effect reversible?	Effect on adhesion formation?	Detaches preformed adhesions?	Effect on KCIL?
	25,26,40,57]				
	Antisera to Ly-2				
	No [64]				
	Antisera to target *H-2*				
	In, + [8,13,14, 15,16,20,22, 26,65,81]	Not immediately: [8]	*In (MK)* [38,81]	*Pa* [81]	*No (SR)* [81]: *(AD)* [4,8]
	In,Tr [28]				
	Antisera to Thy-1 or T cells				
	No [34]				
	Atropine				
	10^{-12} M *No* [71]				
	10^{-6}–10^{-5} M				
	Au [71]				
	Azathioprine				
	20 μg *No* [61]				
En	Azide				
	1.5×10^{-3} M *In*,+ [2]	Yes (37°C) [2]	*In (CC,*22°C) [2]	No (*CC,*24°C) [2]	*No (SR)* [2]
	1×10^{-2} M *In*,+ [80]	Yes (24°C) [80] *Pa* (37°C) [80]	*In (MK,*24°C) [80]	No (*MK,*24°C) [80]	
	4×10^{-2} M *In*,+ [31]	Yes (37°C) [31]	*Pa (FMK,*37°C) [31]	No (*FMK,*37°C) [3]	*No (ED)* [31]
En	Azide (prekilling of target cells)				
	10^{-1} M 60 min 37°C		*In*(MK)77		
LA	Benzyl alcohol				
	1.3×10^{-3} M *In*,+ [44,45]	*Ra* [44]	*In (Di)* [51]		*No (SR)* [44]
CN	8-Bromo cyclic guanosine monophosphate				
	10^{-7}–5×10^{-6} M *Au* [68,74] *No* [36]				
AH	Burimamide (antagonizes *In* by histamine [58]):				
	10^{-4} M *No* [58]				
	10^{-3} M *In* [58]				

(Cont'd)

Table IV (Cont'd)

Agent category ↓	Agent, concentration, and effect	Is effect reversible?	Effect on adhesion formation?	Detaches preformed adhesions?	Effect on KCIL?
LA	Butanol 3.4×10^{-2} M *In* [44]				
CN	Carbamylcholine 10^{-14}–10^{-11} M *Au* [67] *No* [89]; *Au,Tr* [68,74]				
CI	Carrageenin *No* [5,20]				
	Catalase 0.1 mg *No* [51]				
	Cerium (Ce³⁺) 1 mM *No* [51]				
	Chloroquin 10µg *In,Pa* [12]	Yes [12]	*No (MK)* [12]		
AH	Chlorpheniramine maleate 10^{-4} M *In,Pa* [58]				
LA	Chlorpromazine 5×10^{-6} M *In,Pa* [44]				
CN	Cholera enterotoxin 1 ng *In,+* [48]	No [48]			
	1–100 ng *In,Pa* [42]	No [42]			
	2 µg *In,Pa*67,68	No [67]			
	Chondroitin sulfate 1 mg *No* [51,55]				
CI	Cobra venom factor *No* [5,20]				
	Colchicine 10^{-5}–10^{-3} M	*No* [43,59,69]	*No (MA)* [38]		
	In,+ [42, 59]				
	In,Pa [19,69]		*In (CC)* [51]		
	Complement *No* [20,54]				
	Concanavalin A 5 µg *Au* [6,66]				
	Cortisone *No* [16,57]				

Table IV (Cont'd)

Agent category	Agent, concentration, and effect	Is effect reversible?	Effect on adhesion formation?	Detaches preformed adhesions?	Effect on KCIL?
En	Cyanide 1.5×10^{-3} M *In* [2]	Yes (37°C) [2]	*In (CC,*22°C) [2]	No *(CC,*24°C) [2]	No *(SR)* [2]
CN	Cyclic adenosine monophosphate 10^{-5}–10^{-3} M *In,Pa* [41]				
AH	Cyclizine HCl 10^{-4} M *In,Pa* [58]				
	Cycloheximide 10 µg *In.Pa* [15,57,73]	*Ra* [15]			
	Cysteine <1 mg *No* [51]				
	Cytochalasin A 3 µg *In,* + [18,73]	*No [18]*	*In (MA)* [18]		
	Cytochalasin B 5–10 µg *In,*+ [18,19,21,24,30, 31,39,59,73,76]	*Ra* [18,21,24,31, 39,59,63]	*In (MK)*[18,38, 76] *(MA)* [18]; *(Di)* [63]; *(FMK)* [31]	*No (Di)* [63] : *(FMK)* [31]	*No(Ad)* [21,37, 59] ; *(DD)* [63]; *(ED)* [31]
	Cytosine arabinoside 10µg *No* [61]				
En	2-Deoxyglucose 5×10^{-2} M *In,*+ [73]				
	Deuterium oxide 50% *No* [69] 75% *In,Pa* [69]				
	Dextran 4–12% *In* [29, 31,37]				*In* [29,37]; *(ED)* [31]
	Dextran sulfate 30 µg *In,Pa* [83] 1 mg *In,*+ [51,55]				
	Dibutyryl cyclic adenosine mono- phosphate: 10^{-5}–10^{-3} M *In,*+ [41,67]		*In (Di)* [51]		
	Dicumarol 10^{-3} M In,+ [51]				

Table IV (Cont'd)

Agent category ↓	Agent, concentration, and effect	Is effect reversible?	Effect on adhesion formation?	Detaches preformed adhesions?	Effect on KCIL?
LA?	Dimethyl sulfoxide 4–6% In,+ [24, 31,51,87]	*Ra* [51,87]; Yes: [31]	*In* (*Di*) [51]; (*FMK*) [31]	Yes (*Di*) [51]; No (*FMK*) [31]	No (*Ad,SR*) [8 (*ED*) [31]
En	Dinitrophenol 5×10^{-4} M *In*,+ [2,80]	*Ra* (37°C) [2], (24°C) [80]	*In*(*MK*, 24°C) [80]	No (*CC*, 24°C) [2]; *Pa,Sl* (*MK*, 24°C) [80]	No (*SR*) [2]
AH	Diphenhydramine 10^{-5}–10^{-4} M *In,Pa* [58]	Yes [58]			
	EDTA: exceeding $Ca^{2+} + Mg^{2+}$	*Ra* [16,24,39,52, 57,75]		*Ra*(*MK*) [75]; (*CC*) [52]	*Au* rate (*AC*) [56]; *No*(*Ad*) 39,50,54,57]
	In,+ [16,24,39, 50,75] *In*,++ [53,54, 56,57]				
	EGTA: exceeding Ca *In,Pa* [51] (Section V.E.2)	*Ra* [51]	See Section IV.C	No (*Di*) [51]	
	Emetine ⩾10^{-5} M *In*,+ [42]	*No* [42]			
LA	Ethanol 0.25 M *In,Pa* [44]				
	Ethanol prekilling of target cells 60% 5 min 25°C		*In* (MK) [77]		
	Formaldehyde prekilling of target cells 0.2% 24 hr 7°C		*No* (*MK*) [77]		
	1% 24 hr 7°C		*In* (*MK*) [77]		
	Fructose 1 mg *No* [46]				
	FUdR (5 fluorodeoxyuridine) 2×10^{-4} M *No* [57]				

Table IV (Cont'd)

Agent category ↓ Agent, concentration, and effect	Is effect reversible?	Effect on adhesion formation?	Detaches preformed adhesions?	Effect on KCIL?
Galactose				
1 mg *No* [46]				
Glucose (in				
phosphate-buf-				
fered saline)				
1 mg *Au* [46]				
Glutaraldehyde pre-				
treatment of				
target cells				
0.15% 10 sec		*No (MK)* [77]		
No [19]				
0.25% 5 min		*No (MK)* [33]		
0.4% 10 sec *In*		*In (MK)* [77]		
[19]	No [19]			
Glycerol				
10% *In,*+ [51]				
H-2 antigen, sub-				
cellular, from				
target cells:				
Au [17]		*No (MA)* [82]		
No [1,15,82]				
In [7,84]				
In (non-				
specific) [82]				
Heparin				
1 U/ml *Au*				
[45]				
100 U/ml				
In,+ [11,12]	Yes [11,12,55]	*No (MK)* [11,12]		
100–300 U/ml				
In, +, Tr [55]				
10–500 U/ml				
No [45]				
CN Histamine				
$10^{-5}-10^{-3}$ M				
In,Pa [41,58,60]				
Hyaluronic acid				
0.5 mg *No* [51,55]				
Hydrocortisone				
In [27]				
10 μg *No* [16]				
Hypotonic prekill-				
ing of target cell:				

(Cont'd)

Table IV (Cont'd)

Agent category ↓	Agent, concentration, and effect	Is effect reversible?	Effect on adhesion formation?	Detaches preformed adhesions?	Effect on KCIL?
	30 mOsm 60 min 25°C		*In* [77]		
CN	Imidazole 10^{-8}–10^{-7} M *Au* [68,70]				
	Inosine *No* [88]				
CN	Insulin 10^{-8}–10^{-11} M *Au,Tr* [72]				
	Interferon *Au* [49]	*No* [49]			
En	Iodoacetamide 10^{-3} M *In*,+ [51]				
En	Iodoacetate (cf. pyruvate) 10^{-4} M *In*, + [31]	*No* [31]			*No* (*ED*) [31]
	2.5×10^{-3} M *In*,+ [2]	Yes [2]			
	Ionophore A23187 10^{-6} M *No* [31]				
CN	Isoproterenol 10^{-7}–10^{-4} M *In,Pa,Tr* [41,68]				
LA	Lidocaine 1.9×10^{-3} M *In,Pa* [44]				
	5×10^{-3} M *In*,+ [63]	Yes [63]	*In,Pa* (*Di*) [63]	*Ra* (*Di*) [63]	*Au* rate (*DD*) [63
	2-Mercaptoethanol 2×10^{-4} M *No* [51]				
LA	Methanol 1.2 M *In*,+ [44, 51]	Yes [51]	*In* (*Di*) [51]		
	Mitomycin C 25 μg *No* [73]				
	Neuraminidase pretreatment of CTL: 50 U/ml 30 min 37°C	*Sl* [86]	*Au* (*MK*) [10,11, 12]		

Table IV (Cont'd)

Agent category / Agent, concentration, and effect	Is effect reversible?	Effect on adhesion formation?	Detaches preformed adhesions?	Effect on KCIL?
Au [10,11,12, 43,86]				
Neuraminidase pre-treatment of target cells 100 U/ml 60 min 37°C *No*: 79,86				
Nicotinamide adenine dinucleotide (reduced, NADH) 5×10⁻⁴ M *No* [51]				
p-Nitrophenol 5×10⁻⁴ M *In,*+ [30], *Pa* [51]	Yes [30]			
Oligomycin 10 μg *In,*+ [73]	*No* [73]			
Organophosphonates (serine esterase inhibitors) 10⁻³ M *In,Pa* [30]	Yes: 30			
Organophosphorous fluoridates (serine esterase inhibitors) 10⁻⁴ M *In,Pa* [30]; *In,*+ [73]	No or *Sl* [30,73]			
Ouabain 10⁻⁴ M *No* [73]				
Pactamycin 10⁻⁷–10⁻⁶ M *No* [42, 78] ≥10⁻⁵ M *In,*++ [24,42]	No [42]			No (*AD*) [24]
pH 3 prekilling of target cells 60 min 25°C		*In* (*MK*) [77]		
pH 5.5 *In,*+ [75]	Yes [75]		Yes (*MK*) [75]	

En (agent category)

(Cont'd)

Table IV (Cont'd)

Agent category Agent, concentration, and effect	Is effect reversible?	Effect on adhesion formation?	Detaches preformed adhesions?	Effect on KCIL?
LA Phenol 3.5×10⁻³ M *In,Pa* [44] 10⁻² M *In,+* [31]	Yes [31]	*In (FMK)* [31]	*No (FMK)* [31]	*No (ED)* [31]
Phenyl methyl sulfonyl fluoride (protease inhibitor): 10 μg *No* [51]				
Phosphatidyl serine 10–300 μg *No* [51]				
Phospholipase A <1 μg *No* [11,12]				
Phospholipase C ≤10μg *No* [10,11,12,43]				
Phytohemagglutinin 10 μg *Au* [6]				
Poly (A:U) *No* [85]				
Polyanethole sulfonate 1 mg *In,++* [51, 55]	Yes [51]			
Polyglutamic acid 3 mg *No* [51]				
Polyvinyl sulfate 1 mg *In* [51,55]				
Prednisolone 1–10 μg *In,Pa* [12,27,62]	Yes [12,62]	*No (MK)* [12]		*No (AD)* [62]
LA Procaine 2.3×10⁻³ M *In,Pa* [44]				
Propranolol (antagonizes inhibition by isoproterenol [41]: 10⁻⁵ M *No* [41]				
CN Prostaglandins A1, A2,B2,F2α 10⁻⁵ M *In,Pa* [35]				

Table IV (Cont'd)

Agent category ↓	Agent, concentration, and effect	Is effect reversible?	Effect on adhesion formation?	Detaches preformed adhesions?	Effect on KCIL?
CN	Prostaglandin E1 $10^{-8}-3\times10^{-5}$ M In,+ [41] $1-3\times10^{-4}$ M In,Pa [35,38,67, 68]		Slight In (MK) [38]		
CN	Prostaglandin E2 $10^{-7}-3\times10^{-5}$ M $In;Pa$ [41] 10^{-4} M	Ra [39]			
	Prostaglandin F1α 10^{-4} M No [41]				
	Proteases, pre-treating CTL <0.1 mg <30 min Au [43] >1 mg >30 min In,+ [5,10,11, 12,43,57]	Sl [5,10,11, 12,43,57]	⏐ In (MK) [10,11, 12]	Yes [3,32]	
	Proteases, pre-treating target cells (papain, pronase) 5 mg 60 min 37°C In, Pa [79]	Sl [79]			
	Proteases, pre-treating target cells (trypsin) 5 mg 60 min 37°C No [79]				
	Proteins, various soluble No [5]				
	Puromycin ≥12 µg In,+ [9,73]		In (MK) [9]		
AH	Pyrilamine maleate 10^{-4} M In,Pa [58]				
	Pyruvate (4×10^{-2} M no effect on In by iodoacetate 10^{-4} M [31])				

(Cont'd)

Table IV (Cont'd)

Agent category	Agent, concentration, and effect	Is effect reversible?	Effect on adhesion formation?	Detaches preformed adhesions?	Effect on KCIL?
LA	Salicyl alcohol 1.3×10⁻³ M In,+ [44]	Yes [44]			
	Serum 1–10% Au [5,46] >10% In,Pa [55]				
	Serum, dialyzed (in glucose-free saline), 2% In,+ [46]	No [46]			
	Sucrose 1 mg No [46]				
CN	Tetramethyl-ammonium 10⁻¹⁰–10⁻⁵ M Au,Tr [71]				
CN	Theophylline 10⁻³ M In; Pa [35,41,67] 10⁻² M In, + [31]	Yes [31]	In,Pa (FMK) [31]	No (FMK) [31]	No (ED) [31]
	Trypan blue 50 μg In,Pa [12] 500 μg In,+ [51]	Yes [12] Yes [51]	No (MK) [12] In,Pa (Di) [51]		
	Vinblastine 10⁻⁶–10⁻⁴ M In,+ [7,42] In:Pa69	No [42,69]			
	Vi polysaccharide 200 μg In, Pa [11,12]				

Key to References

[1] Berke and Amos (1973)
[2] Berke and Gabison (1975)
[3] Berke and Levey (1972)
[4] Berke and Sullivan (1973)
[5] Berke et al. (1972a)
[6] Bevan and Cohn (1975)
[7] Bonavida (1974a)
[8] Bonavida (1974b)
[9] Brondz (1969)
[10] Brondz (1972)
[11] Brondz et al. (1971)

[12] Brondz et al. (1973)
[13] Brunner et al. (1966)
[14] Brunner et al. (1967)
[15] Brunner et al. (1968)
[16] Brunner et al. (1969)
[17] Brunner et al. (1971)
[18] Bubbers and Henney (1975a)
[19] Bubbers and Henney (1975b)
[20] Canty and Wunderlich (1970)
[21] Cerottini and Brunner (1972)
[22] Cerottini and Brunner (1974)

[23] Cerottini et al. (1971)
[24] Cerottini et al. (1974)
[25] Chapuis and Brunner (1971)
[26] Cohen and Feldman (1971)
[27] Cohen et al. (1970)
[28] Faanes et al. (1973)
[29] Ferluga and Allison (1974)
[30] Ferluga et al. (1972)
[31] Golstein and Smith (Chapter 8)
[32] Golstein et al. (1971)
[33] Golstein et al. (1972b)
[34] Golstein et al. (1972a)
[35] Henney (1973b)
[36] Henney (1973c)
[37] Henney (1974)
[38] Henney and Bubbers (1973b)
[39] Henney and Bubbers (1973a)
[40] Henney et al. (1972b)
[41] Henney et al. (1972a)
[42] Henney et al. (1974)
[43] Kedar et al. (1974)
[44] Kemp and Berke (1973b)
[45] Kemp and Berke (1973a)
[46] Kemp et al. (1974)
[47] Kimura (1974)
[48] Lichtenstein et al. (1973)
[49] Lindahl et al. (1972)
[50] MacDonald (1975)
[51] Martz (unpublished data)
[52] Martz (1975a)
[53] Martz (1975b)
[54] Martz and Benacerraf (1973b)
[55] Martz and Benacerraf (1973a)
[56] Martz et al. (1974)
[57] Mauel et al. (1970)
[58] Plaut et al. (1973b)
[59] Plaut et al. (1973a)
[60] Plaut et al. (1973c)
[61] Röllinghoff et al. (19730
[62] Sanderson and Franks (1975)
[63] Shain and Martz (1976)
[64] Shiku et al. (1975)
[65] Sinclair et al. (1975)
[66] Stavy et al. (1972)
[67] Strom et al. (1972)
[68] Strom et al. (1973c)
[69] Strom et al. (1973a)
[70] Strom et al. (1973b)
[71] Strom et al. (1974)
[72] Strom et al. (1975)
[73] Strom et al. (1976a)
[74] Strom et al. (1976b)
[75] Stulting and Berke,(1973b)
[76] Stulting et al. (1973)
[77] Stulting et al. (1975)
[78] Thorn and Henney (1976)
[79] Todd (1975a)
[80] Todd (1975b)
[81] Todd et al. (1973)
[82] Todd et al. (1975)
[83] Vachek and Kölsch (1975)
[84] Wagner and Boyle (1972)
[85] Wagner and Cone (1974)
[86] Weiss and Cudney (1972)
[87] Wolberg et al. (1973)
[88] Wolberg et al. (1975)

ACKNOWLEDGMENTS

These studies were initiated with the guidance and collaboration of Professor Baruj Benacerraf, and I am grateful for his continuing advice and encouragement. I also thank many colleagues too numerous to name for helpful discussions and for sharing unpublished data.

I thank Lenny Colarusso for his skillful and dedicated performance of the recent experiments described, David Archibald, Elizabeth Mellin, and Mark Drogin for additional technical assistance, and Ms. Sharon Smith for excellent secretarial assistance.

This work was supported by Grant CA-14723 from the National Institutes of Health.

IX. REFERENCES

Basten, A., Miller, J.F.A.P., and Abraham, R., 1975, Relationship between Fc receptors, antigen-binding sites on T and B cells, and *H-2* complex-associated determinants, *J. Exp. Med.* **141**:547.

Berke, G., and Amos, D.B., 1973, Mechanism of lymphocyte-mediated cytolysis. The LMC cycle and its role in transplantation immunity, *Transplant. Rev.* **17**:71.

Berke, G., and Gabison, D., 1975, Energy requirements of the binding and lytic steps of T lymphocyte-mediated cytolysis of leukemic cells *in vitro, Eur. J. Immunol.* **5**:671.

Berke, G., and Levey, R.H., 1972, Cellular immunoabsorbents in transplantation immunity. Specific *in vitro* deletion and recovery of mouse lymphoid cells sensitized against allogeneic tumors, *J. Exp. Med.* **135**:972.

Berke, G., and Sullivan, K.A., 1973, Temperature control of lymphocyte-mediated cytotoxicity *in vitro, Transplant. Proc.* **5**:421.

Berke, G., Ax, W., and Feldman, M., 1969, Graft reaction in tissue culture. II. Quantification of the lytic action on mouse fibroblasts by rat lymphocytes sensitized on mouse embryo monolayers, *Immunology* **16**:643.

Berke, G., Sullivan, K.A., and Amos, B., 1972a, Rejection of ascites tumor allografts. I. Isolation, characterization, and *in vitro* reactivity of peritoneal lymphoid effector cells from BALB/c mice immune to EL4 leukosis, *J. Exp. Med.* **135**:1334.

Berke, G., Sullivan, K.A., and Amos, D.B., 1972b, Rejection of ascites tumor allografts, II. A pathway for cell-mediated tumor destruction *in vitro* by peritoneal exudate lymphoid cells, *J. Exp. Med.* **136**:1594.

Berke, G., Gabison, D., and Feldman, M., 1975, The frequency of effector cells in populations containing cytotoxic T lymphocytes, *Eur. J. Immunol.* **5**:813.

Bernstein, I.D., Thor, D.E., Zbar, B., and Rapp, H.J., 1971, Tumor immunity: Tumor suppression *in vivo* initiated by soluble products of specifically stimulated lymphocytes, *Science* **172**:729.

Bevan, M.J., 1975, The major histocompatibility complex determines susceptibility to cytotoxic T cells directed against minor histocompatibility antigens, *J. Exp. Med.* **142**:1349.

Bevan, M.J., and Cohn, M., 1975, Cytotoxic effects of antigen- and mitogen-induced T cells on various targets, *J. Immunol.* **114**:559.

Bonavida, B., 1974a, Studies on the induction and expression of T cell-mediated immunity. I. Blocking of cell-mediated cytolysis by membrane antigens, *J. Immunol.* **112**:926.

Bonavida, B., 1974b, Studies on the induction and expression of T cell-mediated immunity. II. Antiserum blocking of cell-mediated cytolysis, *J. Immunol.* **112**:1308.

Borle, A.B., 1968, Calcium metabolism in HeLa cells and the effect of parathyroid hormone, *J. Cell Biol.* **36**:567.

Brondz, B.D., 1968, Complex specificity of immune lymphocytes in allogeneic cell cultures. *Folia Biol. (Prague)* **14**:115.

Brondz, B.D., 1969, Effect of actinomycin D and puromycin on the *in vitro* cytotoxic activity of lymphocytes, *Transplant. Proc.* **1**:416.

Brondz, B.D., 1972, Lymphocyte receptors and mechanisms of *in vitro* cell-mediated immune reactions, *Transplant. Rev.* **10**:112.

Brondz, B.D., Snegiröva, A.E., Rassulin, Y.A., and Shamborant, G., 1971, Effect of some enzymes, polysaccharides, and lysosome-active drugs on interaction of immune lymphocytes with allogenic target cells, in. *Progress in Immunology 1*, pp. 447–460 (B. Amos, ed.), Academic Press, New York.

Brondz, B.D., Snegiröva, A.E., Rassulin, Y.A. and Shamborant, O.G., 1973, Modification of in vitro immune lymphocyte–target cell interaction by some biologically active drugs, *Immunochemistry* 10:175.

Brondz, B.D., Egorov, I.K., and Drizlikh, G.I., 1975, Private specificities of *H-2K* and *H-2D* loci as possible selective targets for effector lymphocytes in cell-mediated immunity, *J. Exp. Med.* 141:11.

Brunner, K.T., and Cerottini, J.C., 1971, Cytotoxic lymphocytes as effector cells of cell-mediated immunity, in: *Progress in Immunology I,* pp. 385–398 (B. Amos, ed.), Academic Press, New York.

Brunner, K.T., Mauel, J., and Schindler, R., 1966, *In vitro* studies of cell-bound immunity; cloning assay of the cytotoxic action of sensitized lymphoid cells on allogeneic target cells, *Immunology* 11:499.

Brunner, K.T., Mauel, J., and Schindler, R., 1967, Inhibitory effect of isoantibody on *in vivo* sensitization and on the *in vitro* cytotoxic action of immune lymphocytes, *Nature (London)* 213:1246.

Brunner, K.T., Mauel, J., Cerottini, J.-C., and Chapuis, B., 1968, Quantitative assay of the lytic action of immune lymphoid cells on ^{51} Cr-labelled allogeneic target cells *in vitro;* inhibition by isoantibody and by drugs, *Immunology* 14:181.

Brunner, K.T., Mauel, J., Rudolf, H., and Chapuis, B., 1969, Homograft immunity: Mechanisms of immunologic enhancement and of the cellular immune reaction *in vitro,* in: *Cellular Recognition,* pp. 243–250 (R.T. Smith and R.A. Good, eds.), Appleton-Century-Crofts, New York.

Brunner, K.T., Nordin, A.A., and Cerottini, J.-C., 1971, *In vitro* studies of sensitized lymphocytes and alloantibody-forming cells in mouse allograft immunity. Cellular interactions in the immune response, in: *2nd International Convocation of Immunologists,* Buffalo, New York, 1970, pp. 220–230, S. Karger, Basel.

Bubbers, J., and Henney, C.S., 1975a, Studies on the mechanism of lymphocyte-mediated cytolysis. V. The use of cytochalasins A and B to dissociate glucose transport from the lytic event, *J. Immunol.* 115:145.

Bubbers, J.E., and Henney, C.S., 1975b, Studies on the synthetic capacity and antigenic expression of glutaraldehyde-fixed target cells, *J. Immunol.* 114:1126.

Burakoff, S.J., Martz, E., and Benacerraf, B., 1975, Is the primary complement lesion insufficient for lysis? Failure of cells damaged under osmotic protection to lyse in EDTA or at low temperature after removal of osmotic protection, *Clin. Immunol. Immunopathol.* 4:108.

Burakoff, S.J., Germain, R.N., Dorf, M.E., and Benacerraf, B., 1976, Inhibition of cell-mediated cytolysis of trinitrophenyl derivatized target cells by alloantisera directed to the products of the *K* and *D* loci of the *H-2* complex, *Proc. Natl. Acad. Sci. U.S.A.* 73:625.

Cantor, H., and Boyse, E.A., 1975, Functional subclasses of T lymphocytes bearing different Ly antigens. I. The generation of functionally distinct T cell subclasses is a differentiative process independent of antigen, *J. Exp. Med.* 141:1376.

Canty, T.G., and Wunderlich, J.R., 1970, Quantitative *in vitro* assay of cytotoxic cellular immunity, *J. Natl. Cancer Inst.* 45:761.

Cerottini, J.-C., and Brunner, K.T., 1972, Reversible inhibition of lymphocyte-mediated cytotoxicity by cytochalasin B, *Nature (London) New Biol.* 237:272.

Cerottini, J.-C., and Brunner, K.T., 1974, Cell-mediated cytotoxicity, allograft rejection, and tumor immunity, *Adv. Immunol.* 18:67.

Cerottini, J.-C., and Brunner, K.T., 1977, Mechanism of T and K cell-mediated cytolysis, in: *B and T Cells in Immune Recognition* (F. Loor and G.E. Roelants, eds.), Wyley and Sons, Chichester, England, in press.

Cerottini, J.-C., Nordin, A.A. and Brunner, K.T., 1971, Cellular and humoral response to transplantation antigens. I. Development of alloantibody-forming cells and cytotoxic lymphocytes in the graft-vs-host reaction, *J. Exp. Med.* **134**:553.

Cerottini, J.-C., MacDonald, H.R., Engers, H.D., Thomas, K., and Brunner, K.T., 1974, Mechanisms of cell-mediated immunologic injury, *Adv. Biosci.* **12**:47.

Chapuis, B., and Brunner, K.T., 1971, Cell-mediated immune reactions *in vitro*. Reactivity of lymphocytes from animals sensitized to chicken erythrocytes, tuberculin or transplantation antigens, *Int. Arch. Allergy* **40**:321.

Cohen, I.R., and Feldman, M., 1971, The lysis of fibroblasts by lymphocytes sensitized *in vitro*: Specific antigen activates a nonspecific effect, *Cell. Immunol.* **1**:521.

Cohen, I.R., Stavy, L., and Feldman, M., 1970, Glucocorticoids and cellular immunity *in vitro*, *J. Exp. Med.* **132**:1055.

Davies, H.G., Marsden, N.V.B., Ostling, S.G., and Zade-Oppen, A.M.M., 1968, The effect of some neutral macromolecules on the pattern of hypotonic hemolysis, *Acta Physiol. Scand.* **74**:577.

Doherty, P.C., and Zinkernagel, R.M., 1975, *H-2* compatibility is required for T-cell-mediated lysis of target cells infected with lymphocytic choriomeningitis virus, *J. Exp. Med.* **141**:502.

Faanes, R.B., Choi, Y.S., and Good, R.A., 1973, Escape from isoantiserum inhibition of lymphocyte-mediated cytotoxicity, *J. Exp. Med.* **137**:171.

Ferluga, J., and Allison, A.C., 1974, Observations on the mechanism by which T-lymphocytes exert cytotoxic effects, *Nature (London)* **250**:673.

Ferluga, J., Asherson, G.L. And Becker, E.L., 1972, The effect of organophosphorus inhibitors, *p*-nitrophenol and cytochalasin B on cytotoxic killing of tumour cells by immune spleen cells and the effect of shaking, *Immunology* **23**:577.

Freedman, L.R., Cerottini, J.-C., and Brunner, K.T., 1972, *In vivo* studies of the role of cytotoxic T cells in tumor allograft immunity, *J. Immunol.* **109**:1371.

Gately, M.K., Mayer, M.M., and Henney, C.S., 1976, Effect of antilymphotoxin on cell-mediated cytotoxicity, *Cellular Immunol.* **27**:82.

Golstein, P., 1974, Sensitivity of cytotoxic T cells to T-cell mediated cytotoxicity, *Nature (London)* **252**:81.

Golstein, P., and Blomgren, H., 1973, Further evidence for autonomy of T cells mediating specific *in vitro* cytotoxicity: Efficiency of very small amounts of highly purified T cells, *Cell. Immunol.* **9**:127.

Golstein, P., and Fewtrell, C., 1975, Functional fractionation of human cytotoxic cells through differences in their cation requirements, *Nature (London)* **255**:491.

Golstein, P., and Smith, E.T., 1976, The lethal hit stage of mouse T and non-T cell-mediated cytolysis—differences in cation requirements and characterization of an analytical "cation pulse" method, *Eur. J. Immunol.*, in press.

Golstein, P., Svedmyr, E.A.J., and Wigzell, H., 1971, Cells mediating specific *in vitro* cytotoxicity. I. Detection of receptor-bearing lymphocytes, *J. Exp. Med.* **134**:1385.

Golstein, P., Wigzell, H., Blomgren, H., and Svedmyr, E.A.J., 1972a, Cells mediating specific *in vitro* cytotoxicity. II. Probable autonomy of thymus-processed lymphocytes (T cells) for the killing of allogeneic target cells, *J. Exp. Med.* **135**:890.

Golstein, P., Svedmyr, E.A.J., and Blomgren, H., 1972b, Specific adsorption of cytoxic thymus-processed lymphocytes (T cells) on glutaraldehyde-fixed fibroblast monolayers, *Eur. J. Immunol.* **2**:380.

Green, H., and Goldberg, B., 1960, The action of antibody and complement on mammalian cells, *Ann. N. Y. Acad. Sci.* **87**:352.

Green, H., Barrow, P., and Goldberg, B., 1959, Effect of antibody and complement on permeability control in ascites tumor cells and erythrocytes, *J. Exp. Med.* **110**:699.

Hämmerling, G.J., and McDevitt, H.O., 1974, Antigen binding T and B lymphocytes. I. Differences in cellular specificity and influence of metabolic activity on interaction of antigen with T and B cells, *J. Immunol.* **112**:1726.

Häyry, P., Andersson, L.C., Nordling, S., and Virolainen, M., 1972, Allograft response *in vitro, Transplant. Rev.* **12**:91.

Henney, C., 1973a, Studies on the mechanism of lymphocyte-mediated cytolysis. II. The use of various target cell markers to study cytolytic events, *J. Immunol.* **110**:73.

Henney, C.S., 1973b, On the mechanism of T-cell mediated cytolysis, *Transplant. Rev.* **17**:37.

Henney, C.S., 1973c, Relationships between the cytolytic activity of thymus-derived lymphocytes and cellular cyclic nucleotide concentrations, in: *Cyclic AMP, Cell Growth and the Immune Response,* pp. 195–209 (W. Braun, C.W. Parker, and L.M. Lichtenstein, eds.), Springer-Verlag, New York.

Henney, C.S., 1974, Estimation of the size of a T-cell induced lytic lesion, *Nature (London)* **249**:456.

Henney, C.S., 1975, T cell-mediated cytolysis: Consideration of the role of a soluble mediator, *J. Reticuloendothel. Soc.* **17**:231.

Henney, C.S., and Bubbers, J.E., 1973a, Studies on the mechanism of lymphocyte-mediated cytolysis. I. The role of divalent cations in cytolysis by T lymphocytes, *J. Immunol.* **110**:63.

Henney, C.S., and Bubbers, J.E., 1973b, Antigen–T lymphocyte interactions: Inhibition by cytochalasin B, *J. Immunol.* **111**:85.

Henney, C.S., Bourne, H.R., and Lichtenstein, L.M., 1972a, The role of cyclic 3',5'-adenosine monophosphate in the specific cytolytic activity of lymphocytes, *J. Immunol.* **108**:1526.

Henney, C.S., Clayburgh, J., Cole, G.A., and Prendergast, R.A., 1972b, B lymphocyte mediated cytolysis: A complement independent phenomenon, *Immunol. Commun.* **1**:93.

Henney, C.S., Gaffney, J., and Bloom, B.R., 1974, On the relation of products of activated lymphocytes to cell-mediated cytolysis, *J. Exp. Med.* **140**:837.

Kamat, R., and Henney, C.S., 1975, Studies on T cell clonal expansion. I. Suppression of killer T cell production *in vivo, J. Immunol.* **115**:1592.

Kedar, E., Ortiz de Landazuri, M., and Fahey, J.L., 1974, Enzymatic enhancement of cell-mediated cytotoxicity and antibody-dependent cell cytotoxicity, *J. Immunol.* **112**:26.

Kemp, A., and Berke, G., 1973a, Effects of heparin and benzyl alcohol on lymphocyte-mediated cytotoxicity *in vitro, Cell. Immunol.* **7**:512.

Kemp, A.S., and Berke, G., 1973b, Inhibition of lymphocyte-mediated cytolysis by the local anesthetics benzyl and salicyl alcohol, *Eur. J. Immunol.* **3**:674.

Kemp, A.S., Berke, G., Dawson, J.R., and Amos, D.B., 1974, The influence of normal serum components on lymphocyte-mediated cytolysis *in vitro, Transplantation* **17**:447.

Kennedy, L.J., Jr., Dorf, M.E., Unanue, E.R., and Benacerraf, B., 1975, Binding of poly-GAT by thymic lymphocytes from genetic responder and non-responder mice: Effect of antihistocompatibility serum, *J. Immunol.* **114**:1670.

Kimura, A.K., 1974, Inhibition of specific cell-mediated cytotoxicity by anti-T-cell receptor antibody, *J. Exp. Med.* **139**:888.

Klein, E., and Klein, G., 1972, Specificity of homograft rejection *in vivo,* assessed by inoculation of artifically mixed compatible and incompatible tumor cells, *Cell. Immunol.* **5**:201.

Kuppers, R.C., and Henney, C.S., 1976, Evidence for direct linkage between antigen recognition and lytic expression in effector T cells, *J. Exp. Med.* **143**:684.

Kuppers, R.C., and Henney, C.S., 1977, Studies on the mechanism of lymphocyte-mediated cytolysis. IX. Relationships between antigen recognition and lytic expression in killer T cells, *J. Immunol.*, in press.

Kurth, R., and Medley, G., 1975, A membrane permeability test for the detection of cell surface antigens, *Immunology* **29**:803.

Lauf, P.K., 1975, Immunological and physiological characteristics of the rapid immune hemolysis of neuraminidase-treated sheep red cells produced by fresh guinea pig serum, *J. Exp. Med.* **142**:974.

Lichtenstein, L.M., Henney, C.S., Bourne, H.R., and Greenough, W.B., III, 1973, Effects of cholera toxin on *in vitro* models of immediate and delayed hypersensitivity, *J. Clin. Invest.* **52**:691.

Lindahl, P., Leary, P., and Gresser, I., 1972, Enhancement by interferon of the specific cytotoxicity of sensitized lymphocytes, *Proc. Natl. Acad. Aci. U.S.A.* **69**:721.

MacDonald, H.R., 1975, Early detection of potentially lethal events in T-cell mediated cytolysis, *Eur. J. Immunol.* **5**:251.

Martz, E., 1975a, Early steps in specific tumor cell lysis by sensitized mouse T-lymphocytes. I. Resolution and characterization, *J. Immunol.* **115**:261.

Martz, E., 1975b, Inability of EDTA to prevent damage mediated by cytolytic T lymphocytes, *Cell. Immunol.* **20**:304.

Martz, E., 1976a, Early steps in specific tumor cell lysis by sensitized mouse T lymphocytes. II. Electrolyte permeability increase in the target cell membrane concomitant with programming for lysis, *J. Immunol.* **117**:1023.

Martz, E., 1976b, Sizes of isotopically-labeled molecules released during lysis of tumor cells labeled with ^{51}Cr and [^{14}C]nicotinamide, *Cellular Immunol.* **26**:313.

Martz, E., and Benacerraf, B., 1973a, Inhibition of immune cell-mediated killing by heparin, *Clin. Immunol. Immunopathol.* **1**:533.

Martz, E., and Benacerraf, B., 1973b, An effector-cell independent step in target cell lysis by sensitized mouse lymphocytes, *J. Immunol.* **111**:1538.

Martz, E., and Benacerraf, B., 1974, Crucial events in target cell lysis by sensitized mouse T-lymphocytes: A killer-cell independent, temperature-sensitive step, *Adv. Biosci.* **12**:37.

Martz, E., and Benacerraf, B., 1975, T lymphocyte-mediated cytolysis: Temperature dependence of killer cell dependent and independent phases and lack of recovery from the lethal hit at low temperatures, *Cell. Immunol.* **20**:81.

Martz, E., and Benacerraf, B., 1976, Multiple target cell killing by the cytolytic T lymphocyte and the mechanism of cytotoxicity, *Transplantation* **21**:5.

Martz, E., Burakoff, S.J., and Benacerraf, B., 1974, Interruption of the sequential release of small and large molecules from tumor cells by low temperature during cytolysis mediated by immune T-cells or complement, *Proc. Natl. Acad. Sci. U.S.A.* **71**:177.

Mauel, J., Rudolf, H., Chapuis, B. and Brunner, K.T., 1970, Studies of allograft immunity in mice. II. Mechanism of target cell inactivation *in vitro* by sensitized lymphocytes, *Immunology* **18**:517.

Miller, R.G., and Dunkley, M., 1974, Quantitative analysis of the ^{51}Cr release cytotoxicity assay for cytotoxic lymphocytes, *Cell. Immunol.* **14**:284.

Mintz, B., and Silvers, W.K., 1970, Histocompatibility antigens on melanoblasts and hair follicle cells, *Transplantation* **9**:497.

Plaut, M., Lichtenstein, L.M., and Henney, C.S., 1973a, Studies on the mechanism of lymphocyte-mediated cytolysis. III. The role of microfilaments and microtubules, *J. Immunol.* **110**:771.

Plaut, M., Lichtenstein, L.M., Gillespie, E., and Henney, C.S., 1973b, Studies on the mechanism of lymphocyte-mediated cytolysis. IV. Specificity of the histamine receptor on effector T cells, *J. Immunol.* 111:389.

Plaut, M., Lichtenstein, L.M., and Henney, C.S., 1973c, Increase in histamine receptors on thymus-derived effector lymphocytes during the primary immune response to alloantigens, *Nature (London)* 244:284.

Plaut, M., Bubbers, J.E., and Henney, C.S., 1976, Studies on the mechanism of lymphocyte-mediated cytolysis. VII. Two stages in the T cell-mediated lytic cycle with distinct cation requirements, *J. Immunol.* 116:150.

Portzehl, H., Caldwell, P.C., and Rüegg, J.C., 1964, The dependence of contraction and relaxation of muscle fibers from the crab *Maia squinado* on the interal concentration of free calcium ions, *Biochem. Acta* 79:581.

Röllinghoff, M., Schrader, J., and Wagner, H., 1973, Effect of azathioprine and cytosine arabinoside on humoral and cellular immunity *in vitro*, *Clin. Exp. Immunol.* 15:261.

Rouse, B.T., and Wagner, H., 1972, The *in vivo* activity of *in vitro* immunized mouse thymocytes. II. Rejection of skin allografts and graft-vs-host activity, *J. Immunol.* 109:1282.

Sanderson, C.J., 1976a, The mechanism of T cell mediated cytotoxicity. I. The release of different cell components, *Proc. R. Soc. London Ser. B.* 192:221.

Sanderson, C.J., 1976b, The mechanism of T cell mediated cytotoxicity. II. Morphological studies of cell death by time-lapse microcinematography, *Proc. R. Soc. London Ser. B.* 192:241.

Sanderson, C.J., and Franks, D., 1975, Effect of prednisolone on cell-mediated cytotoxicity *in vitro*, *Int. Arch. Allergy Appl. Immunol.* 48:610.

Sanderson, C.J., and Taylor, G.A., 1975, The kinetics of ^{51}Cr release from target cells in cell-mediated cytotoxicity and the relationship to the kinetics of killing, *Cell Tissue Kinet.* 8:23.

Sears, D.A., Weed, R.I., and Swisher, S.N., 1964, Differences in the mechanism of *in vitro* immune hemolysis related to antibody specificity, *J. Clin. Invest.* 43:975.

Seeman, P., 1972, Macromolecules may inhibit diffusion of hemoglobin from lysing erythrocytes by exclusion of solvent, *Can. J. Physiol. Pharmacol.* 51:226.

Seeman, P., 1974, Ultrastructure of membrane lesions in immune lysis, osmotic lysis, and drug-induced lysis, *Fed. Proc. Fed. Amer. Soc. Exp. Biol.* 33:2116.

Shain, B., and Martz, E., 1976, Early steps in specific tumor cell lysis by sensitized mouse T-lymphocytes. IV. Sites of action of the inhibitors cytochalasin B and lidocaine, in preparation.

Shearer, G.M., Rehn, T.G., and Garbarino, C.A., 1975, Cell-mediated lympholysis of trinitrophenyl-modified autologous lymphocytes. Effector cell specificity to modified cell surface components controlled by the *H-2K* and *H-2D* serological regions of the murine major histocompatibility complex, *J. Exp. Med.* 141:1348.

Shiku, H., Kisielow, P., Bean, M.A., Takahashi, Boyse, E.A., Oettgen, H.F., and Old, L.J., 1975, Expression of T cell differentiation antigens on effector cells in cell-mediated cytotoxicity *in vitro*, *J. Exp. Med.* 141:227.

Sinclair, N.R.St.C., Lees, R.K., Fagan, G., and Birnbaum, A., 1975, Regulation of the immune response. III. Characteristics of antibody-mediated suppression of an *in vitro* cell-mediated immune response, *Cell. Immunol.* 16:330.

Sprent, J., and Miller, J.F.A.P., 1972, Interaction of thymus lymphocytes with histoincompatible cells. III. Immunological characteristics of recirculating lymphocytes derived from activated thymus cells, *Cell. Immunol.* 3:213.

Stavy, L., Treves, A.J., and Feldman, M., 1972, Capacity of thymic cells to effect target cell lysis following treatment with concanavalin A, *Cell. Immunol.* 3:623.

Strom, T.B., Diesseroth, A., Morganroth, J., Carpenter, C.B., and Merrill, J.P., 1972, Alteration of the cytotoxic action of sensitized lymphocytes by cholinergic agents and activators of adenylate cyclase, *Proc. Nat. Acad. Sci. U.S.A.* **69**:2995.

Strom, T.B., Garovoy, M.R., Carpenter, C.B., and Merrill, J.P., 1973a, Microtubule function in immune and non-immune lymphocyte-mediated cytotoxicity, *Science* **181**:171.

Strom, T.B., Diesseroth, A., Morganroth, J., Carpenter, C.B., and Merrill, J.P., 1973b, Regulatory role of the cyclic nucleotides in alloimmune lymphocyte-mediated cytotoxicity. Effect of imidazole, *Transplant. Proc.* **5**:425.

Strom, T.B., Carpenter, C.B., Garovoy, M.R., Austen, K.F., Merrill, J.P., and Kaliner, M., 1973c, The modulating influence of cyclic nucleotides upon lymphocyte-mediated cytotoxicity, *J. Exp. Med.* **138**:381.

Strom, T.B., Sytkowski, A.J., Carpenter, C.B., and Merrill, J.P., 1974, Cholinergic augmentation of lymphocyte-mediated cytotoxicity. A study of the cholinergic receptor of cytotoxic T lymphocytes, *Proc. Natl. Acad. Sci. U.S.A.* **71**:1330.

Strom, T.B., Bear, R.A., and Carpenter, C.B., 1975, Insulin-induced augmentation of lymphocyte-mediated cytotoxicity, *Science* **187**:1206.

Strom, T.B., Garovoy, M.R., Bear, R.A., Gribik, M., and Carpenter, C.B., 1976a, A comparison of the effects of metabolic inhibitors upon direct and antibody-dependent lymphocyte mediated cytotoxicity, *Cell. Immunol.* **20**:247.

Strom, T.B., Lundin, A.P., III, and Carpenter, C.B., 1976b, The role of cyclic nucleotides in lymphocyte activation and function, *Prog. Clin. Immunol.,* in press.

Stulting, R.D., and Berke, G., 1973a, The use of ^{51}Cr release as a measure of lymphocyte-mediated cytolysis *in vitro, Cell. Immunol.* **9**:474.

Stulting, R.D., and Berke, G., 1973b, Nature of lymphocyte–tumor interaction. A general method for cellular immunoabsorbtion, *J. Exp. Med.* **137**:932.

Stulting, R.D., Berke, G., and Hiemstra, K., 1973, Evaluation of the effects of cytochalasin B on lymphocyte-mediated cytolysis, *Transplantation* **16**:684.

Stulting, R.D., Todd, R.F., III, and Amos, D.B., 1975, Lymphocyte-mediated cytolysis of allogeneic tumor cells *in vitro*. II. Binding of cytotoxic lymphocytes to formaldehyde-fixed target cells, *Cell. Immunol.* **20**:54.

Sullivan, K.A., Berke, G., and Amos, B., 1972, ^{51}Cr leakage from and uptake of trypan blue by target cells undergoing cell-mediated destruction, *Transplantation* **13**:627.

Thorn, R.M., and Henney, C.S., 1976, Studies on the mechanism of lymphocyte-mediated cytolysis. IV. A reappraisal of the requirement for protein synthesis during T cell-mediated lysis, *J. Immunol.* **116**:146.

Todd, R.F., III, 1975a, Lymphocyte-mediated cytolysis of allogeneic tumor cells *in vitro*. III. Enzyme sensitivity of target cell antigens, *Cell. Immunol.* **20**:257.

Todd, R.F., III, 1975b, Inhibition of binding between cytolytic (T) lymphocytes and tumor target cells by inhibitors of energy metabolism, *Transplantation* **20**:350.

Todd, R.F., III, Stulting, R. D., and Berke, G., 1973, Mechanism of blocking by hyperimmune serum of lymphocyte-mediated cytolysis of allogeneic tumor cells, *Cancer Res.* **33**:3203.

Todd, R.F., III, Stulting, R.D., and Amos, D.B., 1975, Lymphocyte-mediated cytolysis of allogeneic tumor cells *in vitro*. I. Search for target antigens in subcellular fractions, *Cell. Immunol.* **18**:304.

Vachek, H., and Kölsch, E., 1975, Dextran sulfate stimulates the induction but inhibits the effector phase in T cell-mediated cytotoxicity, *Transplantation* **19**:183.

Wagner, H., and Boyle, W., 1972, Subcellular mouse alloantigens: Cytotoxic immune responses and specific blocking *in vitro, Nature (London) New Biol.* **240**:92.

Wagner, H., and Cone, R.E., 1974, Adjuvant effect of poly (A:U) upon T cell-mediated *in vitro* cytotoxic allograft responses, *Cell. Immunol.* **10**:394.

Wagner, H., and Röllinghoff, M., 1974, T cell-mediated cytotoxicity: Discrimination between antigen recognition, lethal hit, and cytolysis phase, *Eur. J. Immunol.* 4:745.

Weiss, L., and Cudney, T.L., 1971, Some effects of neuraminidase on the *in vitro* interactions between spleen and mastocytoma (P815) cells, *Int. J. Cancer* 7:187.

Wigzell, H., 1965, Quantitative titrations of mouse *H-2* antibodies using ^{51}Cr-labelled target cells, *Transplantation* 3:423.

Wilson, D.B., 1965, Quantitative studies on the behavior of sensitized lymphocytes *in vitro*, *J. Exp. Med.* 122:143.

Wisniewski, H.M., and Bloom, B.R., 1975, Primary demyelination as a nonspecific consequence of a cell-mediated immune reaction, *J. Exp. Med.* 141:346.

Wolberg, G., Hiemstra, K., Burge, J.J., and Singler, R.C., 1973, Reversible inhibition of lymphocyte-mediated cytolysis by dimethyl sulfoxide (DMSO), *J. Immunol.* 111:1435.

Wolberg, G., Zimmerman, T.P., Hiemstra, K., Winston, M., and Chu, L.C., 1975, Adenosine inhibition of lymphocyte-mediated cytolysis: Possible role of cyclic adenosine monophosphate, *Science* 187:957.

Zagury, D., Bernard, J., Theirness, N., Feldman, M., and Berke, G., 1975, Isolation and characterization of individual functionally reactive cytotoxic T lymphocytes: Conjugation, killing and recycling at the single cell level, *Eur. J. Immunol.* 5:818.

Zbar, B., Wepsic, H.T., Borsos, T., and Rapp, H.J., 1970, Tumor graft rejection in syngeneic guinea pigs: Evidence for a two-step mechanism, *J. Natl. Cancer Inst.* 44:473.

Chapter 10

Functional Analysis of Distinct Human T-Cell Subsets Bearing Unique Differentiation Antigens

Leonard Chess and Stuart F. Schlossman

Division of Tumor Immunology
Sidney Farber Cancer Institute and
Department of Medicine
Harvard Medical School
Boston, Massachusetts

I. INTRODUCTION

The majority of peripheral blood lymphocytes have differentiated under the influence of the thymus gland to express a number of distinct immunologic functions. Direct analysis of human peripheral T-cell functions *in vitro* has shown that T cells proliferate and elaborate mediators in response to specific soluble antigens, respond to nonspecific polyclonal mitogens (Geha *et al.*, 1973a; Chess *et al.*, 1974a; Rocklin *et al.*, 1974), proliferate and differentiate into specifically cytotoxic killer cells after triggering by allogeneic target cells (Sondel *et al.*, 1975), and serve as helper or suppressor cells regulating both T-cell functions and the B-cell production of antibody (Waldman *et al.*, 1974; Shou *et al.*, 1976; Friedman *et al.*, 1976). Precise dissection of the cellular mechanisms and interactions involved in these diverse T-cell functions has been facilitated by recent advances in three related areas: (1) the identification of human-lymphocyte subpopulations bearing unique surface determinants; (2) the development of new techniques for the isolation of highly purified subpopulations of human T cells; and (3) the development of *in vitro* techniques to discriminate the functional behavior of the isolated subsets. In this chapter, we will briefly review some recent findings relative to the isolation and surface characterization of human peripheral T lymphocytes and their subsets, and then focus our attention on the differentiation pathways and the functional heterogeneity among the human T-cell subsets.

II. SURFACE PROPERTIES OF HUMAN LYMPHOCYTE SUBSETS

It is now generally agreed that at least three types of peripheral circulating human lymphocytes can be defined on the basis of surface binding with fluorescent antiimmunoglobulin reagents, rosetting with sheep erythrocytes (E rosettes), and rosetting with antibody- and complement-coated sheep erythrocytes (EAC rosettes) (Froland and Natvig, 1973). The majority of human T cells are Ig-negative, EAC-rosette-negative, and E-rosette-positive, whereas human B cells are surface-immunoglobulin-positive, bear complement receptors, and are E-rosette-negative. In addition, a third population of cells termed Null cells are Ig-negative, E-rosette-negative, and have been shown to be heterogeneous with respect to EAC binding.

The ability to characterize these distinct human-lymphocyte subpopulations with conventional techniques has allowed for their quantitation in peripheral blood and other lymphoid tissues in both normal individuals and patients during their natural history of disease and during clinical intervention. Moreover, these analytical techniques have permitted the development of several methods relying on cell-surface properties that permit the isolation of these lymphocyte subpopulations for functional studies.

While these conventional techniques have been extremely useful, however, they are still relatively crude, and a number of problems still exist. In particular, the rosetting techniques (both E and EAC) have been difficult to quantitate, and they vary enormously because of factors that include serum source, contamination with red cells, time, source and age of sheep cells, incubation temperature, and even the mechanical force used in resuspension of the rosettes. Perhaps of greater importance, these techniques do not deal with the extraordinary heterogeneity that exists within the T-, B-, and Null-cell populations. Further dissection of the heterogeneity within these subsets will be important in the analysis of the functional properties of lymphocytes and necessary for an understanding of the maturation and differentiation of lymphocytes. With these goals in mind, several laboratories have sought more precise approaches to the identification and characterization of human lymphocyte subsets.

Particular attention has been focused on the identification of surface-membrane determinants on human-lymphocyte subpopulations analogous to the

TL, Ly, Thy-1, and Ia determinants present on murine lymphocyte subpopulations. For example, in recent studies, an antiserum has been prepared that identifies surface determinant(s) on thymocytes that are not detected on "mature" normal peripheral blood human T cells or B cells (Schlossman et al., 1976). This antiserum (anti-H_{TL}) was prepared by immunizing rabbits with E-rosette-positive blast cells from a child with acute lymphatic leukemia (ALL) and subsequently absorbed with an autologous lymphoblastoid B-cell line obtained from the patient while clinically in remission. The H_{TL} antiserum reacts not only with thymocytes, but in addition is reactive with the leukemic cells from approximately 20% of patients with ALL. This subgroup of ALL patients often presents with a high white cell count, thymic mass, and clinically tends to do poorly with respect to chemotherapy (Sallan et al., 1976), and can be clinically distinguished from the H_{TL}-unreactive ALL patients. Of importance, the H_{TL}-unreactive patients bear Ia-like molecules on the surfaces of their cells. Since the anti-H_{TL} serum reacts only with thymocytes, fetal thymocytes, and T-cell-derived neoplastic cells, it is clearly analogous to other TL antisera defined in the mouse. The failure to detect H_{TL} antigen on "mature" peripheral T cells suggests that the antiserum defines a state of differentiation of the T-cell pool.

To approach the heterogeneity of the more differentiated T cell, several anti-human-T-cell antisera have been developed. Most attempts to prepare antibodies specific for human-T-cell determinants have relied heavily on absorption of heteroantisera with allogeneic bone marrow, fetal liver, adult B cells, B-cell lines, and chronic lymphatic leukemia (CLL) cells; these antisera are relatively specific for T cells in cytotoxicity studies (Aiuti and Wigzell, 1973; Smith et al., 1973; Brown and Greaves, 1974; Woody et al., 1975; Brouet and Toben, 1976), but in general have not been specific with respect to fluorescence and have not been useful for detailed functional analyses. We have sought to overcome some of these problems by using highly purified (see Section III) human T cells for immunization, and have absorbed the antiserum generated with autologous but not allogeneic B cells (Evans et al., 1977). The use of autologous lymphoblastoid-line cells for absorption of heteroantisera has been found to be of importance both with respect to the removal of antibodies directed at species, major histocompatability complex (MHC), or fetal antigens and with respect to the efficiency of absorption. For example, rabbits immunized with highly purified T cells and subsequently absorbed with human red cells and with as few as 200×10^6 autologous B lymphoblastoid cells eliminated detectable reactivity on peripheral B cells and B leukemic cells (CLL cells). In contrast, the reactivity on peripheral T cells or thymocytes plateaued at 60 and 90%, respectively, and could not be absorbed by as many as 1×10^9 B cells. Serial dilution of the absorbed antiserum demonstrated that maximum killing of peripheral T cells (50–60%) occurred at dilutions (1:10 to 1:40) at which 90–100% of thymocytes

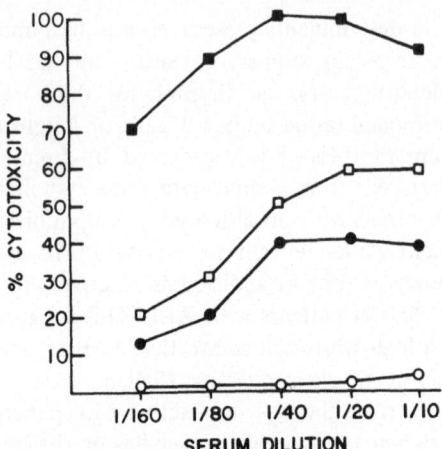

Fig. 1. Specificity of anti-T_{H1} for thymus-derived cells. Thymocytes (■), peripheral T cells (□), unfractionated lymphocytes (●), and peripheral B cells (○) were reacted with anti-T_{H1} + C, and the percentage cytotoxicity was measured by ^{51}Cr release.

were lysed (Fig. 1). No further increase in peripheral-T-cell killing was obtained by a second treatment with antiserum and complement, suggesting that the discrete subset of T cells was recognized. For the present studies, we have designated the antigens recognized on T cells as T_{H1} and the absorbed hetero-antiserum *anti-T_{H1}*. Importantly, peripheral B cells are not lysed by anti-T_{H1} at any dilution tested. The specificity of the absorbed antiserum for T cells could be demonstrated equally well by immunofluorescence utilizing a sandwich technique with FITC-goat-anti-rabbit F(ab)$_2$ and analysis on a Fluorescence Activated Cell Sorter (FACS). Figure 2 shows a histogram of the binding of this absorbed antiserum with purified T- and B-cell populations. B-cell binding is no different from background staining with normal rabbit serum, whereas the T-cell population is brightly stained.

Taken together, the H_{TL} and T_{H1} antigens permit a preliminary view of the differentiation of human T cells from adult thymocytes. As shown in Fig. 3, thymocytes bear receptors for sheep erythrocytes, H_{TL}, and the T_{H1} antigens. With differentiation, the sheep-cell receptor remains intact, whereas the H_{TL} antigen is lost from all detectable peripheral T cells. In contrast, the T_{H1} antigen is readily detected on a subset of peripheral T cells conprising 60% of the total, but is significantly reduced on the remaining 40% of T cells. As will be defined below, both T_{H1}^+ and T_{H1}^- cells define functionally distinct subsets of T lymphocytes (Evans *et al.*, 1976).

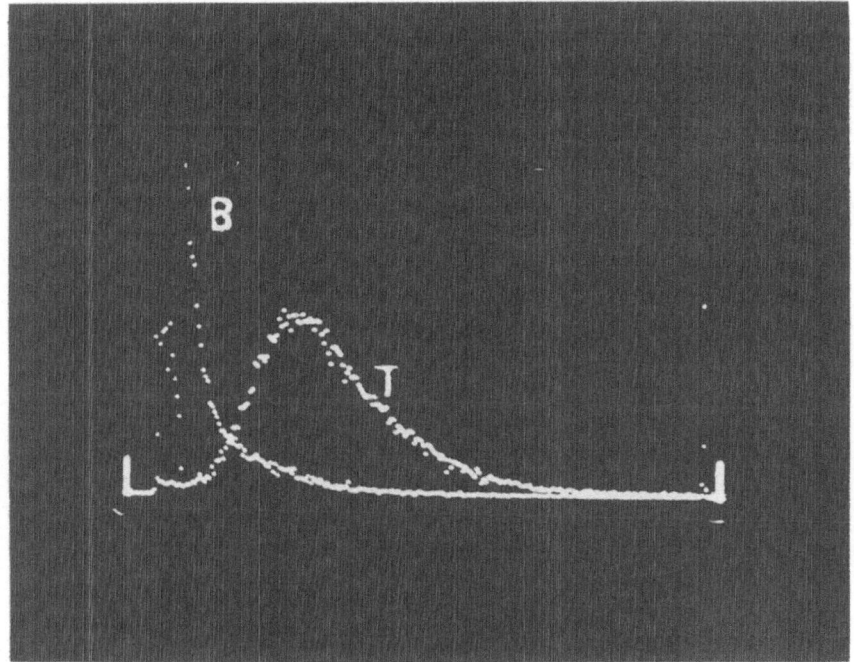

Fig. 2. Fluorescence distribution of anti-T_{H1} on peripheral T and B cells.

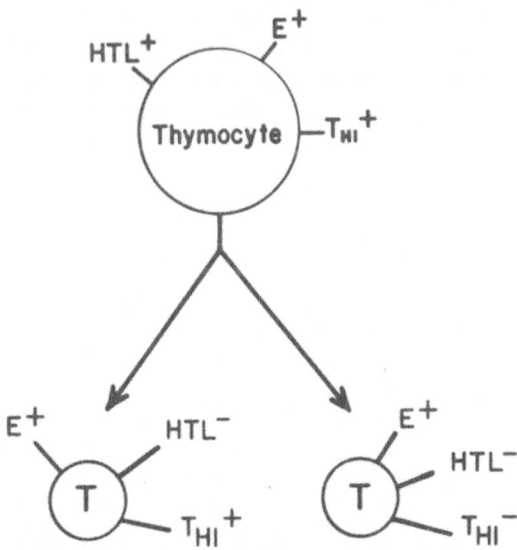

Fig. 3. Differentiation antigens on human T cells.

In contrast to the T-cell and thymocyte antigens described above, a number of new human-B-cell determinants have recently been defined that are distinct from the complement and Fc receptors, surface immunoglobulins, EBV receptors, HLA antigens, and B2 microglobulin. Of particular interest are the recently described anti-human Ia-like sera that detect molecules that functionally and genetically appear similar to murine Ia antigens (Winchester *et al.*, 1975; Humphreys *et al.*, 1976). These sera do not react in complement-dependent cytotoxicity assays or by immunofluorescence to any significant degree with T cells. It is possible, however, that Ia determinants are "masked" on human T cells and can be detected only by careful functional studies directed at the inhibition of selected T-cell function. Alternatively, the expression of Ia on T cells may require alteration of the cell surface by standard techniques including enzyme treatment (i.e., trypsin or neuraiminidase) or perhaps mitogen triggering. We have recently analyzed an antiserum prepared against a polypeptide–antigen complex (p23,30) isolated and purified from membranes from a human B lymphoblastoid cell line (IM1). Rabbit antisera to this complex (anti-p23,30) are unreactive with T cells by either complement-mediated or fluorescent assays. In contrast, the antiserum is highly reactive with B lymphocytes and B-cell lines to dilutions of 1/4,000. In addition, anti-p23,30 can detect the subset of Null lymphocytes (E-rosette-negative, Ig-negative and EAC-positive), which are likely to be B-cell precursors. Interestingly, the p23,30 antigen resembles the structure of murine Ia antigens, and functionally the antiserum raised to p23,30 has properties in common with anti-Ia murine antisera (Humphreys *et al.*, 1976; Chess *et al.*, 1976). For example, the anti-p23,30 serum can be shown to inhibit the mixed lymphocyte reaction and antibody-dependent cytotoxic functions, both of which are also inhibited by murine anti-Ia sera. More important, like murine anti-Ia serum, anti-p23,30 can markedly inhibit the differentiation of B cells into plaque-forming and antibody-producing cells *in vitro* (Friedman *et al.*,

Table I. Surface Properties of Human Peripheral Lymphocyte Subsets and Thymocytes

Lymphocyte subpopulation	Surface determinants					
	E Rosette	EAC Rosette	SmIg	H_{TL}	H_{T1}	Ia-like (p23,30)
T	+	−	−	−	+[a]	−
B	−	+	+	−	−	+
Null	−	+[b]	−	−	−	+[b]
Thymocyte	+	−	−	+	+	−

[a] H_{T1} is present on 50–60% of peripheral T cells and approximately 90% of thymocytes.
[b] Null cells are heterogeneous with respect to EAC receptors and p23,30, with the same 20–30% of cells reacting with each.

1976). Genetically, the p23,30 antigen appears to be linked to *HLA*, since cytotoxic alloantisera that recognize *HLA*-linked B-cell alloantigens are inhibited by p23,30 antigens isolated from the appropriate cell lines. Thus, the evidence is compelling that human Ia-like antigens can be isolated and antisera to them readily prepared. As suggested above, the role of Ia antigens with respect to human T-cell functions remains an important avenue of future study.

In Table I, we have summarized the precise surface properties of human peripheral (T, B, and Null) lymphocytes and thymocytes with respect to the "classic" and newer surface determinants.

III. METHODS FOR THE ISOLATION OF HUMAN T CELLS AND THEIR SUBSETS

Previously, it was shown that human peripheral lymphocytes could be quantitatively separated into surface Ig^+ and Ig^- subsets by Sephadex G-200 anti-Fab cellular immunoabsorbent chromatography (Chess *et al.*, 1974b). Human B cells will bind to the Sephadex anti-Fab as a consequence of intrinsic or adsorbed surface immunoglobulin, whereas non-Ig-bearing cells (T + Null cells) do not bind. The bound Ig^+ cells can be recovered by competitive antigen elution with human immunoglobulins. The cells passing directly through the column contain less than 1% Ig-bearing lymphocytes. Nevertheless, this population is heterogeneous with respect to E-rosetting, since only 70–80% of this population forms E rosettes. The cells binding to and eluted from the column contain greater than 98% Ig^+ cells and less than 2% E-rosetting cells. It should be emphasized that the separated populations are functionally intact, can be recovered with minimum loss, and maintain their surface properties *in vitro*.

From a technical point of view, the column immunoabsorbent techniques can be utilized both to isolate and to deplete cells with antisera directed at cell-surface antigens other than Ig. For example, goat anti-rabbit $F(ab)_2$ columns can be utilized to isolate cell populations coated with specific rabbit antisera directed at unique T- and B-surface determinants and the cells recovered by competitive elution with rabbit γ-globulins. This "sandwich" column technique has permitted the specific depletion and recovery of the T_{H1}^+ subset of human T cells as well as the p23,30$^+$ and p23,30$^-$ subsets of Null cells.

In addition, the FACS-I has recently been used to identify and separate subpopulations of human lymphocytes. The FACS can analyze single-cell suspensions quantitatively with espect to two parameters, i.e., size as measured by light-scattering, and fluorescence. The output of the FACS provides a histogram of the number of fluorescent cells stained against the intensity of fluorescence per cell. Arbitrary criteria for defining specific subpopulations can be made using these histograms and the machine programmed to isolate high- and low-density fluorescent-binding subpopulations for functional analysis. Detailed methodology, analysis, and cell-separation capability of this machine have been described (Hulett *et al.*, 1969). We would emphasize that the sensitivity of the FACS is greater than that obtained with standard fluorescent microscopy, and, perhaps more important, specifically stained cells can be isolated and subjected to functional characterization (see below).

Rosette depletion techniques have also been widely utilized in a number of laboratories to primarily isolate subpopulations enriched in either T or B cells. Thus, depleting an unfractionated population of E-rosetting cells results in a population of cells that, although heterogeneous, is highly enriched in B cells and Null cells. Alternatively, depletion of EAC-rosetting cells from an unfractionated population eliminates most of the B lymphocytes, and in addition a subset of Null cells, yielding a resulting population that is predominantly E-rosette-positive and surface-immunoglobulin negative. We have utilized rosette-depletion techniques primarily to further purify populations of cells isolated by immunoabsorbent chromatography. For example, the non-immunoglobulin-bearing population isolated by anti-F(ab)$_2$ chromatography can be incubated with EAC cells and the EAC-rosetting cells depleted by ficoll–hypaque to yield a highly purified T-cell population that is Ig^-, E^+ ($> 90\%$), p23,30$^-$, and EAC$^-$. Alternatively, the E-rosetting cells can be depleted from the Ig^- population by ficoll–hypaque sedimentation using analogous methods. In this case, the resulting population is Null cells (MacDermott *et al.*, 1975). As noted above, this population is Ig^- and E^-, and is heterogeneous with respect to EAC-binding cells and, perhaps more important, with respect to the p23,30 antigen. The 20–30% of cells bearing p23,30 and EAC receptors develop cell-surface Ig and secrete immunoglobulins in cell culture. Precisely the same subset of cells is active in ADCC. The remaining 70–80% of cells within the Ig^-, which are E-rosette-negative and p23,30-negative, have been the subject of recent investigations. One subgroup of this population can be shown to develop the capacity to form E rosettes in cell culture, and most likely represents a precursor pool of T lymphocytes. In fact, it is likely that the Null-cell population within the peripheral-lymphocyte pool represents subsets of precursor cells with the capacity to differentiate into more mature T and B cells, phagocytes, and even granulocyte-colony-forming cells.

IV. FUNCTIONAL PROPERTIES OF ISOLATED HUMAN LYMPHOCYTE SUBSETS

During the last few years, the functional properties of isolated T-, B-, and Null-cell populations have been analyzed with respect to a number of *in vitro*

Table II. Immunologic Functions of Human–Lymphocyte Subsets *in Vitro*[a]

Immune functions	T	B	Null
Proliferative Responses			
Soluble antigen-triggered proliferation	+	−	−
Response to alloantigens in MLC	+	−	−
Stimulating capacity in MLC	+	++	++
Mediator Production			
Migration inhibitory factor (MIF) production	+	+	N.T.[b]
Leukocyte inhibitory factor (LIF)	+	+	N.T.
Lymphocyte mitogenic factor (LMF)	+	−	−
Cytotoxic Responses			
Cell-mediated lympholysis (CML) of allogeneic cells	+	−	−
Antibody-dependent cellular cytotoxicity (ADCC)	−	−	+
Mitogen-induced nonspecific cytotoxicity	+	+	+
Antibody Production			
Capacity for Ig synthesis in cell culture	−	+	+
Plaque-forming cells	−	+	N.T.
Miscellaneous Functions			
Precursors of granulocyte-forming cells, B cells, and T cells	−	−	+
Proliferative response to EB virus	−	+	−

[a]The results presented in this table are largely documented in the text, with appropriate references given.
[b]N.T.: Not tested.

assays of cell-mediated immunity. Many of these studies have been published, and the results are summarized in Table II. For the purpose of this review, we will describe several newer aspects of the functional properties of human T cells, with particular focus on the initial characterization of discrete subsets of T cells using the anti-T_{H1} serum described above.

A. Proliferative Responses to Soluble and Cellular Antigens: Role of T_{H1}^+ and T_{H1}^- Subsets

It is known that T cells but not B cells from individuals previously sensitized to relatively complex antigens (e.g., PPD, mumps, tetanus toxoid) respond by proliferation and [^{3}H] thymidine incorporation to the specific soluble antigens *in vitro*. Moreover, T cells but not B cells are the alloreactive cells that are triggered to proliferate in the mixed leukocyte cultures (Chess *et al.*, 1974a). To determine whether these functions were a property of all T cells or reflected properties of a subset of T lymphocytes, we analyzed the T_{H1}^+ and T_{H1}^- T-cell subsets. In early experiments, it was found that anti-T_{H1} + C treatment of unfractionated lymphocyte populations abrogated the MLC response, but did not affect the proliferative response to soluble antigens. To further analyze this point in detail, T cells from individuals known to proliferate in response to tetanus toxoid, PPD, and mumps antigens were treated in the presence of complement with media alone, normal rabbit serum, anti-T_{H1} or antilymphocyte serum (ALS). ALS reacts with both T_{H1}^+ and T_{H1}^- lymphocytes and was used in this and subsequent experiments as a positive complement-mediated lysis control. After treatment, the T cells were cultured either in the presence or in the absence of soluble antigens and pulsed with [^{3}H]thymidine after 6 days. A representative experiment is shown in Fig. 4. The anti-T_{H1} reagent killed 60% of T cells, but had no significant effect on the antigen-induced proliferative response. More important, however, when identical aliquots of treated T cells were cocultivated with mitomycin-treated allogeneic cells in an MLC assay, anti-T_{H1} serum eliminated the proliferative response. These data suggest that the T_{H1}^+ cell but not the T_{H1}^- cell is MLC-responsive, whereas the T_{H1}^- cell is still capable of responding to soluble antigens.

To determine whether T_{H1}^+ cells could also proliferate in response to soluble antigen, both T_{H1}^+ and T_{H1}^- cells were isolated. To obtain T_{H1}^+ and T_{H1}^- cells, the whole population of T cells was reacted with anti-T_{H1} in the absence of complement, washed, incubated with FITC F(ab)$_2$-goat anti-rabbit F(ab)$_2$, and analyzed on the FACS. The fluorescent profile obtained indicated a gaussian distribution for T_{H1} binding that was arbitrarily divided into weak

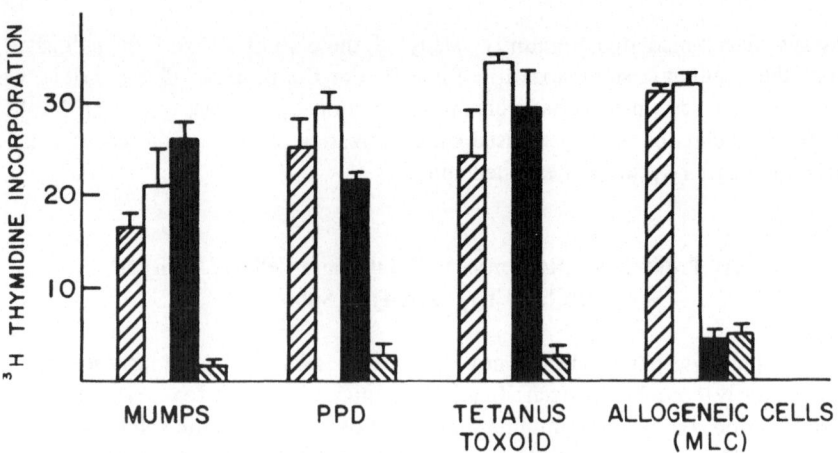

Fig. 4. Effect of depleting T_{H1}^+ cells on functional responses to soluble antigens and to allogeneic cells in MLC. T cells were either untreated (▨), or treated with NRS (□), anti-T_{H1} (■), or ALS (▨) in the presence of complement, washed, and cultured with soluble antigens or allogeneic cells. [^{3}H]Thymidine incorporation was measured, and the results were expressed as cpm×10^{-3}.

binding (lowest 25%) and strong binding (highest 25%). The machine was then programmed to isolate the low-density and the high-density fluorescent cells. The individual populations were collected and analyzed for their proliferative response to both soluble antigens and allogeneic cells in MLC. The cells with low-density staining with anti-T_{H1} were capable of mounting an excellent response to soluble antigen, but did not react to any appreciable degree in MLC, and thus were functionally similar to the T_{H1}^- subset resistant to lysis by anti-T_{H1} + complement. In contrast, the T_{H1}^+ subset that had a high density of staining with anti-T_{H1} were MLC-responsive cells, but did not react with soluble antigens. These data strongly suggest that anti-T_{H1} was in fact dissecting two unique subgroups of human T cells, one reactive in MLC and the other capable of response to soluble antigens.

B. Mediator Production by T-Cell Subsets

It is known that antigen-stimulated T lymphocytes from sensitive donors elaborate lymphocyte mitogenic factor (LMF), which can induct nonsensitized T and B lymphocytes to proliferate and incorporate [^{3}H]thymidine (Geha et al., 1973b). In previous studies, it was shown that purified T cells but not B cells could be induced by antigen to produce LMF (Rocklin et al., 1974). As shown above, the T_{H1}^- cell population responded maximally in soluble antigen-induced proliferation. To determine whether the same population of T_{H1}^- cells was responsible for both antigen-induced proliferation and LMF production, T cells were treated with anti-T_{H1} plus complement and cultured in the presence of tetanus toxoid for 48 hr, and the LMF production was measured (Table III). The supernatants from cultures were examined for LMF activity on indicator cells from tetanus-toxoid-negative individuals. Some cultures were continued for 6 days, and the [^{3}H]thymidine incorporation was measured. Treatment of lymphocytes with anti-T_{H1} and complement did not abolish the proliferative response of these cells to tetanus toxoid. Nevertheless, supernatants from these same cultures did not contain LMF activity when tested on tetanus-toxoid-negative cells. Control supernatants from T lymphocytes treated with normal rabbit serum .and complement had no effect either on the [^{3}H]thymidine incorporation or on their capacity to elaborate LMF. These results further support the view that the antigen-induced proliferating T-cell population is distinct and can be differentiated from the T-lymphocyte subset that elaborates soluble mediators in response to triggering by the same antigen. Although it remains a possibility that at least some degree of proliferation is required to initiate mediator production, it is clear that mediator production need not correlate directly with proliferation.

The effect of anti-T_{H1} lysis on the production of migration inhibitory

Table III. Effect of Anti-T$_{H1}$ Lysis on Mitogenic Factor Production by T Cells

Cell cultures	[³H] Thymidine incorporation	Supernatant effect on tetanus-toxoid-negative indicator cells [³H] thymidine incorporation	Mitogenic factor index[a]
T lymphocytes + media	2,476± 872	563± 32	
T lymphocytes + tetanus toxoid (10µg/ml)	24,361±2,571	4,566±232	8.1
T lymphocytes (treated with NRS + C) + media	3,339± 168	428±132	
T lymphocytes (treated with NRS + C) + tetanus toxoid (10 µg/ml)	27,312± 315	5,350±398	12.5
T lymphocytes (treated with anti-T$_{H1}$ + C) + media	436 ± 121	312± 75	
T lymphocytes (treated with anti-T$_{H1}$ + C) + tetanus toxoid (10 µg/ml)	25,371±3,121	843±131	2.7

[a]Calculated by dividing the mitogenic activity of the antigen-stimulated supernatant by the mitogenic activity of the control supernatant.

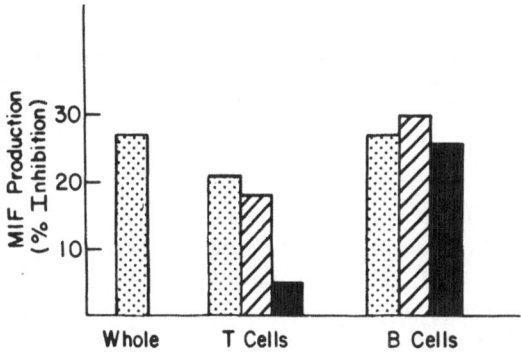

Fig. 5. Effect of depleting T_{H1}^+ cells on MIF production. Lymphocyte subpopulations from a candida sensitive donor were either untreated (▨), or treated in the presence of complement with NRS (▨) or anti-T_{H1} (■). The resulting populations were cultured with candida, and the MIF was measured after 48 hr. (These studies were performed in collaboration with Dr. R. Rocklin.)

factor (MIF) was also investigated. It has previously been shown that both T and B cells isolated from immunoabsorbent columns can produce MIF in response to specific soluble antigen, that B- and T-cell MIF had similar molecular weights as defined by chromatography on G-150 Sephadex, and that B cells made quantitatively more MIF than similar numbers of T cells (Rocklin *et al.*, 1974). As described above for LMF production, lymphocyte subsets were isolated and treated with anti-T_{H1} plus complement, antigen was added, and MIF production was measured (Fig. 5). As for LMF, anti-T_{H1} eliminated the MIF production by the isolated T-cell populations without affecting the proliferative response. Perhaps more important, anti-T_{H1} had no effect on antigen-induced MIF production by B cells. Thus, these data show that the T_{H1}^+ cells account for both LMF and MIF production by T cells. In addition, the results provide additional evidence for the view that antigen-induced B-cell MIF production is not secondary to contaminating T cells.

Thus far, the functional data indicated that T_{H1}^+ cells are active in MLC responses, LMF production, and MIF production. Further, the T_{H1}^+ cell can be distinguished from the T_{H1}^- cell, which responds by proliferation to soluble antigens. Since the T cells responsible for MLC response, delayed hypersensitivity, and possibly mediator production in the mouse bear Ly-1 phenotypes (Cantor and Boyse, 1975a,b; Cantor *et al.*, 1976; Huber *et al.*, 1976; Jandinski *et al.*, 1976), it was possible that human T_{H1}^+ cells represented an analogous subset. This relationship between Ly-1 and T_{H1} is further strengthened if one views LMF as a "helper factor" and MIF as important in delayed hypersensitivity. Moreover, if this were the case, then one might predict that T_{H1}^- cells would express functions similar to the murine Ly-2,3 cells, i.e., killer-cell activity or suppression (Jandinski *et al.*, 1976). To explore this possibility, we analyzed the effect of the anti-T_{H1} on human-cell-mediated lympholysis.

C. Cell-Mediated Lympholysis

In previous studies, it was demonstrated that T cells but not B or Null cells could be triggered by allogeneic cells to differentiate into specifically cytotoxic killers (Sondel *et al.*, 1975). Evidence that the killer cells themselves were T_{H1}^- was provided in the following experiment: T cells were sensitized with allogeneic mitomycin-treated lymphocytes for 6 days, and the putative killer cells were isolated. Aliquots of killer cells were then treated with either media, normal rabbit serum, anti-T_{H1}, or ALS, and tested on ^{51}Cr targets identical to the sensitizing cells. The ALS reagent completely abolished the cytotoxic activity, and anti-T_{H1} had the same effect. These studies indicate that cytotoxic T cells bear the T_{H1}^+ phenotype. More definitive proof of the relationship of the anti-T_{H1}-resistant cell population to cells with functional properties of Ly-2,3 cells, murine cells, awaits further functional analysis of this subset with respect to suppression and, perhaps more important, the preparation of antisera that will specifically detect antigenic determinants on T_{H1}^- cells not present on the T_{H1}^+ cell populations. The data to date suggest, however, that a parallelism may exist between murine and human T-cell subsets with respect to these functions. Table IV is a "preliminary" table showing the relationships between the Ly and T_{H1} surface determinants.

Last, additional insight into the heterogeneity of human T-cell function has

Table IV. Functional Relationship Between Human and Murine T-Cell Subsets

Functional property	Human phenotype		Murine phenotype	
	T_{H1}^+	T_{H1}^-	Ly-1	Ly-2,3
Mitogen responsiveness (PHA, Con A)	+	+	+	+
MLC response to MHC-related antigens	+	−	+	−
Mediator function regulating B cells (LMF in man, helper activity in mouse)	+	−	+	−
MIF production and/or delayed hypersensitivity	+	−	+	−
Proliferative response to soluble antigens	−	+	N.T.[a]	N.T.
Allogeneic killer activity	+	−	−	+
Suppressor activity	N.T.	N.T.	−	+

[a]N.T.: Not tested.

developed from studies of the Ig^-,E^- subset (Null cell) of lymphocytes. First, as described above, within the E-rosette-negative, Ig^- subset of lymphocytes (Null cells), there exists a p23,30-bearing pool of precursor cells capable of differentiating into B cells. Data have only recently begun to accumulate on the residual population of $p23,30,Ig^-,E^-$ Null cells. It has been shown, for example, that a subset of Ig^-,E^- lymphocytes can differentiate into E^+ cells. Moreover, it has been shown that defects on the differentiation of E^- T cells may be of importance in the pathogenesis of some forms of agammaglobulinemia. Furthermore, evidence is accumulating suggesting that this Null population, although incapable of being triggered by allogeneic cells in MLC or CML, may be triggered by autologous blast cells to differentiate into killer cells effecting the destruction of autologous blast. The relationship of these cells to either the natural killer cells or the subset of T cells that recognize altered MHC in murine models remains an important avenue for future studies in man.

V. CONCLUSIONS

The evidence described in this review suggests that an extraordinary degree of heterogeneity exists among the circulating human peripheral blood lymphocytes, and in particular the human T cells. This heterogeneity is reflected not only by distinct cell-surface determinants, but also, and perhaps more importantly, by the distinct functional properties of the defined subclasses. For example, the presence of T_{H1} cell-surface antigens on T cells defines functional subsets important in MLC responses and mediator production. In contrast, these T_{H1}^+ cells do not account for the bulk of cells proliferating in response to specific soluble antigens. Cells bearing T_{H1} are required for the recognition of foreign-MHC-controlled cell-surface determinants and for the cell-mediated destruction of allogeneic cells. We would expect that these T_{H1}^- cells will soon be distinguished by other, as yet to be defined surface molecules. The functional relationships demonstrated in these studies between the isolated human T_{H1}^+ and T_{H1}^- subsets and the described subsets of murine T cells with respect to Ly (Cantor and Boyse, 1976) is intriguing, and suggests evolutionary pressures to maintain a defined pattern of T-cell functional differentiation in mammals. It should be emphasized that it is probably not by chance alone that the dissection of functionally discrete T-cell subsets has emerged as a consequence of the recognition of distinct differentiation determinants on the cell surface. One might expect these molecular determinants, themselves, to play an important functional role in the subsets they define.

Although the precise mechanisms and biological significance of these modes of T-cell differentiation are unknown, the evidence suggests that these pathways may have evolved, on the one hand, to homeostatically control the immune response and, on the other hand, to adapt efficient mechanisms of recognition of self and non-self determinants. If this proves to be the case, then it is likely that further studies of these and other distinct T-cell subsets in man will permit more precise analysis of clinical disorders in which defects arise either in the differentiation of T cells or in the functional capacity to regulate the immune response to bacterial, viral, or tumor antigens and to recognize altered-self.

Finally, the biological role of antigens similar to H_{TL} that distinguish surface structures on human thymocytes and T-cell leukemias that are absent from the more mature circulating T cells remains an important avenue of investigation. They may, for example, control the further differentiation of thymocytes or perhaps play a role in the homing properties of precursor cells destined to undergo thymus-dependent differentiation. In addition, it is of enormous interest that it is precisely that subgroup of H_{TL}^+ acute lymphatic leukemic cells that lacks the human Ia-like determinants (p23,30). Patients with H_{TL}^+, 23,30⁻ leukemic blasts represent a clinically distinct subgroup of patients relatively resistant to therapy, in contrast to the H_{TL}^-, p23,30⁺ group of patients, who maintain prolonged survival even after therapy is discontinued. Whether the functional properties of these surface determinants on tumor cells in fact dictate the natural history of disease in these patients is currently a major question yet to be resolved.

ACKNOWLEDGMENTS

L. C. was supported by Contracts CB43964 and CB53881 from the National Cancer Institute. S. F. S. was supported by USPHS Grant RO1 AI-12069 from the National Institute of Allergy and Infectious Diseases.

VI. REFERENCES

Aiuti, F., and Wigzell, H., 1973, *Clin. Exp. Immunol.* 13:171.
Brouet, J.C., and Toben, H., 1976, *J. Immunol.* 116:1041.
Brown, G., and Greaves, M.F., 1974, *Eur. J. Immunol.* 4:302.
Cantor, H., and Boyse, E.A., 1975a, *J. Exp. Med.* 141:1376.
Cantor, H., and Boyse, E.A., 1975b, *J. Exp. Med.* 141:1390.
Cantor, H., and Boyse, E.A., 1976, *in*: Proceedings of the 41st Cold Spring Harbor Symposium, *Origins of Lymphocyte Diversity,* in press.
Cantor, H., Shen, F., and Boyse, E.A., 1976, *J. Exp. Med.* 143:1391.
Chess, L., MacDermott, R.P., Sondel, P.M., and Schlossman, S.F., 1974a, *Prog. Immunol. II* 3:125.

Chess, L., MacDermott, R.P., and Schlossman, S.F., 1974b, *J. Immunol.* **113**:1113.

Chess, L., MacDermott, R.P., and Schlossman, S.F., 1974c, *J. Immunol.* **113**:1122.

Chess, L., Evans, R., Humphreys, R.E., Strominger, J.L., and Schlossman, S.F., 1976, *J. Exp. Med.* **143**.

Evans, R., Schlossman, S.F., and Chess, L., 1977, *J. Exp. Med.* **145**:221.

Friedman, S.M., Breard, J., and Chess, L., 1976, *J. Immunol.* **117**:2021.

Froland, S.S., and Natvig, J.B., 1973, *Transplant. Rev.* **16**:114.

Geha, R.S., Rosen, F.S., and Merler, E., 1973a, *J. Clin. Invest.* **52**:1726.

Geha, R.S., Schneeberger, E., Rosen, F.S., and Merler, E., 1973b, *J. Exp. Med.* **138**:1230.

Huber, B., Devinsky, O., Gershon, R.K., and Cantor, H., 1976, *J. Exp. Med.* **143**:1534.

Hulett, H.R., Bonner, W.A., Barrett, J., and Herzenberg, L.A., 1969, *Science* **166**:747.

Humphreys, R.E., Chess, L., Schlossman, S.F., and Strominger, J., 1976, *J. Exp. Med.* **144**:98.

Jondal, M., Wigzell, H., and Aiuti, F., 1973, *Transplant. Rev.* **16**:163.

MacDermott, R.P., Chess, L., and Schlossman, S.F., 1975, *Clin. Immunol. Immunopathol.* **4**:415.

Rocklin, R.E., MacDermott, R.P., Chess, L., Schlossman, S.F., and David, J.R., 1974, *J. Exp. Med.* **140**:1303.

Sallan, J., Sherwood, G., Schlossman, S.F., and Chess, L., 1977, submitted for publication.

Schlossman, S.F., Chess, L., Humphreys, R.E., and Strominger, J.L., 1976, *Proc. Natl. Acad. Sci. U.S.A.* **73**:1288.

Shou, L., Schwartz, S.A., and Good, R.A., 1976, *J. Exp. Med.* **143**:1160.

Smith, R.W., Terry, W.D., Buell, D.N., and Sell, K.W., 1973, *J. Immunol.* **110**:884.

Sondel, P.M., Chess, L., MacDermott, R.P., and Schlossman, S.F., 1975, *J. Immunol.* **114**:982.

Waldman, T.A., Durm, M., Broder, S., Blackman, M., Blaese, R.M., and Strober, W., 1974, *Lancet* **2**:609.

Winchester, R.J., Fu, S.M., Wernet, P., Kunkel, H.G., Dupont, B., and Jersild, C., 1975, *J. Exp. Med.* **141**:924.

Woody, J.N., Ahmed, A., Knudsen, R.C., Strong, D.M., and Sell, K.W., 1975, *J. Clin. Invest.* **55**:956.

Index